The Orthodontic Mini-Implant Clinical Handbook

The Orthodontic Mini-Implant Clinical Handbook

Second Edition

Richard Cousley
Consultant Orthodontist
The Priestgate Clinic
Peterborough
UK;
Honorary Consultant Orthodontist
Peterborough City Hospital
The North West Anglia NHS Foundation Trust
Peterborough
UK

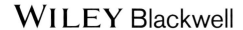

This edition first published 2020
© 2020 John Wiley & Sons Ltd

Edition History
John Wiley & Sons (1e, 2013)

Registered Offices
John Wiley & Sons, Inc., 111 River Street, Hoboken, NJ 07030, USA
John Wiley & Sons Ltd, The Atrium, Southern Gate, Chichester, West Sussex, PO19 8SQ, UK

Editorial Office
9600 Garsington Road, Oxford, OX4 2DQ, UK

For details of our global editorial offices, customer services, and more information about Wiley products visit us at www.wiley.com.

Wiley also publishes its books in a variety of electronic formats and by print-on-demand. Some content that appears in standard print versions of this book may not be available in other formats.

Library of Congress Cataloging-in-Publication Data

Names: Cousley, Richard, author.
Title: The orthodontic mini-implant clinical handbook / Richard Cousley.
Description: Second edition. | Hoboken, NJ : Wiley-Blackwell, 2020. |
    Includes bibliographical references and index.
Identifiers: LCCN 2019045151 (print) | LCCN 2019045152 (ebook) | ISBN
    9781119509752 (hardback) | ISBN 9781119509721 (adobe pdf) | ISBN
    9781119509745 (epub)
Subjects: MESH: Orthodontic Anchorage Procedures | Dental Implantation |
    Dental Implants | Miniaturization
Classification: LCC RK667.I45 (print) | LCC RK667.I45 (ebook) | NLM WU
    400 | DDC 617.6/93–dc23
LC record available at https://lccn.loc.gov/2019045151
LC ebook record available at https://lccn.loc.gov/2019045152

Cover Design: Wiley
Cover Images: Courtesy of Richard Cousley

Set in 9.5/12.5pt STIX Two Text by SPi Global, Pondicherry, India
Printed and bound in Singapore by Markono Print Media Pte Ltd

10   9   8   7   6   5   4   3   2   1

Contents

Preface to Second Edition

In some respects, it seems relatively early for a second edition to be published seven years after the first one. However, the subject of mini-implants in orthodontics is a dynamic and rapidly evolving field in terms of research publications, clinical techniques, collective comprehension and clinical insight. Some of these refinements appear subtle, but nevertheless represent clinically significant refinements in both our comprehension and applications. Therefore, this second edition has arisen from the realisation that both experienced orthodontists and those new to mini-implant anchorage will benefit from an updated appraisal of this progressive field and its ever-increasing applications in clinical orthodontics.

For example, our understanding of the nature of three-dimensional control of target tooth movements has greatly increased in the last 10 years. This has resulted from the initial recognition and then comprehension of biomechanical side-effects observed during the early years of mini-implant usage (and described in Chapter 1). This increased understanding has been matched with the introduction of relatively simple but effective clinical adjuncts such as powerarms (as described in Chapters 7 and 9). These have greatly enhanced our biomechanical control of anterior and posterior tooth movements. Consequently, we are now much more able to control not only anchorage but the delivery of bodily tooth movements in all three dimensions. However, it is important to acknowledge that mini-implants do not provide 'miracle' solutions since orthodontics still has to overcome biological limitations such as the severe alveolar bone deficiencies in hypodontia cases (discussed in Chapter 9).

Over the last 10 years, existing clinical techniques have been refined, and become more standardised and evidence based, as exemplified by protocols for molar intrusion in the treatment of anterior openbites (Chapter 10). The outer envelope of achievable orthodontic treatments has also been further expanded. This is amply illustrated by the inclusion of a new chapter in this edition on mini-implanted anchored maxillary expansion (Chapter 13). Last, but not least, orthodontic diagnostic imaging options have changed dramatically in recent years with the dissemination of lower dose cone beam computed tomography (CBCT) machines and software. This has had a positive impact on the use of mini-implants with the introduction of 3D imaging and planning techniques (described in Chapter 5).

However, one key theme has been continued from the first edition. The second edition still provides a combination of pragmatic clinical advice on common orthodontic clinical problems, based on a synthesis of the literature evidence base, judgement, experience and clinical insight. Therefore, I hope that you enjoy reading this textbook and that I have done service to my orthodontic peers and, indeed, to Sir Isaac Newton, the physics-based father of anchorage concepts.

Richard Cousley
2019

1

Orthodontic Mini-implant Principles and Potential Complications

This chapter could alternatively have been titled 'the advantages and disadvantages' or, more trendily, 'the pros and cons' of mini-implants, since it describes what we have to gain and possibly lose from their use. However, before we embark on these details, it's important to summarise what is meant by *orthodontic mini-implants* and how we've arrived at current clinical applications.

1.1 The Origins of Orthodontic Bone Anchorage

Orthodontic-specific skeletal fixtures were developed from two distinct sources:

- restorative implants
- maxillofacial surgical plating kits [1].

Orthodontic *implants* were first produced in the 1990s by modification of dental implant designs, making them shorter (e.g. 4–6 mm length) and wider (e.g. 3 mm diameter). However, they retained the crucial requirement for osseointegration, which is a direct structural and functional union of bone with the implant surface causing clinical ankylosis of the fixture. In contrast, orthodontic *miniplates* and *mini-implants* (miniscrews) are derived from bone fixation technology, and primarily rely on mechanical retention rather than osseointegration. In effect, modification of the maxillofacial bone plate design, adding a transmucosal neck and intraoral head, resulted in the miniplate, whilst adaption of the fixation screw design produced the mini-implant. Since the start of this millennium, a wide variety of customised orthodontic mini-implants have been produced and these are now used in the vast majority of orthodontic bone anchorage applications. Orthodontic implants are no longer in standard use and the invasive nature of miniplates tends to limit their use to orthopaedic traction (e.g. Class III) cases or occasionally where the alveolar and palatal sites are too limited for mini-implant usage (as exemplified in Chapter 8).

1.2 The Evolution of Mini-implant Biomechanics

Hindsight is a wonderful tool, especially with new treatment modalities such as orthodontic mini-implants. Much has changed in my clinical practice since I first used mini-implants, back in 2003. And when one looks at the early texts on mini-implants (including the first edition of this textbook), the evolution of techniques is also very apparent. The mini-implant evolution in the 10 years from circa 2005 to 2015 may be best summarised as shown in Table 1.1.

1.3 3D Anchorage Indications

This gradual refinement of mini-implant techniques has been accompanied by a substantial increase in the range of clinical applications for mini-implants. The proportion of these uses will vary between orthodontists, depending on their individual caseloads, and even on financial and cultural influences. Overall, it's best to subdivide modern anchorage control according to each of the three dimensions and 'other' applications, with common examples for each category listed below.

Anchorage dimension

Anteroposterior	• Incisor retraction and torque
	• Molar distalisation
	• Molar advancement
Vertical	• Single/multiple teeth intrusion
	• Tooth extrusion
Transverse	• Centreline corrections
	• Altering occlusal plane
	• Rapid maxillary expansion (RME)
Other	• Intermaxillary fixation (IMF) and traction
	• Temporary dental restorative abutment

Table 1.1 The clinical evolution of orthodontic mini-implant anchorage is subdivided into three chronological stages, with a description of the main focus at each stage along with representative clinical examples and associated side-effects

Stage of evolution	Clinical focus	Technique examples	Side-effects
1	Reliable anchorage	Direct anchorage, from alveolar sites	Vertical effects of oblique traction, e.g. lateral openbites and uncontrolled incisor movements
		Indirect anchorage, especially palatal sites	Hidden anchorage loss due to failings of connecting anchorage components
2	Minimised side-effects	Traction powerarms	Prevention of incisor extrusion/retroclination
		Rigid transpalatal auxiliaries	Prevention of molar buccal/palatal tipping movements during intrusion
3	Optimised target tooth movements (in addition to anchorage control)	Controlled 3D tooth movements during: • incisor retraction • molar distalisation • molar intrusion	Bodily movement of target teeth, e.g. • torque control during incisor retraction, bodily distalisation of molars, vertical molar intrusion movements

1.4 Using the Right Terminology

Unfortunately, a misleading array of terms has been used for bone anchorage devices (BADs) and their applications in both journals and the commercial literature. Essentially, it is best to encompass all types of fixtures which provide skeletal anchorage under the umbrella terms BADs or temporary anchorage devices (TADs), although the latter term does not indicate the essential role of bone in this anchorage. This book covers only one of the three types of BADs: mini-implants. Whilst the terms *mini-implant* and *miniscrew* are used interchangeably in the literature, it is erroneous to use the terms *microscrews* or *microimplants* since these fixtures are small (mini) and not *micro*scopic. I prefer the term mini-implant since it conveys the small size and implantable nature of these temporary fixtures.

Second, there appears to be much misunderstanding over whether mini-implants osseointegrate. Most mini-implants are made from either titanium or titanium alloy and histological studies show variable levels of bone–implant contact (BIC) [2,3]. However, it is misleading to refer to this as osseointegration. Rather, clinical usage and percussion indicate that mini-implants are mechanically retained (like bone fixation screws) rather than forming a clinically discernible ankylotic union with the bone (which occurs with restorative implants secondary to the initial BIC phase). Hence, mini-implants can be immediately loaded and easily unscrew, usually without anaesthetic, at any time after insertion. This may be because of their relatively smooth surface and possibly because the surface contact is more a physical phenomenon than a biochemical one.

> Mini-implants are mechanically retained (like bone fixation screws) rather than forming a clinically discernible ankylotic union with the bone.

1.5 Principal Design Features

Most mini-implants have three constituent parts: the head, neck and body (Figure 1.1), and are fabricated from a titanium alloy such as surgical grade 5 (Ti-6Al-4V). Grade 5 machined (smooth) titanium alloy is a good choice for mini-implants because it supports rapid cell proliferation and has good cytocompatibility (which is better than stainless steel) and cell adhesion [4,5]. The head is the platform which connects to orthodontic appliances or elastic traction. The neck is the part that traverses the mucosa. The body is the endosseous section with threads around a core and a tapered tip. Mini-implants were initially available only in self-tapping (non-drilling) forms whereby a full-depth pilot hole had to be drilled before mini-implant insertion. However, many self-drilling screws are now available. These have a tapered body shape with sharp tips and threads, and are inserted in a corkscrew-like manner. Full-depth predrilling is avoided, although shallow perforation of the cortex is still advantageous where the cortex is thick or dense, for example the posterior mandible and palate.

1.6 Clinical Indications for Mini-implants

Mini-implant usage may be broadly divided according to the case application and form of anchorage.

1.6.1 Routine Cases

- Cases with high anchorage demands, such as retraction of prominent upper incisors or centreline correction (especially where unilateral anchorage only is required). Orthodontists new to mini-implant use may find it easiest to introduce them into their clinical practice in such

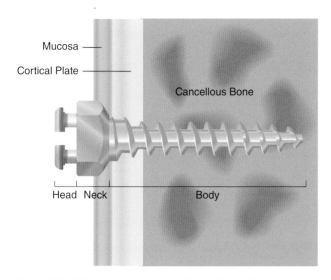

Figure 1.1 The three principal sections of a mini-implant: the head superficial to the tissues, the neck traversing the mucosa, and the threaded body within the cortical and cancellous bone.

Mucosa

Cortical Plate

Cancellous Bone

Head Neck   Body

cases since the other aspects of the treatment are usually uncomplicated, enabling the orthodontist to readily recognise the anchorage effects and gain experience.

- Adults and older adolescents who wouldn't comply well with other anchorage options, especially headgear.
- Where extrusive tooth movements would be unfavourable (risking an anterior openbite or vertical excess).

1.6.2 Complex Cases

- Where conventional biomechanics would be limited, for example molar intrusion to correct an anterior openbite.
- Where conventional dental anchorage is limited by an inadequate number of anchor teeth (due to tooth loss or hypodontia) or periodontal support.

1.6.3 Direct and Indirect Anchorage

Direct loading is when traction is applied from the mini-implant's head to an appliance, typically with elastic chain or nickel titanium (NiTi) coil springs (Figure 1.2a). Indirect loading involves using the mini-implant to reinforce anchor teeth, from which traction is applied (Figure 1.2b,c). The most commonly shown example of this involves mid-palatal mini-implant(s) anchorage of the first molars. This approach is advocated because of the high success rates of parasagittal mini-implants, even in adolescents. For example, a retrospective study of 384 parasagittal mini-implants inserted by Dr Björn Ludwig (in Germany) gave a 98% success rate [6]. Whilst indirect anchorage also has a potential advantage of avoiding some potential biomechanical side-effects (discussed later in this chapter), it carries the

risk of insidious anchorage loss through flexing of the intermediary wire connection and undetected tipping or bodily translation of the mini-implant. This has been reported to cause up to 0.5 mm of movement (anchorage loss) of the anchor tooth, in any one plane, when it is connected by a short piece of 0.019×0.025 in steel wire to a mini-implant [7], and 1–1.4 mm mean anteroposterior mesial drift of indirect molars in cases treated with bimaxillary incisor retraction [8].

Becker et al. [9] recently published a meta-analysis of *en masse* retraction treatments involving direct (buccal mini-implants) and indirect (palatal) anchorage [9]. Their results show that direct traction techniques provided better anchorage control than indirect anchorage approaches in both anteroposterior and vertical planes. This appears to have been due to occult mesial migration of some palatal mini-implants and bending of the transpalatal arch (TPA) component. Therefore, it was recognised that direct anchorage provides better outcomes in terms of anchorage control despite the possibility of higher mini-implant stability in midpalate sites. Interestingly, the favourable biomechanical effects of direct anchorage, such as controlled bodily movement of target teeth, were not studied in this meta-analysis, but represent an additional clinical benefit of direct anchorage usage [10–14]. This aspect will be discussed in detail at the end of this chapter.

In summary, I prefer to use direct anchorage wherever possible and this will be elucidated in the clinical scenario chapters. A key exception to this rule occurs in young patients whose bone immaturity means that the higher success rates of midpalate sites negates the biomechanical limitations of indirect anchorage. In effect, direct anchorage prioritises biomechanical considerations and indirect anchorage focuses on anatomical factors.

> Direct anchorage provides better outcomes in terms of anchorage control despite the possibility of higher mini-implants stability in midpalate sites.

1.7 Benefits and Potential Mini-implant Complications

Mini-implants have been shown to provide maximum anchorage along with the following benefits.

- No need for additional patient compliance (over and above the compliance required for fixed appliance treatment).
- Flexible timing for anchorage control, such that mini-implant anchorage may be 'switched' on and off at virtually

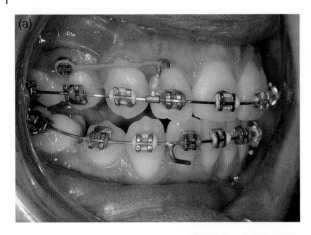
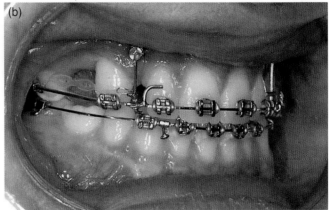
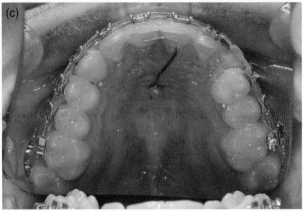

Figure 1.2 (a) Direct anchorage where this grey elastomeric attachment provides traction from the mini-implant head to a powerarm on the fixed appliance for *en masse* retraction of the anterior teeth. (b) The maxillary mini-implant provides indirect anchorage for molar protraction in this hypodontia case. Horizontal traction is applied, using elastomeric chain connected to a vertical auxiliary wire via a ligature wire. The auxiliary wire is joined to both the main archwire, using a cross-tube attachment, and the mini-implant head (where its position is secured by composite resin). (c) Indirect anchorage of the upper incisors during unilateral molar protraction, using an elastomeric chain on the fixed appliance. This involves a 0.019 × 0.025 stainless steel auxiliary wire from the midpalatal mini-implant's head to the central incisors' palatal surfaces, secured to both with composite resin.

any stage in treatment. This differs from conventional options where the anchorage, such as headgear, needs to be applied at the outset and is very difficult to add later in treatment.

- Greater predictability of both the treatment mechanics and clinical outcomes. For example, one can now confidently retract the labial segment without anchorage or torque loss in a controlled manner (as described in Chapter 7).
- Reduced treatment time, especially where it's more efficient to move groups of teeth rather than subdivide movements in an attempt to spare anchorage demands. This is exemplified by *en masse* retraction of the canine and incisor teeth in a single phase, rather than two-phase retraction of the canines then incisors. A randomised trial showed a four-month time saving in this respect [15].
- 3D anchorage control. Traditionally, orthodontists think of anchorage reinforcement in the anteroposterior

dimension, with much less emphasis on vertical and transverse anchorage. However, now that it's feasible to control anchorage in all three dimensions, orthodontics can truly aim to correct 3D malocclusion traits.

However, a number of risks and side-effects have been observed over the years with mini-implant clinical usage and in the research literature. Fortunately, these are reversible in most clinical situations, but it is important to consider them in an effort to maximise mini-implant treatment success and to provide informed patient consent. The main risks are described in the following sections.

1.8 Mini-implant Success and Failure

Failure of a mini-implant is the 'risk' that one ought to focus on most in day-to-day clinical terms. Mini-implant failure means that it cannot be used for its intended clinical loading/anchorage purposes. Conversely, mini-implant success is generally defined as the fixture remaining stable under continuous orthodontic loading for a minimum period of six months, although many studies have used one year as the minimum observation time. One of the most recent overviews of success rates has been provided by a meta-analysis of 3250 mini-implants, which showed a combined rate of 86% [16]. When the effect of insertion site is analysed, there is a consensus in the literature that the success rate varies according to the jaw involved, at approximately 80% and 90% for alveolar sites in the mandible and maxilla respectively, and up to 99% in the midpalate [17–30]. Conversely, success rates for infrazygomatic sites are relatively low, at 78%, as reported in a study of 30 consecutive Caucasian patients [31]. This may seem counterintuitive since the mandible is generally regarded as the stronger jaw bone, but the reasons for this paradox will be explained in Chapter 2.

Interestingly, mini-implants with minor mobility may still be graded as successful. This is evident clinically by slight rotational or lateral movement of the mini-implant on manipulation. This is painless and consequently asymptomatic for the patient. It is easily resolved by tightening the mini-implant, usually by a clockwise turn (insertional rotation), provided that this does not submerge the head, and without the need for anaesthesia. Notably, for Infinitas mini-implants, one complete turn equates to 0.7 mm further insertion. However, if the mini-implant displays obvious lateral mobility with light digital pressure then this indicates failure and the mini-implant should be removed.

Fortunately, most mini-implant failures become clinically evident within the first few months of insertion [20,24,25], enabling early replacement or a modification to the treatment plan. However, it important to realise that replacement mini-implants still have much lower success rates than primary insertions [32,33]. For example, a recent study of 471 mini-implants showed primary and secondary (replacement) success rates of 85% and 58% for maxillary buccal sites and 79% and 77% respectively for midpalate sites [33]. This marked drop in success rates for buccal, but not palatal, insertion sites suggests that the midpalate ought to be considered if a maxillary buccal mini-implant fails unless there has been an obvious and rectifiable explanation for the failure. Therefore, it is important to determine the likely reason for failure and undertake remedial clinical steps, such as root divergence, to favourably alter the chances of success for a secondary buccal site insertion. On the plus side, when a mini-implant feels firm after two months *in situ* then normal orthodontic forces may be applied with confidence.

Mini-implant failures are staged according to the time taken for this to manifest after insertion.

- Primary failure occurs when a mini-implant is clinically mobile at the time of insertion. This is due to inadequate cortical bone support in terms of its thickness and density, or close mini-implant proximity to an adjacent tooth root or incorrect insertion technique. These factors will be fully discussed in the relevant sections.
- Secondary failure refers to a situation where the mini-implant is initially stable but then exhibits mobility, usually after 1–2 months. This delayed instability is due to bone necrosis around the mini-implant threads, which may result from thermal bone damage (during pilot drilling), excessive insertion torque, excessively close proximity to a tooth root, traction overload, or a combination of these.

> Most mini-implant failures become clinically evident within the first few months of insertion, enabling early replacement.

1.9 Medical Contraindications

There are no absolute medical contraindications which specifically apply to orthodontic mini-implants. Conditions, such as diabetes mellitus and immunosuppression, which are relative contraindications to orthodontic treatment in general must be considered in terms of soft tissue hyperplasia and infection risks. However, if the patient has good oral hygiene then comprehensive treatment may proceed as normal. Older, especially female, patients with osteoporosis may present problems in terms of reduced bone support and hence mini-implant stability, but this can be accounted for in terms of insertion site and force application considerations. The increasing number of older patients on bisphosphonate drug treatment are a specific group which may limit orthodontic treatment, especially against tooth extractions (because of osteonecrosis risks). Whilst I have successfully treated patients taking oral bisphosphonates with routine orthodontic treatment (e.g. alignment), I have no experience of using mini-implants in this group of patients and am unaware of any literature published on this.

1.10 Root/Periodontal Damage

Multiple clinical and animal studies have been conducted with the aim of intentionally inflicting damage on tooth roots, using both pilot drills and self-drilling mini-implants [34–42]. Fortunately, these studies have consistently shown that traumatised root surfaces are repaired within 12 weeks by cellular cementum and periodontal regeneration, provided that there is no infection portal present (which is usually the case). The cementum repair even occurred when root dentine was fully exposed [34]. Orthodontists can also be reassured that there are no known reports of tooth ankylosis or loss arising from mini-implant use. This may be because, in normal clinical usage, if a self-drilling mini-implant contacts a root then the insertion stalls and its tip will become blunt, preventing extensive penetration of the root tissues. Furthermore, the patient is likely to complain of pain (from periodontal pain receptors) even before root contact occurs. If the root is actually contacted then the orthodontist is also likely to feel a sharp increase in insertion torque [43].

So if a mini-implant doesn't actually contact a root surface, is there still scope for indirect damage? A recent finite element analysis study indicated that less than 1 mm of separation of the mini-implant and the adjacent root surface may still risk root resorption because a transfer of stress through the thin layer of bone causes an osteoclastic reaction beside the root surface [44]. However, this has not been validated by animal or clinical studies, and the reciprocal effect on bone remodelling around the mini-implant is more likely to have a negative impact. For example, a histological analysis of mini-implants inserted in a dog model showed a significant reduction in BIC where the implant body contacted the root or even just the bundle bone (around the periodontal ligament) [45]. Therefore, it is reasonable to conclude that any irreversible effect from close proximity of a mini-implant and a tooth root will be on the mini-implant: it will have an increased risk of failure (by becoming mobile) rather than the tooth being irreversibly damaged [43,46–50].

> Any irreversible effect from mini-implant–tooth proximity is on the mini-implant: it fails (by becoming mobile), *not* the tooth.

1.11 Perforation of Nasal and Maxillary Sinus Floors

Concerns have been raised in the literature that mini-implant perforation of the nasomaxillary cavities (Figure 1.3) may result in either infection or the creation of a fistula. However, the consensus based on dental implant research is that a soft tissue lining rapidly forms over the end of a perforating fixture, and that mini-implant sites heal by bone infill because of the narrow width of the explantation hole. Motoyoshi et al. [51] investigated clinical effects in a retrospective study where 82 mini-implants had been inserted mesial and buccal to the maxillary first molar [51].

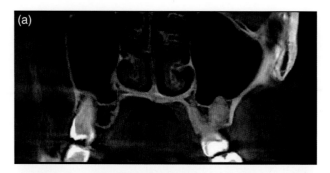

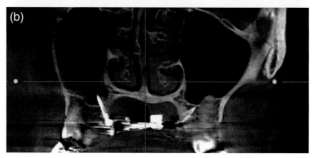

Figure 1.3 Coronal slice views of a CBCT scan of the maxilla (a) before and (b) one month after insertion of mini-implants in palatal alveolar sites. The mini-implant, sited distal to the right maxillary first molar, has been inserted at a relatively vertical inclination and has perforated the maxillary sinus, as seen in (b). However, this was asymptomatic and there has been no change in the clarity of the maxillary sinus.

They found perforation of the maxillary sinus in 10% of the sites, but with no sinusitis symptoms, nor differences in insertion torque and secondary stability. In contrast, a study of infrazygomatic insertions showed that 78% penetrated the maxillary sinus at this site [52]. Whilst these were apparently asymptomatic, mucosal thickening was seen on cone beam computed tomography (CBCT) in 88% of these sites where the mini-implant penetrated by at least 1 mm. Therefore, in order to maximise bone engagement and minimise both patient discomfort and possible sinus disease, it is generally recommended that maxillary alveolar insertion sites should be within 8 mm of the alveolar crest in dentate areas, and at a more coronal level where maxillary molars are absent. The infrazygomatic crest is not recommended for this reason.

1.12 Damage to Neurovascular Tissues

Disruption of the inferior dental, mental or greater palatine nerves and blood vessels is highly unlikely given their relative distance from standard insertion sites. The nasopalatine nerve is closer to potential anterior palatal insertion sites, but this can be readily avoided if recommended midpalatal insertion procedures are followed; for example, midpalatal insertion sites ought to be distal to the transverse level of the maxillary canines.

1.13 Mini-implant Fracture

Mini-implant fracture is thankfully a rare occurrence nowadays since most mini-implant materials and designs do not easily fracture within the normal torque limits in clinical practice [53,54]. However, some studies, aimed at fracturing mini-implants in hard acrylic blocks, have failed to allow for the low insertion torques experienced with many designs and especially in the case of self-drilling body versions. Therefore, fractures due to poor clinical technique may be attributed incorrectly to mini-implant weakness.

Fracture may occur during insertion, but also on removal if the mini-implant has been preweakened. Fracture of the mini-implant tip may occur when a root is inadvertently contacted (i.e. the insertion position and/or angle is incorrect) or when the insertion angle is altered with the mini-implant partially inserted through the cortical plate. This is most likely to occur due to incorrect technique and/or clinical inexperience. Fracture of the main section of a mini-implant body is a particular risk, on either insertion or removal, with mini-implants which feature a narrow diameter and cylindrical body design (Figure 1.4) [55,56] or when excessive insertion torque occurs (e.g. in the posterior mandible with dense, thick cortical bone). If a mini-implant fractures on removal, flush with the bone surface, and the retained part is unlikely to impede any remaining tooth movements, then it may be left *in situ* because of the biocompatibility of titanium alloy (Figure 1.4c). In the rare event that removal of a fractured part is indicated then this involves creating access by raising a small mucoperiosteal flap, trephination of a narrow collar of bone around the mini-implant end, and then derotation of the fractured fragment using a Weingarts or mosquitos-like instrument.

1.14 Pain

There is often an expectation that high levels of pain will occur but the opposite is true, such that some patients appear to feel virtually no discomfort during and after insertion [57,58]. The majority of patients appear to experience mild pressure-related pain at the time of insertion and up to 24 hours of low-level pain thereafter. This is self-limiting, controlled by simple analgesics (e.g. paracetamol or ibuprofen) and comparable (but of shorter duration) to other orthodontic experiences, such as the effects of separators and aligning archwires [59], and certainly much less than premolar tooth extractions [60]. The latter comparison is beneficial when it comes to explaining the likely pain experience to patients who already have a fixed appliance *in situ*.

Assuming that the superficial soft tissues have been adequately anaethetised, mini-implant insertions cause dental pain because of the pressure wave generated by insertion of a rigid fixture into a confined bone space. While there are no pain receptors within the bone tissues, if the pressure dissipates further it will reach the periodontal tissues of adjacent teeth, and hence stimulate their periodontal pain receptors. The patient will feel this as dental pain in the affected tooth. Fortunately, I think that it's within the orthodontist's scope to proactively reduce the level of pressure discomfort by diverging the roots of adjacent teeth prior to insertion (as described in Chapter 5). This creates more interproximal space and hence a greater distance between the mini-implant site and the adjacent periodontal pain receptors. While there is no clinical evidence to support (or refute) this hypothesis, my experience is that patients with increased interproximal spaces complain of less pain both at the time of insertion and afterwards.

When it comes to mini-implant removal, local anaesthesia is usually not required and indeed, patients find that the injection sensation is worse than the actual discomfort of

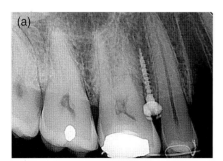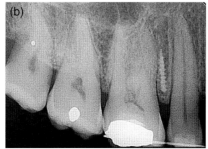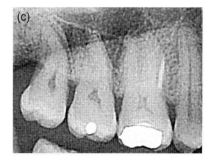

Figure 1.4 Intraoral radiographs taken after (a) insertion of a cylindrically shaped mini-implant mesial to the maxillary first molar, and (b) its fracture near the coronal end of the body. The initial fracture line is visible in the intact mini-implant. (c) Sectional orthpantomograph (OPG) showing the (asymptomatic) retained mini-implant body over five years later.

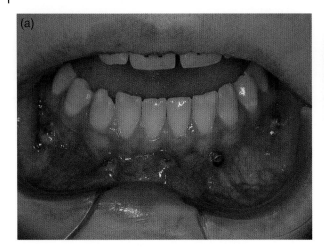
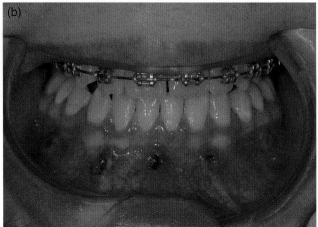

Figure 1.5 Overgrowth of the labial sulcular tissues caused by these mandibular mini-implant insertions within loose mucosa in this orthognathic surgical case (a). Local anaesthetic infiltration injections were required for the hyperplastic tissue to be peeled off the implant heads for their removal (b).

explanation [61]. An exception to this rule may occur when a mini-implant is being removed from the anterior region where there has been some soft tissue overgrowth of the mini-implant head, especially when it has been inserted in loose mucosa (Figure 1.5). For all removal procedures, it is essential that the mini-implant is unwound the entire way out of the implant hole since any attempt to pull it out will result in soft tissue pain where the threads catch on the mucosa. In addition, the orthodontist should ensure that the screwdriver is fully engaged on the mini-implant at the start of explantation, since premature disengagement during the removal process will cause pain because of the implant's mobility within the soft tissue envelope.

> The majority of patients appear to experience mild pressure-related pain at the time of insertion.

1.15 Soft Tissue Problems

The most common soft tissue issue related to mini-implant usage is chronic low-grade peri-implant inflammation. This is analogous to gingivitis around the mini-implant neck, and is usually superficial and self-limiting. It is more likely if the mini-implant is either inserted into an area of mobile mucosa (Figure 1.6) or overinserted (partially submerged) in attached gingiva (Figure 1.7). If tissue hyperplasia fails to resolve with oral hygiene measures, and either interferes with use of the mini-implant or causes patient discomfort, then the mini-implant should be removed. Fortunately, acute infections are rarely seen. For example, an audit of my first 500 mini-implant insertions confirmed that only one patient had returned to clinic

within several days with a painful, inflamed soft tissue swelling around a mini-implant. This episode of acute infection was readily resolved by immediate explantation of the mini-implant, without the need for antibiotics.

It is also unlikely that peri-implant colonisation by specific pathogenic bacteria is responsible for infection problems in failed mini-implants, as demonstrated by microbiological studies (comparing successful and failed mini-implant flora) [62–65]. Instead, soft tissue causes of failure are probably related to generalised inflammation effects. Even then, it is likely that the soft tissue influences on stability are small compared with other factors such as root proximity.

The labial or buccal mucosa adjacent to a mini-implant head may occasionally be traumatised, manifesting as a mucosal ulcer (Figure 1.8). This is most likely to occur if the mini-implant has a prominent profile (a long head and neck distance from the tissue surface) or sharp edges, or it is inserted in or near loose mucosa. Conversely, mucosal hyperplasia or ulceration may occur if the traction auxiliary (in direct anchorage scenarios) impinges excessively on the underlying mucosa, especially in the presence of poor oral hygiene (Figure 1.9).

1.16 Mini-implant Migration

This depends on the head (and neck) to body ratio, on the degree of bone support (stability), and on the relative force level. In effect, both self-tapping and self-drilling mini-implants may tip and/or translate bodily in the direction of the applied force [66–70]. This is problematic if it causes the mini-implant head to approximate an adjacent bracket or crown and cause soft tissue impingement or difficulty in utilising the mini-implant head.

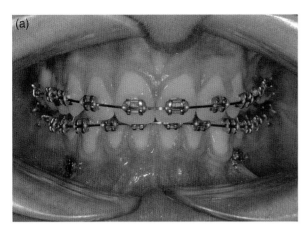
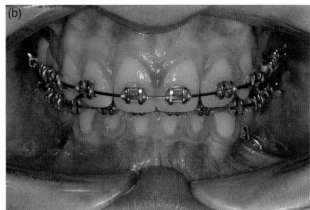
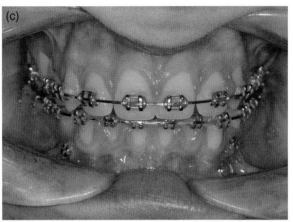

Figure 1.6 (a) Photograph of lower anterior mini-implants immediately after insertion. (b) Hyperplasia of the loose sulcular mucosa around the right mini-implant one month after insertion. (c) Effective oral hygiene measures have resolved the hyperplastic tissue problem on the right side eight weeks later, enabling the continued use of this mini-implant.

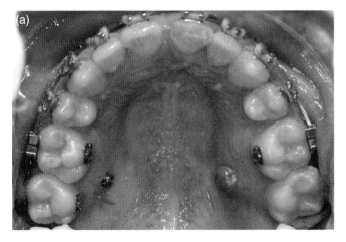
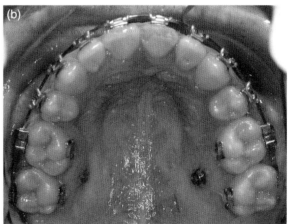

Figure 1.7 (a) Hyperplasia of the palatal mucosa covering an overinserted mini-implant in the palatal alveolar site between the left molars. (b) Normal tissue appearance after simple excision of the hyperplastic tissue and replacement of this mini-implant. Minor peri-implant hyperplasia is seen on the right side.

1.17 Biomechanical Side-effects

In many respects, conventional fixed appliances often only exhibit subtle biomechanical side-effects such as frictional binding, tooth tipping and anchorage loss, because these effects are usually localised to single teeth or a group of several teeth. For example, traction applied at the coronal level (to a bracket) may result in tipping and poorly controlled bodily movement of that tooth. Since the adjunctive use of mini-implants provides more profound anchorage, active in all three dimensions and extrinsic to the fixed appliance, the side-effects may also be more strongly expressed and affect the entire arch (when continuous arch mechanics are utilised).

Two pertinent examples of this occur if oblique traction is applied from a mini-implant directly to a canine bracket for anterior segment retraction, with either a flexible or a rigid archwire in place. In the first instance, this oblique vector of traction encourages the canine to tip distally causing the flexible archwire to exhibit a 'rollercoaster' bowing phenomenon (Figure 1.10a). In the latter situation, the oblique traction causes a rigid archwire to rotate the entire arch (around its centre of rotation near the premolar apices), causing a combination of incisor extrusion and retroclination and molar intrusion (Figure 1.10b). This manifests clinically as a molar openbite, with development of a vertical step between the first and second molar teeth (if the second molar is unconnected).

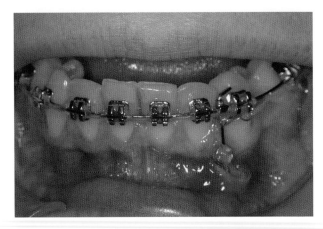

Figure 1.8 Labial ulceration caused by this mandibular mini-implant's insertion at the mucogingival junction and by the active movement of the adjacent labial sulcus.

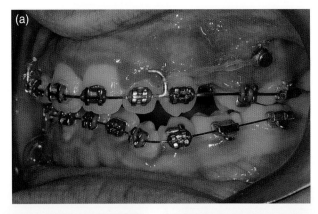

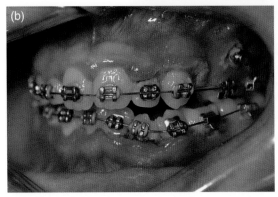

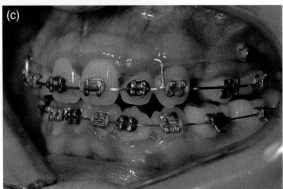

Figure 1.9 (a) Elastomeric traction auxiliary in contact with the alveolar mucosa following insertion of maxillary buccal mini-implants. (b) Maxillary alveolar ulcerative gingivitis after one month with the powerchain *in situ*, along with generalised gingival hyperplasia resulting from poor oral hygiene. (c) Photograph taken a further four months later with new traction applied following an improvement in oral hygiene.

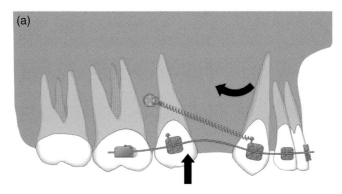
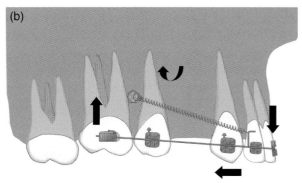

Figure 1.10 Diagrams showing the vertical side-effects of an oblique vector of traction from a buccal mini-implant to the anterior teeth on (a) flexible and (b) rigid archwires. Distal tipping of the canine and a rollercoaster bowing of the archwire occur in scenario (a), whilst predominantly molar intrusion occurs in (b).

1.18 Factors Affecting Mini-implant Success

A large number of mini-implant research papers have been published in the orthodontic (and to a lesser extent the surgical and dental implant) literature at an ever-increasing rate since the start of this millennium. This collective evidence provides a sound basis for mini-implant usage, although it may be difficult for orthodontists and dental colleagues to keep track of all this new information. Consequently, Chapters 2–4 aim to collate and summarise the essential findings of the most relevant scientific and clinical research papers, in order that orthodontists may both understand and maximise their clinical usage of mini-implants. In general, the factors determining success may be divided into three categories and these will be discussed sequentially in the next three chapters.

1) Patient (anatomical) factors (Chapter 2)

- Macro – somatic and general patient factors
- Mini – insertion site anatomy
- Micro – bone characteristics

2) Mini-implant design factors (Chapter 3)

- Materials and surface characteristics
- Dimensions

3) Clinical factors (Chapter 4)

- Insertion technique
- Force application

On balance, the risk–benefit relationship for mini-implants appears to be highly favourable for patients with high or atypical anchorage requirements. This means that the consent process (discussed in Chapter 4) should focus on tangible limitations, such as mini-implant instability and pain, rather than on more theoretical risks of tissue damage.

References

1 Prabhu, J. and Cousley, R.R.J. (2006). Bone anchorage devices in orthodontics. *J. Orthod.* 33: 288–307.

2 Serra, G., Morais, L.S., Elias, C.N. et al. (2008). Sequential bone healing of immediately loaded mini-implants. *Am. J. Orthod. Dentofac. Orthop.* 134: 44–52.

3 Vannet, B.V., Sabzevar, M.M., Wehrbein, H., and Asscherickx, K. (2007). Osseointegration of miniscrews: a histomorphometric evaluation. *Eur. J. Orthod.* 29: 437–442.

4 Galli, C., Piemontese, M., Ravanetti, F. et al. (2012). Effect of surface treatment on cell responses to grades 4 and 5 titanium for orthodontic mini-implants. *Am. J. Orthod. Dentofac. Orthop.* 141: 705–714.

5 Malkoc, S., Ozturk, F., Orek, B.C. et al. (2012). Real-time cell analysis of the cytotoxicity of orthodontic mini-implants on human gingival fibroblasts and mouse osteoblasts. *Am. J. Orthod. Dentofac. Orthop.* 141: 419–426.

6 Karagkiolidou, A., Ludwig, B., Pazera, P. et al. (2013). Survival of palatal miniscrews used for orthodontic appliance anchorage: a retrospective cohort study. *Am. J. Orthod. Dentofac. Orthop.* 143: 767–772.

7 Jang, W., Choi, Y.J., Hwang, S. et al. (2019). Anchorage loss assessment of the indirect anchor tooth during adjunctive orthodontic treatment. *Am. J. Orthod. Dentofac. Orthop.* 155: 347–354.

8 Monga, N., Kharbanda, O.P., and Samrit, V. (2016). Quantitative and qualitative assessment of anchorage loss during en masse retraction with indirectly loaded miniscrews in patients with bimaxillary protrusion. *Am. J. Orthod. Dentofac. Orthop.* 150: 274–282.

9 Becker, K., Pliska, A., Busch, C. et al. (2018). Efficacy of orthodontic mini implants for en masse retraction in the maxilla: a systematic review and meta-analysis. *Int. J. Implant Dent.* 4: 35.

10 Ammar, H.H., Ngan, P., Crout, R.J. et al. (2011). Three-dimensional modelling and finite element analysis in treatment planning for orthodontic tooth movement. *Am. J. Orthod. Dentofac. Orthop.* 139: e59–e71.

11 Kojima, Y., Kawamura, J., and Fukui, H. (2012). Finite element analysis of the effect of force directions on tooth movement in extraction space closure with miniscrew sliding mechanics. *Am. J. Orthod. Dentofac. Orthop.* 142: 501–508.

12 Lai, E.H., Yao, C.J., Chang, J.Z. et al. (2008). Three-dimensional dental model analysis of treatment outcomes for protrusive maxillary dentition: comparison of headgear, miniscrew, and miniplate skeletal anchorage. *Am. J. Orthod. Dentofac. Orthop.* 134: 636–645.

13 Sung, S.J., Jang, G.W., Chun, Y.S., and Moon, Y.S. (2010). Effective en-masse retraction design with orthodontic mini-implant anchorage: a finite element analysis. *Am. J. Orthod. Dentofac. Orthop.* 137: 648–657.

14 Yao, C.J., Lai, E.H., Chang, J.Z. et al. (2008). Comparison of treatment outcomes between skeletal anchorage and extraoral anchorage in adults with maxillary dentoalveolar protrusion. *Am. J. Orthod. Dentofac. Orthop.* 134: 615–624.

15 Al-Sibaie, S. and Hajeer, M.Y. (2014). Assessment of changes following en-masse retraction with mini-implants anchorage compared to two-step retraction with conventional anchorage in patients with class II division 1 malocclusion: a randomized controlled trial. *Eur. J. Orthod.* 36: 275–283.

16 Alharbi, F., Almuzian, M., and Bearn, D. (2018). Miniscrews failure rate in orthodontics: systematic review and meta-analysis. *Eur. J. Orthod.* 40: 519–530.

17 Antoszewska, J., Papadopoulos, M.A., Park, H.S., and Ludwig, B. (2009). Five-year experience with orthodontic miniscrew implants: a retrospective investigation of factors influencing success rates. *Am. J. Orthod. Dentofac. Orthop.* 136: 158.e1–158e10.

18 Berens, A., Wiechmann, D., and Dempf, R. (2006). Mini- and micro-screws for temporary skeletal anchorage in orthodontic therapy. *J. Orofac. Orthop.* 67: 450–458.

19 Chen, Y., Chang, H.H., Lin, H.Y. et al. (2008). Stability of miniplates and miniscrews used for orthodontic anchorage: experience with 492 temporary anchorage devices. *Clin. Oral Implants Res.* 19: 1188–1196.

20 Kim, Y.H., Yang, S., Kim, S. et al. (2010). Midpalatal miniscrews for orthodontic anchorage: factors affecting clinical success. *Am. J. Orthod. Dentofac. Orthop.* 137: 66–72.

21 Lim, H.J., Eun, C.S., Cho, J.H. et al. (2009). Factors associated with initial stability of miniscrews for orthodontic treatment. *Am. J. Orthod. Dentofac. Orthop.* 136: 236–242.

22 Luzi, C., Verna, C., and Melsen, B. (2009). Guidelines for success in placement of orthodontic mini-implants. *J. Clin. Orthod.* 43: 39–44.

23 Manni, A., Cozzani, M., Tamborrino, F. et al. (2011). Factors influencing the stability of miniscrews. A retrospective study on 300 miniscrews. *Eur. J. Orthod.* 33: 388–395.

24 Moon, C., Lee, D., Lee, H. et al. (2008). Factors associated with the success rate of orthodontic miniscrews placed in the upper and lower posterior buccal region. *Angle Orthod.* 78: 101–106.

25 Moon, C., Park, H., Nam, J. et al. (2010). Relationship between vertical skeletal pattern and success rate of orthodontic mini-implants. *Am. J. Orthod. Dentofac. Orthop.* 138: 51–57.

26 Park, H., Jeong, S., and Kwon, O. (2006). Factors affecting the clinical success of screw implants used as orthodontic anchorage. *Am. J. Orthod. Dentofac. Orthop.* 130: 18–25.

27 Suzuki, E.Y. and Suzuki, B. (2011). Placement and removal torque values of orthodontic miniscrew implants. *Am. J. Orthod. Dentofac. Orthop.* 139: 669–678.

28 Wu, T., Kuang, S., and Wu, C. (2009). Factors associated with the stability of mini-implants for orthodontic anchorage: a study of 414 samples in Taiwan. *J. Oral Maxillofac. Surg.* 67: 1595–1599.

29 Melo, A.C.M., Andrighetto, A.R., Hirt, S.D. et al. (2016). Risk factors associated with the failure of miniscrews - a ten-year cross sectional study. *Braz. Oral Res.* 30: e124.

30 Di Leonardo, B., Ludwig, B., Lisson, J.A. et al. (2018). Insertion torque values and success rates for paramedian insertion of orthodontic miniimplants. *J. Orofac. Orthop.* 79: 109–115.

31 Uribe, F., Mehr, R., Mathur, A. et al. (2015). Failure rates of mini-implants placed in the infrazygomatic region. *Prog. Orthod.* 16: 31.

32 Uesugi, S., Kokai, S., Kanno, Z., and Ono, T. (2017). Prognosis of primary and secondary insertions of orthodontic miniscrews: what we have learned from 500 implants. *Am. J. Orthod. Dentofac. Orthop.* 152: 224–231.

33 Uesugi, S., Kokai, S., Kanno, Z., and Ono, T. (2018). Stability of secondarily inserted orthodontic miniscrews after failure of the primary insertion for maxillary anchorage: maxillary buccal area vs midpalatal suture area. *Am. J. Orthod. Dentofac. Orthop.* 153: 54–60.

34 Ahmed, K.S., Rooban, T., Krishnaswamy, N.R. et al. (2012). Root damage and repair in patients with

temporary skeletal anchorage devices. *Am. J. Orthod. Dentofac. Orthop.* 141: 547–555.

35 Brisceno, C.E., Rossouw, P.E., Carrillo, R. et al. (2009). Healing of the roots and surrounding structures after intentional damage with miniscrew implants. *Am. J. Orthod. Dentofac. Orthop.* 135: 292–301.

36 Chen, Y., Chang, H., Chen, Y. et al. (2008). Root contact during insertion of miniscrews for orthodontic anchorage increases the failure rate: an animal study. *Clin. Oral Implants Res.* 19: 99–106.

37 Hembree, M., Buschang, P.H., Carrillo, R. et al. (2009). Effects of intentional damage of the roots and surrounding structures with miniscrew implants. *Am. J. Orthod. Dentofac. Orthop.* 135: 280e1–280e9.

38 Kadioglu, O., Buyukyilmaz, T., Zachrisson, B.U., and Maino, B.G. (2008). Contact damage to root surfaces of premolars touching miniscrews during orthodontic treatment. *Am. J. Orthod. Dentofac. Orthop.* 134: 353–360.

39 Lee, Y., Kim, J., Baek, S. et al. (2010). Root and bone response to the proximity of a mini-implant under orthodontic loading. *Angle Orthod.* 80: 452–458.

40 Maino, B.G., Weiland, F., Attanasi, A. et al. (2007). Root damage and repair after contact with miniscrews. *J. Clin. Orthod.* 41: 762–766.

41 Renjen, R., Maganzini, A.L., Rohrer, M.D. et al. (2009). Root and pulp response after intentional injury from miniscrew placement. *Am. J. Orthod. Dentofac. Orthop.* 136: 708–714.

42 Ghanbarzadeh, M., Heravi, F., Abrishamchi, R. et al. (2017). Cementum and dentin repair following root damage caused by the insertion of self-tapping and self-drilling miniscrews. *J. Orthod. Sci.* 6: 91–96.

43 Motoyoshi, M., Uchida, Y., Inaba, M. et al. (2016). Are assessments of damping capacity and placement torque useful in estimating root proximity of orthodontic anchor screws? *Am. J. Orthod. Dentofac. Orthop.* 150: 124–129.

44 Albogha, M.H. and Takahashi, I. (2019). Effect of loaded orthodontic miniscrew implant on compressive stresses in adjacent periodontal ligament. *Angle Orthod.* 89: 235–241.

45 Oh, H., Cha, J., Yu, H., and Hwang, C. (2018). Histomorphometric evaluation of the bone surrounding orthodontic miniscrews according to their adjacent root proximity. *Korean J. Orthod.* 48: 283–291.

46 Asscherickx, K., Vande Vannet, B., Wehrbein, H., and Sabzevar, M.M. (2008). Success rate of miniscrews relative to their position to adjacent roots. *Eur. J. Orthod.* 30: 330–335.

47 Dao, V., Renjen, R., Prasad, H.S. et al. (2009). Cementum, pulp, periodontal ligament, and bone response after direct injury with orthodontic anchorage screws: a histomorphologic study in an animal model. *J. Oral Maxillofac. Surg.* 67: 2440–2445.

48 Iwai, H., Motoyoshi, M., Uchida, Y. et al. (2015). Effects of tooth root contact on the stability of orthodontic anchor screws in the maxilla: comparison between self-drilling and self-tapping methods. *Am. J. Orthod. Dentofac. Orthop.* 147: 483–491.

49 Kang, Y.G., Kim, J.Y., Lee, Y.J. et al. (2008). Stability of miniscrews invading the dental roots and their impact on the paradental tissues in beagles. *Angle Orthod.* 79: 248–255.

50 Motoyoshi, M., Uemura, M., Ono, A. et al. (2010). Factors affecting the long-term stability of orthodontic mini-implants. *Am. J. Orthod. Dentofac. Orthop.* 137: 588.

51 Motoyoshi, M., Sanuki-Suzuki, R., Uchida, Y. et al. (2015). Maxillary sinus perforation by orthodontic anchor screws. *J. Oral Sci.* 57: 95–100.

52 Jia, X., Chen, X., and Huang, X. (2018). Influence of orthodontic mini-implant penetration of the maxillary sinus in the infrazygomatic crest region. *Am. J. Orthod. Dentofac. Orthop.* 153: 656–661.

53 Smith, A., Hosein, Y.K., Dunning, C.E., and Tassid, A. (2015). Fracture resistance of commonly used self-drilling orthodontic mini-implants. *Angle Orthod.* 85: 26–32.

54 Assad-Loss, T.F., Kitahara-Céia, F.M.F., Silveira, G.S. et al. (2017). Fracture strength of orthodontic mini-implants. *Dental Press J. Orthod.* 22: 47–54.

55 Chen, C.H., Chang, C.S., Hsieh, C.H., and Tseng, Y.C. (2006). The use of microimplants in orthodontic anchorage. *J. Oral Maxillofac. Surg.* 64: 1209–1213.

56 Park, H., Jeong, S., and Kwon, O. (2006). Factors affecting the clinical success of screw implants used as orthodontic anchorage. *Am. J. Orthod. Dentofac. Orthop.* 130: 18–25.

57 Lee, T.C.K., McGrath, C.P.J., Wong, R.W.K., and Rabie, A.B.M. (2008). Patients' perceptions regarding microimplant as anchorage in orthodontics. *Angle Orthod.* 78: 228–233.

58 Lehnen, S., McDonald, F., Bourauel, C., and Baxmann, M. (2011). Patient expectations, acceptance and preferences in treatment with orthodontic mini-implants. A randomly controlled study. Part I: Insertion techniques. *J. Orofac. Orthop.* 72: 93–102.

59 Kuroda, S., Sugawara, Y., Deguchi, T. et al. (2007). Clinical use of miniscrew implants as orthodontic anchorage: success rates and postoperative discomfort. *Am. J. Orthod. Dentofac. Orthop.* 131: 9–15.

60 Ganzer, N., Feldmann, I., and Bondemark, L. (2016). Pain and discomfort following insertion of miniscrews and premolar extractions: a randomized controlled trial. *Angle Orthod.* 86: 891–899.

61 Lehnen, S., McDonald, F., Bourauel, C. et al. (2011). Expectations, acceptance and preferences of patients in treatment with orthodontic mini-implants. Part II: Implant removal. *J. Orofac. Orthop.* 72: 214–222.

62 De Freitas, A.O.A., Alviano, C.S., and Alviano, D.S. (2012). Microbial colonization in orthodontic mini-implants. *Braz. Dent. J.* 23: 422–427.

63 Tortamano, A., Dominguez, G.C., Haddad, A.C.S.S. et al. (2012). Periodontopathogens around the surface of mini-implants removed from orthodontic patients. *Angle Orthod.* 82: 591–595.

64 Alves, C.B.C., Segurado, M.N., Dorta, M.C.L. et al. (2016). Evaluation of cytotoxicity and corrosion resistance of orthodontic mini-implants. *Dental Press J. Orthod.* 21: 39–46.

65 Andrucioli, M.C.D., Matsumoto, M.A.N., Saraiva, M.C.P. et al. (2018). Successful and failed mini-implants: microbiological evaluation and quantification of bacterial endotoxin. *J. Appl. Oral Sci.* 26: e20170631.

66 Alves, M., Baratieri, C., and Nojima, L.I. (2011). Assessment of mini-implant displacement using cone beam computed tomography. *Clin. Oral Implants Res.* 22: 1151–1156.

67 El-Beialy, A.R., Abu-El-Ezz, A.A., Attia, K.H. et al. (2009). Loss of anchorage of miniscrews: a 3-dimensional assessment. *Am. J. Orthod. Dentofac. Orthop.* 136: 700–707.

68 Liou, E.J.W., Pai, B.C.J., and Lin, J.C.Y. (2004). Do miniscrews remain stationary under orthodontic forces? *Am. J. Orthod. Dentofac. Orthop.* 126: 42–47.

69 Liu, H., Ly, T., Wang, N. et al. (2011). Drift characteristics of miniscrews and molars for anchorage under orthodontic force: 3-dimensional computed tomography registration evaluation. *Am. J. Orthod. Dentofac. Orthop.* 139: e83–e89.

70 Wang, Y. and Liou, E.J.W. (2008). Comparison of the loading behaviour of self-drilling and predrilled miniscrews throughout orthodontic loading. *Am. J. Orthod. Dentofac. Orthop.* 133: 38–43.

2

Maximising Mini-implant Success

Patient (Anatomical) Factors

The influences on mini-implant success rates are generally subdivided into three categories: patient, mini-implant (design), and technique factors. These will be discussed accordingly in this book, beginning with patient factors in this chapter.

Patient factors may be subdivided as:

- macro – somatic and general patient factors
- mini – insertion site anatomy
- micro – bone characteristics.

There is now a consensus in the literature that mini-implant success tends to be unaffected by patient gender, anteroposterior (Class I, II, or III) skeletal relationship, dental crowding, periodontal, and temporomandibular status. Therefore, these factors will not be discussed in detail. Having said that, my clinical experience is that gender may have an indirect influence in individual cases in terms of male–female variations in bone characteristics since these factors clearly do affect stability.

The basis and clinical consequences of these bone influences are summarised below. However, it's first worth defining some of the relevant terminology.

- Primary stability – the initial support for the mini-implant, due to its physical engagement in the cortical and cancellous bone. This is clinically reflected by the final insertion torque. Its influence reduces over several weeks as secondary stability supersedes it.
- Secondary stability – the long-term bone support for the mini-implant. This is due to (reactive) bone remodelling around the mini-implant body. On one hand, bone resorption leads to a loss of primary stability, whilst emerging bone deposition increases the secondary stability.
- Torque – measured in Newton centimetres (Ncm – the same Sir Isaac Newton who described the fundamentals of anchorage in his third Law). Insertion torque is the rotational resistance to a mini-implant being wound into the bone. A manual screwdriver readily reflects this in terms of how easy or difficult it is to turn/rotate the

screwdriver: low forces mean low primary stability, while high forces indicate high primary stability. Some mini-implant handpieces give a digital read-out of the torque, or allow the orthodontist to set the maximum insertion torque.

2.1 Cortical Bone Thickness and Density

A combination of clinical, animal and artificial bone studies has demonstrated that the most important patient determinants of primary stability are the density and thickness of the maxillary and mandibular cortical plates. This helps to explain the variations seen in clinical studies of mini-implant success rates where both anatomical sites and individuals differ in terms of the cortical bone layer's quantity and quality [1]. The key facts to consider are as follows.

- Cortical bone thickness (depth) is generally regarded as ranging from 1 to 2 mm (Figure 2.1) and generally increases towards the apical aspect of the alveolus. However, a recent micro-computed tomography (CT) study of cadavers has shown frequent areas of the maxillary and anterior buccal cortex with less than 1 mm cortex depth (compared to a mean of 1.3 mm palatal alveolar cortex depth and 2 mm or more in the posterior mandible) [2]. In the maxillary alveolus, cortical thickness peaks both mesial and distal to the canines (in the region of the canine eminence) and the first molars, which partly accounts for the frequent use of these sites for anterior and posterior anchorage points, respectively. Notably, the maxillary alveolar cortex is thicker on the palatal than the buccal side, which contributes to the value of palatal alveolar insertions in anterior openbite correction (discussed in Chapter 10), and the highest alveolar values for both jaws occur in mandibular molar sites [2–10].
- An increase in either the cortical thickness or density leads to an increase in insertion torque (the resistance to rotational insertion movements) [11–17]. Thickness and

The Orthodontic Mini-Implant Clinical Handbook, Second Edition. Richard Cousley.
© 2020 John Wiley & Sons Ltd. Published 2020 by John Wiley & Sons Ltd.

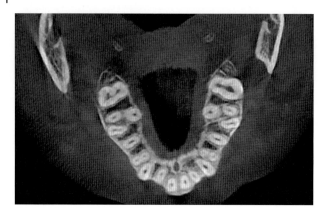

Figure 2.1 An axial cone beam CT where the cortical bone is seen as the peripheral dense white line. Notably, the alveolar cortex is much thinner than the mandibular ramus tissue seen posterolateral to the maxillary alveolus in this image. The positions of the two buccal and single palatal roots of the first molar teeth are also evident.

density are co-dependent factors, with density appearing to be the more influential in terms of mini-implant primary stability [13,14]. The density of the underlying cancellous bone is much less relevant, and hence has less influence on insertion torque [14].

- The ideal range of maximum insertion torque appears to be 5–15 Ncm for alveolar sites [12,18–23]. Interestingly, in my experience, the maximum torque for midpalate sites is often higher, peaking between 15 and 20 Ncm in adults. This has been corroborated by a retrospective study of consecutive midpalate insertions (in adolescents and adults) where 90% had 10–25 Ncm final torque readings [24]. Maximum torque occurs during final seating of the mini-implant and is felt as an increase in resistance on turning a manual screwdriver, such that difficulty in digital rotation typically equates to the top of this torque range. This is clinically valid without it being necessary to measure this in individual patients. In effect, low torque equates to poor *primary* stability (inadequate cortical support) and excessive torque results in *secondary* failure because microscopic bone stress leads to microfractures and subclinical ischaemic necrosis around the mini-implant threads [25]. This manifests clinically as the mini-implant screwing in with little resistance at the low end of the torque scale, and it being difficult to manually turn the screwdriver at the high end. Such excessive torque, especially in posterior mandibular sites, may be avoided by initial perforation of the cortical plate, as described later.

> The most important patient determinants of primary stability are the density and thickness of the cortical plates.

- Cortical bone thickness and density are both greater in the mandible than in the maxilla [26]. Our initial instinctive view is that the mandible provides greater primary stability because we regard it as a 'tougher' bone. However, mandibular success rates (reported in the literature) are less than those for the maxilla. This is because greater amounts of cortical thickness and density cause excessive insertion torque, which reflects high levels of peri-implant bone stress. This localised stress results in microscopic bone necrosis around the threads and hence secondary mini-implant failure [19].
- Cancellous bone, which has a similar density in both jaws [26–28], has often been suggested to have little effect on primary stability, except when the cortex is less than 1 mm. This occurs in some patients' maxillary buccal alveolar sites, and the cortical plate provides inadequate stability on its own [2]. In such sites, engagement of the cancellous bone does contribute to mini-implant stability, as demonstrated in an animal bone study [29]. This may account for the positive association between higher cancellous bone density and mini-implant success rates in a study of 127 maxillary buccal mini-implants [30]. Cancellous bone may also influence secondary stability in the long term, by stabilising the mini-implant body against migration and tipping [15,17,31]. This requires a mini-implant with a relatively longer body (e.g. 9 mm length) to engage sufficient cancellous bone area.

2.2 Interproximal Space

The literature provides data on the *average* amount of interproximal space available for mini-implant insertion, but it is crucial to understand that there is wide individual variation depending on the adjacent teeth's root sizes, shapes (degree of root taper and curvature) and alignment (i.e. root proximity or separation). Arguably, this almost means that 'average' figures are meaningless in individual patients, since each site must be assessed individually for bone volume (Figure 2.2). However, mean measurements do provide useful information such as highlighting that there is more space available on the palatal than the buccal aspect of the posterior maxillary alveolus (e.g. 5 and 3 mm, respectively). This is due to the differential number and shape of the molar roots, specifically the single palatal versus the two buccal roots of the molars (Figure 2.1).

Assuming reasonable tooth alignment, the typical buccal alveolar insertion sites for the maxilla are mesial to the first molar, and adjacent to the canines and central incisors, and for the mandible, adjacent to the molars and premolars [32]. Crucially, limited interproximal space is no longer regarded as a significant barrier since it may be increased

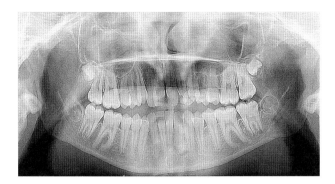

Figure 2.2 A panoramic radiograph which illustrates the typical variations in interproximal spaces, as affected by dental crowding, root length, morphology and tip. For example, the left mandibular first premolar's distal tip has resulted in more than average space between it and the second premolar, but less between it and the canine root.

in clinical practice by both preinsertion root divergence and oblique mini-implant insertion, as described in Chapter 5.

2.3 Soft Tissue and Oral Hygiene

Clinical experience indicates that there are distinct differences in soft tissue thickness according to anatomical location. This has been borne out in a ultrasound study of soft tissue thickness at mini-implant insertion sites, where the midpalate mucosa was the thinnest (mean 0.8 mm), followed by buccal sites (mean 1.3 mm) and palatal alveolar sites (mean 3.1 mm) [33]. In practical terms, these findings support the use of short-neck mini-implants in buccal sites and long-neck versions in palatal alveolar sites. In theory, short-neck mini-implants could be used in the midpalate, but longer neck versions may be helpful here to provide a means of attachment by elevating the head position. However, there is no evidence relating attached tissue thickness and mini-implant success rates *per se*.

What is known is that poor oral hygiene and peri-implant soft tissue inflammation (Figure 2.3) are risk factors for secondary failure [34–39]. Since these problems are more likely to occur in loose (non-keratinised) mucosa, it is almost always recommended that mini-implants are inserted through attached mucosa. This should minimise soft tissue disruption and the destabilising effects of mobile peri-implant tissue. The zone of mucosa which lies immediately around (coronal or just apical to) the mucogingival junction (MGJ) has been popularised by Sebastian Baumgaertel as a potential site, but there are no published data on success rates in this specific area [40,41]. It is likely that the key 'take home' message is that insertions should be sited in attached gingiva sites, with the option of 'straying' into the loose mucosa adjacent to the MGJ, provided that the sulcular tissues are stretched taut. This avoids interference during the insertion stage, by preventing the loose mucosa from wrapping around the mini-implant threads.

> It is almost always recommended that mini-implants are inserted through attached mucosa.

2.4 Maxillomandibular Planes Angle

Patients with a dolichofacial (long face) pattern and a high maxillomandibular planes angle (MMPA) (Figure 2.4) have an increased risk of failure for maxillary buccal mini-implants. This is an anatomical factor, due to their relatively thin maxillary buccal cortical plates (compared with 'short' face, brachyfacial, patients) [34,38,42–45]. However, these dolichofacial patients also typically present with an anterior openbite which may benefit from maxillary molar intrusion. This could affect mini-implant stability in those patients who need mini-implant intrusion for correction

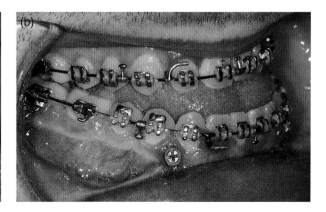

Figure 2.3 Photographs showing typical peri-implant soft tissue inflammation at (a) time of insertion in the right mandibular area and (b) after seven months of elastomeric traction. General problems with oral hygiene and resultant gingival hyperplasia are also evident.

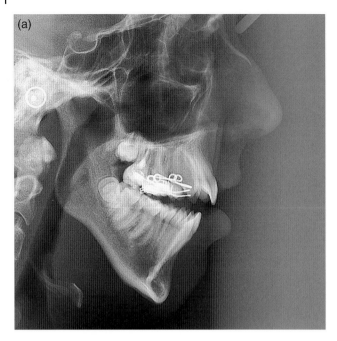 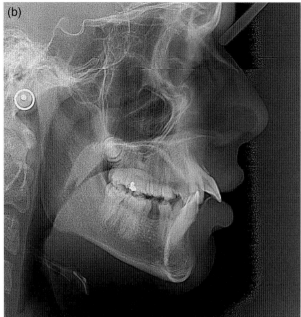

Figure 2.4 Lateral cephalograms of mini-implant anchorage patients exhibiting (a) long and (b) short face patterns. However, note that these images cannot illustrate the cortical bone characteristics.

of an anterior openbite, and this factor will be discussed further in Chapter 10. Fortunately, this problem of poor stability of maxillary buccal mini-implants may be avoided by mini-implant insertion in palatal alveolar sites [11,46].

2.5 Age

While primary stability is readily achieved in adults, adolescent patients have a significantly higher mini-implant failure rate in alveolar sites [47]. This is due to their reduced levels of cortical thickness and density [5,48,49] and higher rates of bone remodelling, which may compromise a mini-implant in terms of both primary and secondary stability. In effect, immature cortical bone is less able to withstand force applications, especially during the first month after insertion. The risk of secondary failure, occurring during the healing phase when bone resorption processes predominate, appears to be much more critical in adolescents than adults because they have lower primary stability to begin with. It then only takes a small drop in bone support to reduce the total mini-implant stability below the threshold for success. Therefore, whilst mini-implants are still successful in adolescents, it is advisable to be cautious and use light loading forces (e.g. 50 g) for the first six weeks after insertion.

Alternatively, the midpalate may be a preferable insertion site in young patients, even if this means accepting the limitations of indirect anchorage, because of its high reported success rates in children [24].

> Whilst mini-implants are still successful in adolescents, it is advisable to be cautious and keep the loading force low (e.g. 50 g) for the initial six weeks.

2.6 Cigarette Smoking

Heavy tobacco consumption is associated with a significantly higher failure rate [50]. Therefore, whilst cigarette smoking is not an absolute contraindication to mini-implant usage, smokers should be warned of the risk and advised to stop before mini-implant insertion.

2.7 Body Mass Index

Ironically, as cigarette smoking appears to be on the decline, we are treating more patients at the upper and lower ends of the body mass spectrum. Is this relevant? Well, my clinical observation has been that adolescent patients with a low Body Mass Index (BMI) have higher failure rates. This has recently been evidenced by a CT study of maxillary cortical bone thickness and density in relation to BMI and chronological age [49]. There was a statistically significant increase in both bone parameters with an increase in both BMI and patient age. Therefore, it is reasonable to assume that young patients with a low BMI will have higher failure rates for mini-implants. This may be partly negated by the use of midpalate sites in adolescents, assuming that indirect palate anchorage is feasible,

References

1 Lemieux, G., Hart, A., Cheretakis, C. et al. (2011). Computed tomographic characterization of mini-implant placement pattern and maximum anchorage force in human cadavers. *Am. J. Orthod. Dentofac. Orthop.* 140: 356–365.

2 Laursen, M.G., Melsen, B., and Cattaneo, P.M. (2013). An evaluation of insertion sites for mini-implants. A micro-CT study of human autopsy material. *Angle Orthod.* 83: 222–229.

3 Baumgaertel, S. and Hans, M.G. (2009). Buccal cortical bone thickness for mini-implant placement. *Am. J. Orthod. Dentofac. Orthop.* 136: 230–235.

4 Deguchi, T., Nasu, M., Murakami, K. et al. (2006). Quantitative evaluation of cortical bone thickness with computed tomographic scanning for orthodontic implants. *Am. J. Orthod. Dentofac. Orthop.* 129: 721. e7–e12.

5 Farnsworth, D., Rossouw, P.E., Ceen, F., and Buschang, P.H. (2011). Cortical bone thickness at common miniscrew implant placement sites. *Am. J. Orthod. Dentofac. Orthop.* 139: 495–503.

6 Lim, J., Lim, W.H., and Chun, Y.S. (2008). Quantitative evaluation of cortical bone thickness and root proximity at maxillary interradicular sites for orthodontic mini-implant placement. *Clin. Anat.* 21: 486–491.

7 Martinelli, F.L., Luiz, R.R., Faria, M., and Nojima, L.I. (2010). Anatomic variability in alveolar sites for skeletal anchorage. *Am. J. Orthod. Dentofac. Orthop.* 138: 252e1–e9.

8 Monnerat, C., Restle, L., and Mucha, J.N. (2009). Tomographic mapping of mandibular interradicular spaces for placement of orthodontic mini-implants. *Am. J. Orthod. Dentofac. Orthop.* 135: 428e1–e9.

9 Ono, A., Motoyoshi, M., and Shimizu, N. (2008). Cortical bone thickness in the buccal posterior region for orthodontic mini-implants. *Int. J. Oral Maxillofac. Surg.* 37: 334–340.

10 Park, J. and Cho, H.J. (2009). Three-dimensional evaluation of interradicular spaces and cortical bone thickness for the placement and initial stability of microimplants in adults. *Am. J. Orthod. Dentofac. Orthop.* 136: 314e1–314e12.

11 Biavati, A.S., Tecco, S., Migliorati, M. et al. (2011). Three-dimensional tomographic mapping related to primary stability and structural miniscrew characteristics. *Orthod. Craniofac. Res.* 14: 88–99.

12 Cha, J.Y., Takano-Yamamoto, T., and Hwang, C.J. (2010). The effect of miniscrew taper on insertion and removal torque in dogs. *Int. J. Oral Maxillofac. Implants* 25: 777–783.

13 Holm, L., Cunningham, S.J., Petrie, A., and Cousley, R.R.J. (2012). An in vitro study of factors affecting the primary stability of orthodontic mini-implants. *Angle Orthod.* 82: 1022–1028.

14 Marquezan, M., Lau, T.C.L., Mattos, C.T. et al. (2012). Bone mineral density. Methods of measurement and its influence on primary stability of miniscrews. *Angle Orthod.* 82: 62–66.

15 Motoyoshi, M., Yoshida, T., Ono, A., and Shimizu, N. (2007). Effect of cortical bone thickness and implant placement torque on stability of orthodontic mini-implants. *Clin. Oral Implants Res.* 22: 779–784.

16 Wilmes, B. and Drescher, D. (2011). Impact of bone quality, implant type, and implantation site preparation on insertion torques of mini-implants used for orthodontic anchorage. *Int. J. Oral Maxillofac. Surg.* 40: 697–703.

17 Wilmes, B., Rademacher, C., Olthoff, G., and Drescher, D. (2006). Parameters affecting primary stability of orthodontic mini-implants. *J. Orofac. Orthop.* 67: 162–174.

18 Suzuki, E.Y. and Suzuki, B. (2011). Placement and removal torque values of orthodontic miniscrew implants. *Am. J. Orthod. Dentofac. Orthop.* 139: 669–678.

19 Kim, K., Yu, W., Park, H. et al. (2011). Optimization of orthodontic microimplant thread design. *Korean J. Orthod.* 41: 25–35.

20 Motoyoshi, M., Hirabayashi, M., Uemura, M., and Shimizu, N. (2006). Recommended placement torque when tightening an orthodontic mini-implant. *Clin. Oral Implants Res.* 17: 109–114.

21 Motoyoshi, M., Uemura, M., Ono, A. et al. (2010). Factors affecting the long-term stability of orthodontic mini-implants. *Am. J. Orthod. Dentofac. Orthop.* 137: 588. e1–588.e5.

22 Wilmes, B. and Drescher, D. (2009). Impact of insertion depth and predrilling diameter on primary stability of orthodontic mini-implants. *Angle Orthod.* 79: 609–614.

23 McManus, M.M., Qian, F., Grosland, N.M. et al. (2011). Effect of miniscrew placement torque on resistance to miniscrew movement under load. *Am. J. Orthod. Dentofac. Orthop.* 140: e93–e98.

24 Di Leonardo, B., Ludwig, B., Lisson, J.A. et al. (2018). Insertion torque values and success rates for paramedian insertion of orthodontic miniimplants. *J. Orofac. Orthop.* 79: 109–115.

25 Nguyen, M.V., Codrington, J., Fletcher, L. et al. (2018). The influence of miniscrews insertion torque. *Eur. J. Orthod.* 40: 37–44.

26 Park, H., Lee, Y., Jeong, S., and Kwon, T. (2008). Density of the alveolar and basal bones of the maxilla and mandible. *Am. J. Orthod. Dentofac. Orthop.* 133: 30–37.

27 Choi, J., Park, C., Yi, S. et al. (2009). Bone density measurement in interdental areas with simulated placement of orthodontic miniscrew implants. *Am. J. Orthod. Dentofac. Orthop.* 136: 766 e1–766 e12.

28 Chun, Y.S. and Lim, W.H. (2009). Bone density at interradicular sites: implications for orthodontic mini-implant placement. *Orthod. Craniofac. Res.* 12: 25–32.

29 Marquezan, M., Lima, I., Lopes, R.T. et al. (2014). Is trabecular bone related to primary stability of miniscrews? *Angle Orthod.* 84: 500–507.

30 Lee, M.-Y., Jae Hyun Park, J.H., and Sang-Cheol Kim, S.-C. (2016). Bone density effects on the success rate of orthodontic microimplants evaluated with cone-beam computed tomography. *Am. J. Orthod. Dentofac. Orthop.* 149: 217–224.

31 Dalstra, M., Cattaneo, P.M., and Melsen, B. (2004). Load transfer of miniscrews for orthodontic anchorage. *Orthodontist* 1: 53–62.

32 Ludwig, B., Glasl, B., Kinziner, G.S.M. et al. (2011). Anatomical guidelines for miniscrew insertion: vestibular interradicular sites. *J. Clin. Orthod.* 45: 165–173.

33 Parmar, R., Reddy, V., Reddy, S.K., and Reddy, D. (2016). Determination of soft tissue thickness at orthodontic miniscrew placement sites using ultrasonography for customizing screw selection. *Am. J. Orthod. Dentofac. Orthop.* 150: 651–658.

34 Antoszewska, J., Papadopoulos, M.A., Park, H.S., and Ludwig, B. (2009). Five-year experience with orthodontic miniscrews implants: a retrospective investigation of factors influencing success rates. *Am. J. Orthod. Dentofac. Orthop.* 136: 158.e1–158.e10.

35 Park, H., Jeong, S., and Kwon, O. (2006). Factors affecting the clinical success of screw implants used as orthodontic anchorage. *Am. J. Orthod. Dentofac. Orthop.* 130: 18–25.

36 Wu, T., Kuang, S., and Wu, C. (2009). Factors associated with the stability of mini-implants for orthodontic anchorage: a study of 414 samples in Taiwan. *J. Oral Maxillofac. Surg.* 67: 1595–1599.

37 Cheng, S.J., Tseng, I.Y., Lee, J.J., and Kok, S.H. (2004). A prospective study of the risk factors associated with failure of mini-implants used for orthodontic anchorage. *Int. J. Oral Maxillofac. Implants* 19: 100–106.

38 Miyawaki, S., Koyama, I., Inoue, M. et al. (2003). Factors associated with the stability of titanium screws placed in the posterior region for orthodontic anchorage. *Am. J. Orthod. Dentofac. Orthop.* 124: 373–378.

39 Viwattanatipa, N., Thanakitcharu, S., Uttraravichien, A., and Pitiphat, W. (2009). Survival analysis of surgical miniscrews as orthodontic anchorage. *Am. J. Orthod. Dentofac. Orthop.* 136: 29–36.

40 Baumgaertel, S. and Tran, T.T. (2012). Buccal mini-implant site selection: the mucosal fallacy and zones of opportunity. *J. Clin. Orthod.* 46: 434–436.

41 Baumgaertel, S. (2014). Hard and soft tissue considerations at mini-implant insertion sites. *J. Orthod.* 41: S3–S7.

42 Moon, C., Park, H., Nam, J. et al. (2010). Relationship between vertical skeletal pattern and success rate of orthodontic mini-implants. *Am. J. Orthod. Dentofac. Orthop.* 138: 51–57.

43 Horner, K.A., Behrents, R.G., Kim, K., and Buschang, P.H. (2012). Cortical bone and ridge thickness of hyperdivergent and hypodivergent adults. *Am. J. Orthod. Dentofac. Orthop.* 142: 170–178.

44 Ozdemir, F., Tozlu, M., and Germec-Cakan, D. (2013). Cortical bone thickness of the alveolar process measured with cone beam computed tomography in patients with different facial types. *Am. J. Orthod. Dentofac. Orthop.* 143: 190–196.

45 Veli, I., Uysal, T., Baysal, A., and Karadede, I. (2014). Buccal cortical bone thickness at miniscrew placement sites in patients with different vertical skeletal patterns. *J. Orthofac. Orthop.* 74: 417–429.

46 Cousley, R.R.J. (2010). A clinical strategy for maxillary molar intrusion using orthodontic mini-implants and a customised palatal arch. *J. Orthod.* 37: 197–203.

47 Motoyoshi, M., Matsuoka, M., and Shimizu, N. (2007). Application of orthodontic mini-implants in adolescents. *Int. J. Oral Maxillofac. Surg.* 36: 695–699.

48 Cassetta, M., Sofan, A., Altieri, F., and Barbato, E. (2013). Evaluation of alveolar cortical bone thickness and density for orthodontic mini-implant placement. *J. Clin. Exp. Dent.* 5: e245–e252.

49 Ohiomoba, H., Sonis, A., Yansane, A., and Friedland, B. (2017). Quantitative evaluation of maxillary alveolar cortical bone thickness and density using computed tomography imaging. *Am. J. Orthod. Dentofac. Orthop.* 151: 82–91.

50 Bayat, E. and Bauss, O. (2010). Effect of smoking on the failure rates of orthodontic miniscrews. *J. Orthofac. Orthop.* 71: 117–124.

3

Maximising Mini-implant Success
Design Factors

3.1 Mini-implant Design Factors

The endosseous bodies of mini-implants differ within and between different manufacturers' systems in terms of their:

- dimensions – diameter and length
- shape – cylindrical or tapered
- thread design.

It is reasonable to assume that different design characteristics will influence mini-implant stability and success rates. In particular, an increase in mini-implant dimensions (i.e. a larger body) leads to greater contact with the surrounding bone surface area. Crucially, both *in vivo* and *in vitro* research projects have demonstrated that diameter is the most important factor in terms of primary stability because an increase in diameter leads to increased insertion torque [1–6].

An increase in body length has a much less pronounced effect (than an increase in diameter) with only a subtle increase in insertion torque and success rates occurring [7,8]. This is because an increase in length provides greater engagement in the cancellous bone, not the cortex, which is concordant with the fundamental influence of cortical bone on mini-implant stability (as described in Chapter 2). However, increased body length is still likely to be favourable in sites with thin cortical bone (less than 1 mm) where cancellous bone appears to supplement the cortical support. This results in both increased success rates for longer mini-implants with a longer body [9], and especially in reducing the potential long-term movement (tilting/migration) of the mini-implant where the loading force causes excessive peri-implant bone remodelling but not outright failure [10]. Similarly, relatively large-diameter mini-implants are also less likely to be deflected by prolonged loading [11] and, importantly, they are more fracture resistant [12–15].

This begs the question: why are large (e.g. 2 mm) diameter mini-implants not universally used for increased fracture resistance and stability? The answer is simple: 2 mm diameter mini-implants are not easily accommodated in alveolar interproximal spaces so most mini-implants have midbody diameters of around 1.5 mm for these sites. However, 2 mm diameter mini-implants may be used in edentulous alveolar sites and the midpalate (where, conversely, length is limited by anatomical parameters).

> Diameter is the most important factor in terms of primary stability because an increase in diameter leads to increased insertion torque.

The original mini-implant designs had cylindrical body shapes with self-tapping threads, and required predrilling of a full-depth pilot hole. Subsequent designs then favoured tapered (conical) body shapes and these are coincidentally also capable of self-drilling insertion. Both animal and clinical research studies have shown that the latter is more favourable for primary stability since tapered designs have a higher insertion torque than cylindrical ones, and also a higher removal torque during the bone healing phases [1,2,15–19]. This is because self-drilling causes less disruption of the peri-implant bone's original histological architecture and avoids the risk of thermal tissue necrosis (associated with the heat generated by pilot drilling) [6,20–26]. However, predrilling (perforation) of the cortical plate is still valuable in avoiding the generation of excessive torque in thick, dense cortical bone sites, such as in the posterior mandible and midpalate. This is discussed in more detail with regard to insertion technique in Chapter 4.

Finally, the extent of projection of the mini-implant head into the oral cavity is important since the greater the distance between the position of the loading force and the bone surface, then the higher the risk of an unfavourable force (moment) at the mini-implant and bone interface [27–32]. Consequently, it is advisable to use a low-profile mini-implant design in order to avoid an excessive head and neck length combination relative to the body length, and to fully insert mini-implants. This is also favourable from the patient's perspective since excessive prominence of a mini-implant may irritate opposing mucosal and tongue

The Orthodontic Mini-Implant Clinical Handbook, Second Edition. Richard Cousley.
© 2020 John Wiley & Sons Ltd. Published 2020 by John Wiley & Sons Ltd.

tissues. If the mini-implant's point of force application does project out from the surface, then lower forces should be used to avoid excessive cortical bone stress [31].

3.2 The Infinitas™ Mini-implant System

It may be a bewildering task for orthodontists to select a mini-implant kit since a great variety of systems are now available worldwide. These differ from one another in terms of their:

- physical design features
- technique steps (e.g. self-tapping or self-drilling)
- ease of insertion and use (e.g. how traction auxiliaries or wires are attached)
- guidance stent feasibility
- versatility
- size and complexity of the kit
- recommended clinical applications (e.g. direct or indirect anchorage)
- clinical instruction material.

It is unlikely that one system provides dramatically better mini-implant stability rates than all of the others and key principles are widely applicable. However, since the treatments and illustrations in this book mainly involve use of the Infinitas mini-implant system (DB Orthodontics Ltd, UK, www.infinitas-miniimplant.com), it is worth describing both its generic and distinctive features for clarity and reference purposes. The Infinitas mini-implant is unique in several aspects, especially in its head design and customised three-dimensional (3D) guidance stent facility [33]. This chapter describes the key design and clinical features of the Infinitas system's dual clinical and guidance kits.

3.2.1 Infinitas Mini-implant Design Features

Many mini-implant head designs have two separate tiers represented by [1] a channel or 'X'-shaped cross-slots at the top of the head for wire engagement and [2] an external circumferential undercut at a more apical level for the application of traction auxiliaries. In contrast, the Infinitas design has a unique, multipurpose head which combines cross-slots with both external and internal undercuts, all on one vertical level (Figure 3.1). This gives the head a very low profile (intraoral prominence) whilst enabling the direct attachment of all forms of traction auxiliaries and wires (up to 0.021×0.025 in. dimensions). In particular, standard nickel titanium (NiTi) coil springs may be directly engaged, within the internal undercut, on one corner of the bracket-like Infinitas head (Figure 3.2). Aside from patient comfort, this low profile is biomechanically favourable since it reduces the ratio of the head and neck (extra-bony

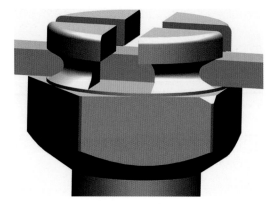

Figure 3.1 Diagram of the Infinitas mini-implant head showing its four bracket-like wings, divided by perpendicular cross-slots, and the external and internal undercuts. A rectangular wire is illustrated within the transverse cross-slot.

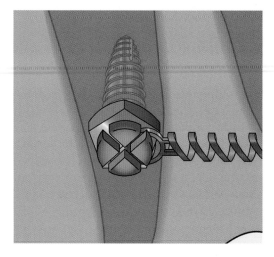

Figure 3.2 Diagram of an obliquely inserted Infinitas mini-implant with a coil spring engaged within the internal undercut of a single wing of its head.

section) to body length, and hence the risk of adverse tipping moments [34].

> The Infinitas design has a unique, multipurpose head which combines cross-slots with both external and internal undercuts, all on one vertical level.

The Infinitas head's precise engineering means that it is a relatively delicate structure. Therefore, the insertion screwdriver achieves a secure connection by engaging the *neck* section, and hence avoids large and potentially deformational forces on the mini-implant head. Consequently, the internal shape of the screwdriver closely matches the pentagonal shape of the coronal part of the neck (Figure 3.1). The more apical section of the neck is tapered to enable mini-implant insertion at both perpendicular and oblique angles to the cortical plate, maximising cortical engagement while minimising compression of the adjacent mucosa (Figure 3.3). There are short (1.5 mm) and long (2.5 mm) neck length versions, to allow for the mucosal depth at typical buccal and palatal insertion sites, respectively [35]. Whilst buccal insertions are routinely performed with a direct transmucosal technique, a reusable circular mucotome (soft tissue punch) is used to remove thick (palatal) gingiva or loose mucosa prior to insertion of a long neck mini-implant. If this is orientated perpendicular to the bone surface then it is easy to achieve a 'clean' cut around the circular edge of the soft tissue punch, for ease of removal of the corresponding piece of tissue.

The Infinitas body has only four size variables: 1.5 and 2.0 mm diameters (as measured in the midbody region) and 6 and 9 mm lengths. In combination with the two neck variables and the multipurpose head design, this means that a range of only five mini-implants provides for all alveolar and palatal insertion options (Table 3.1). This helps to simplify both the clinical decision-making process and inventory. Each mini-implant version is available in both non-sterile and sterile packaging. The latter has the advantage that the mini-implant is ready to use, straight out of the packet (Figure 3.4), whereas the non-sterile versions need to be sterilised in the Infinitas kit prior to use.

All the Infinitas bodies feature a self-drilling tip and threads (Figure 3.5), since self-drilling insertion preserves more original bone than a predrilled technique [20,24]. Engagement of the cortical bone plate, in order to maximise primary stability, is also enhanced by two specific Infinitas design features. First, the thread continues to the coronal end of the body such that it may be fully seated in bone. Second, the 1.5 mm (narrow) Infinitas body version has an additional tapered feature at its coronal end, such that the thread diameter gradually widens from 1.5 to 2 mm before

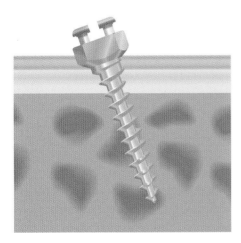

Figure 3.3 Diagram of an obliquely inserted mini-implant where the body traverses the cortical layer at an angle, facilitated by the tapered shape of the neck. Notably, one side of the head is closer to the mucosa than the opposite side.

Table 3.1 The Infinitas mini-implant range and typical insertion sites

Colour code	Diameter	Body length	Neck length	Typical insertion sites and inclinations
	1.5	9	Short	Maxilla: buccal alveolus
				Maxilla: oblique insertions in anterior alveolus
				Mandible: oblique insertions
	1.5	6	Short	Maxilla: perpendicular insertions in anterior alveolus
				Mandible: perpendicular insertions
	1.5	9	Long	Palatal alveolus (maxilla)
	2.0	6	Long	Midpalate
	2.0	9	Long	Edentulous areas

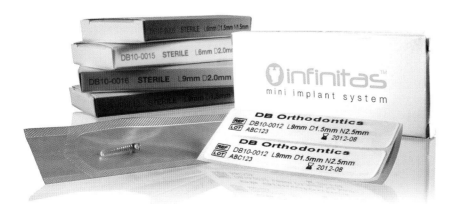

Figure 3.4 Packaging of presterilised Infinitas mini-implants. The mini-implant body is inside a rubber sheath, within the sterile envelope. The operator may pick up the mini-implant by holding this sheath, without the need for sterile gloves, whilst the (sterile) screwdriver is engaged on the mini-implant neck.

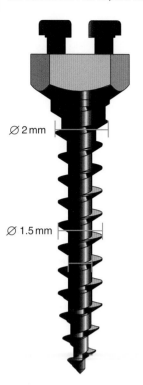

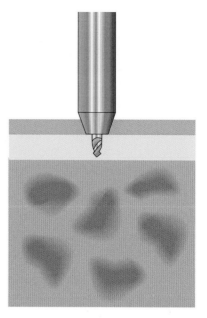

Figure 3.6 Diagram of the Infinitas cortical bone punch traversing the mucosa and inserting into a thick cortical layer.

Figure 3.5 Diagram showing how the body's coronal section tapers out from a 1.5 to 2.0 mm thread diameter.

the junction with the neck (Figure 3.4). This creates a clinically noticeable increase in torque during the final stage of insertion as the body part engaging the cortex widens from the cylindrical to tapered form, with the effect of increasing primary stability [2,36,37]. Another benefit of this additional body taper is that it greatly increases strength in this critical coronal area since a 0.2 mm increase in diameter can increase strength by 50% [37,38]. This helps to minimise the risk of fracture of the body during insertion and removal [39,40].

So why not have a 2 mm diameter over most of the body length? Unfortunately, this would greatly increase the risk of close root proximity in narrow interproximal sites (compared to the 1.5 mm midbody size). Hence, this tapered body design provides a 2 mm diameter superficially where it is most beneficial for strength and stability, but avoids root proximity problems since the narrowest interroot space is frequently 4 mm in from the external bone surface [41].

> This tapered body design provides a 2 mm diameter superficially where it is most beneficial for strength and stability, but avoids root proximity problems.

Excessive insertion torque is most likely to occur in the mandible and palate where the cortex is relatively thick and dense, leading to pressure necrosis of peri-implant bone and subsequent secondary (delayed) failure [24,42–46].

This risk is reduced by pilot drilling, especially within the first 2 mm of drilling depth [43,46]. However, pilot drilling is a nuisance if it requires a low-speed surgical handpiece and saline irrigation (to avoid heat necrosis). Therefore, it is ideal to perforate thick and dense cortical bone in order to avoid excess torque, but avoid drilling deep into the cancellous bone, and to simplify the insertion process by avoiding conventional pilot drilling. The Infinitas system achieves this balance with a customised cortical bone punch (Figure 3.6) which easily perforates dense cortical bone (and the mucosa), with simple slow manual clockwise rotations, up to a maximum depth of 2 mm. Its use is recommended for all posterior mandibular and palatal (alveolar and midpalate) insertion sites in adults, and it is fully compatible with the Infinitas guidance stent. Some orthodontists also prefer to use the punch in buccal sites to initially indent the cortex, without necessarily perforating it. This creates a 'purchase' point and avoids slippage of the mini-implant tip at the start of an oblique insertion.

3.2.2 Infinitas Guidance System

Mini-implant planning involves determination of the optimum mesiodistal and vertical position, and also ideally the vertical and horizontal angles of insertion; that is, 3D planning is required. However, it may still be difficult to accurately position a mini-implant, typically in posterior or palatal locations, because of restricted visual and instrument access. Further discrepancies may arise when the planning and insertion processes are carried out by an inexperienced orthodontist, or especially by different clinicians (e.g. an orthodontist and surgeon). For example, a recent retrospective study of 50 orthognathic cases (where mini-implants were inserted for intermaxillary fixation) showed considerable variation in the surgical mini-implant insertion angles. Perhaps more worryingly for secondary stability was the cone beam computed tomography (CBCT) observation that 41% of these mini-implants had some degree of root contact, even after allowing for the overestimating effect of this on panoramic radiographs [47].

Research has shown that clinical inexperience is associated with greater risks of mini-implant–root proximity and hence increased failure rates [17,29,48,49]. In the situation where the insertion is done by a different clinician, the orthodontist should ideally avoid the need to fully describe the insertion site, angles and clinical plan, and then hope that this plan is both understood and followed. Instead, the 3D positional information should be clearly dictated by a stent, removing the need for educated guesswork or improvisation by the surgeon. Unfortunately, placement of an interproximal wire or custom-made wire guide at the approximate insertion site or on an adjacent fixed appliance usually only indicates the superficial insertion position and not the 3D angles of insertion. This approach is also prone to radiographic parallax errors. Even techniques using a circular guide tube allow excessive lateral play of the insertion instrument [50], and partly rely on visual alignment of the mini-implant with the tube's adjacent edges unless the screwdriver is physically steered by engagement within the guide tube.

These problems can be minimised by the use of a stent capable of reliably transferring the 3D prescription from the planning to the insertion stages, and then physically guiding the insertion process. It is also ideal if relatively little laboratory expertise and cost are required. The Infinitas guidance system meets these requirements by using three simple components: a mini-implant analogue, abutment and guide cylinder which work with a plastic baseplate to form an insertion stent for precise control of insertion instruments (Figure 3.7). There are six simple steps involved in the fabrication of this stent, and these may be carried out by an orthodontist (with access to a vacuum or pressure forming machine) with or without the assistance of an orthodontic technician (following the orthodontist's prescription) as described here.

> A stent is capable of reliably transferring the 3D prescription from the planning to the insertion stages.

1) **Plan the insertion details using a dental model and radiographs**

   For manual stent fabrication, the optimum position and angulations for each mini-implant are determined by

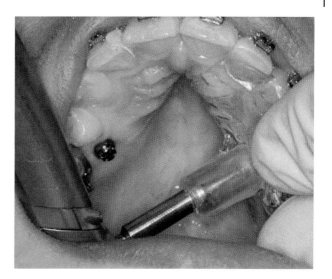

Figure 3.7 Handpiece insertion of an Infinitas mini-implant on the palatal aspect of the alveolus, where the end of the screwdriver insert fits within the 3D stent. The mini-implant's body can be seen through the plastic guidance cylinder.

combining radiographic information (e.g. a periapical or CBCT view of the interproximal space) with the topographical features of a plaster model of the dental arch. In effect, it is much easier to visualise the insertion angles on a model than in the patient's mouth, and the surface contour of the model typically highlights the appropriate insertion space as a concave indentation between tooth roots. In order to preserve as much detail as possible, it is important to avoid waxing/blocking out any fixed appliance brackets near the insertion site when a dental impression is recorded for stent fabrication.

2) **Drill a pilot hole in the model**

   A pilot hole is drilled in the dental model at the planned vertical and mesiodistal insertion point and angles, using a plaster drill and a contra-angle dental handpiece (Figure 3.8). It is recommended that this hole is initially drilled to only half of the analogue length. This gives the option of drilling the remaining depth of the hole at a new insertion angle, should this be appropriate on judging a half-inserted analogue.

3) **Insert the mini-implant analogue into the model**

   The analogue is manually screwed into position in a clockwise direction, using the guidance kit screwdriver. If in doubt, the analogue should only be partially seated until its 3D position has been checked, so that an alteration of the insertion site/directions is easily made by further drilling.

4) **Fit the abutment onto the analogue**

   The abutment is manually fitted onto the head of the analogue and usefully amplifies the analogue's insertion angles (Figure 3.9). If the 3D position of the analogue appears to be suboptimal then it should be removed from the model and the insertion process repeated with different location/angulation details (after filling in the plaster hole as necessary). In particular, it is much easier to refine the position in a dental model at this stage than in the patient's mouth at the insertion visit!

5) **Slide the guide cylinder over the abutment**

   The internal diameter of the cylinder is similar to the external diameter of the abutment, ensuring a close fit between their surfaces.

6) **Form the stent baseplate**

   The assembled combination of dental model, analogue, abutment and guide cylinder components is placed into a pressure or vacuum forming machine such as that used for orthodontic retainer fabrication. The stent baseplate is then formed using a thick (ideally 1.5 mm)

thermoplastic blank. This is much thicker than retainer blanks (which are typically 1 mm), in order to reduce flexing of the stent (if the screwdriver is leant upon). The baseplate, incorporating the guide cylinder, is then trimmed to the desired size, usually incorporating four or more crowns and the insertion site (Figure 3.10). If there are already brackets on the teeth then the baseplate edge should be trimmed clear of them.

All three Infinitas insertion instruments (soft tissue and bone punches, and the screwdriver) fit precisely into the guide cylinder (Figure 3.7) with the same degree of precision as occurs between the guide cylinder and its abutment. The physical guidance provided by the Infinitas stent has several additional benefits. First, it provides a stable insertion point

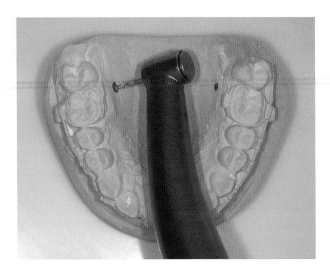

Figure 3.8 Drilling of the palatal aspect of a plaster model, with the drill angled towards the contact point of the molars and at the planned inclination (approximately 90° to the sloping surface).

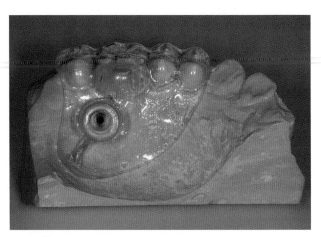

Figure 3.10 A finished insertion stent where the insertion hole in the plaster model is seen in the centre of the guidance cylinder, and the baseplate covers the four posterior teeth and adjacent palatal alveolus.

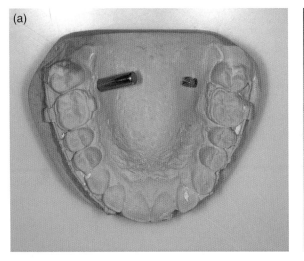

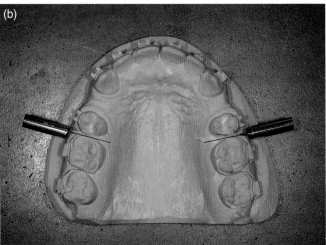

Figure 3.9 (a) Infinitas analogues have been inserted into predrilled holes on both sides of the model and an abutment has been fitted onto the right-sided one. The buccal abutments are being used in (b) to confirm whether the insertion angles pass along the line of the second premolar–first molar contact points.

and avoids slippage of the mini-implant tip during oblique insertion. Second, it reduces directional variation which minimises both flaring of the insertion bed and the risk of fracture of the mini-implant. Finally, it minimises radiographic needs since no additional radiographs are required, either with a guide or a provisional stent *in situ*.

3.3 Digital Stent Fabrication Processes

The manual stent process, described above, has worked well in the last 10 years, but it does involve the process of mentally merging the topographical (model surface) and 2D radiographic information. In the coming years, this process will be superseded by the introduction of digital model technology. For example, it is now possible to produce stents for palatal and alveolar insertion sites using digital CAD-CAM software (Figures 3.11 and 3.12). This enables orthodontists already using virtual orthodontic models to produce a physical stent, using a 3D printed model and the (manual) Infinitas guidance kit. However, whilst digital models provide accurate (tooth and soft tissue) topographical information, they can only offer hints of the underlying root positions. They cannot give us a direct view of what lies below the surface – the skeletal (e.g. cortex and cancellous bone depth and distance to adjacent structures) and dental anatomy in the sites where the mini-implant body will be positioned. These require the additional input of CBCT data for comprehensive 3D planning.

It is becoming feasible to accurately plan mini-implant positions in 3D by merging digital models and CBCT data together [51]. This will unite their topographical and bone/

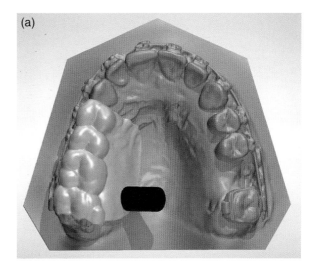

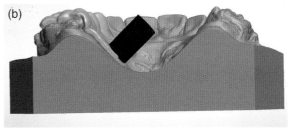

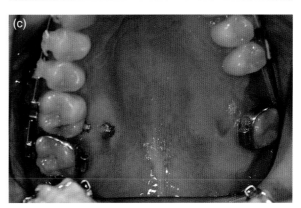

Figure 3.12   (a,b) Illustrations of a unilateral palatal stent designed using 'Appliance Designer' software (www.3shape.com/en/software/ortho-system). The baseplate, shown in light blue, was sculpted on the digital model of the maxillary dentition. The guidance cylinder (*dark blue*) was added and orientated in 3D prior to 3D printing a plastic stent in a biocompatible material. The resultant mini-implant position is shown in (c) immediately after insertion using the stent.

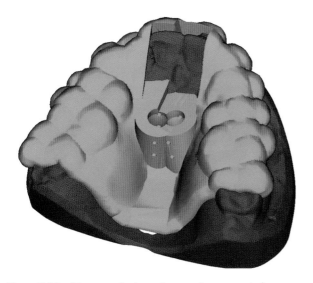

Figure 3.11   Diagram of a (*green*) computer-generated guidance stent, with twin midpalatal cylinders, superimposed on a (*red*) digital model of the maxillary arch.

root positional information, and promises to improve the accuracy of insertions. For example, a 2013 study demonstrated that the use of guidance stents produced from CBCT and digital model data resulted in the avoidance of adjacent tooth roots in 84% of insertions compared with 50% in a control group [52]. At the time of writing this edition, customised software specifically designed for orthodontic mini-implant guidance purposes is being more widely developed (Figure 3.13). Therefore, established

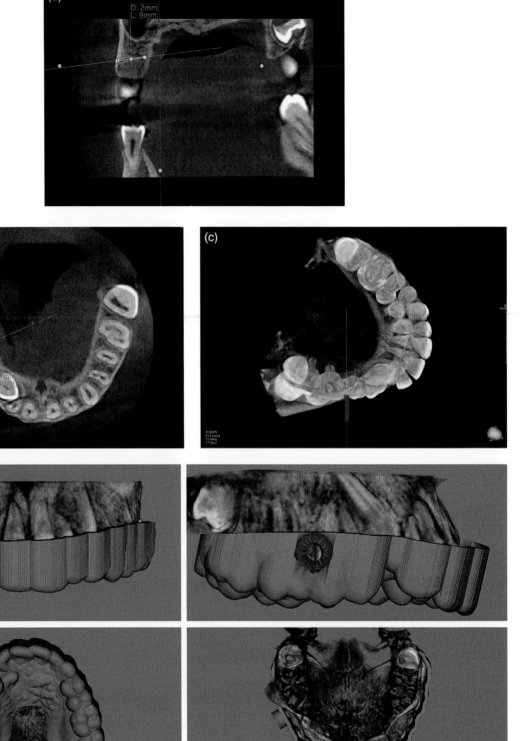

Figure 3.13 (a–c) Diagrams of a CBCT software package being used to plan placement of a (*green*) virtual mini-implant mesial/buccal to the right maxillary first molar, in the three different sectional views plus in a 3D reformatted view. A virtual abutment (shown in red) can be attached to the CBCT mini-implant. This accentuates the 3D angles of insertion. (d) This information is then used to fabricate a virtual guidance stent, produced by 3D printing. Source: The images in (d) were kindly produced using Dolphin® software by Dr Paul Thomas, Scientific Advisor, Dolphin Imaging & Management Solutions (www.dolphinimaging.com).

orthodontic planning packages are likely to incorporate this facility in due course. These will probably feature the ability to computer-design and export a virtual stent for direct 3D printing, without the need to print a working model as an intermediary step. However, those orthodontists who still prefer to have a tactile planning process will be able to 3D print a working model from digital files and then manually drill a pilot hole in a physical model.

References

1 Cha, J.Y., Takano-Yamamoto, T., and Hwang, C.J. (2010). The effect of miniscrew taper on insertion and removal torque in dogs. *Int. J. Oral Maxillofac. Implants* 25: 777–783.

2 Holm, L., Cunningham, S.J., Petrie, A., and Cousley, R.R.J. (2012). An in vitro study of factors affecting the primary stability of orthodontic mini-implants. *Angle Orthod.* 82: 1022–1028.

3 Song, Y., Cha, J., and Hwang, C. (2007). Mechanical characteristics of various orthodontic mini-screws in relation to artificial cortical bone thickness. *Angle Orthod.* 77: 979–985.

4 Wilmes, B., Su, Y., and Drescher, D. (2008). Insertion angle impact on primary stability of orthodontic mini-implants. *Angle Orthod.* 78: 1065–1070.

5 Yano, S., Motoyoshi, M., Uemura, M. et al. (2006). Tapered orthodontic miniscrews induce bone-screw cohesion following immediate loading. *Eur. J. Orthod.* 28: 541–546.

6 Liou, E.J.W., Pai, B.C.J., and Lin, J.C.Y. (2004). Do miniscrews remain stationary under orthodontic forces? *Am. J. Orthod. Dentofac. Orthop.* 126: 42–47.

7 Pithon, M.M., Figueiredo, D.S.F., and Oliveira, D.D. (2013). Mechanical evaluation of orthodontic mini-implants of different lengths. *J. Oral Maxillofac. Surg.* 71: 479–486.

8 Uesugi, S., Kokai, S., Kanno, Z., and Ono, T. (2018). Stability of secondarily inserted orthodontic miniscrews after failure of the primary insertion for maxillary anchorage: maxillary buccal area vs midpalatal suture area. *Am. J. Orthod. Dentofac. Orthop.* 153: 54–60.

9 Melo, A.C.M., Andrighetto, A.R., Hirt, S.D. et al. (2016). Risk factors associated with the failure of miniscrews – a ten-year cross sectional study. *Braz. Oral Res.* 30: e124 1–e124 6.

10 Morarend, C., Qian, F., Marshall, S.D. et al. (2009). Effect of screw diameter on orthodontic skeletal anchorage. *Am. J. Orthod. Dentofac. Orthop.* 136: 224–229.

11 Barros, S.E., Janson, G., Chiqueto, K. et al. (2011). Effect of mini-implant diameter on fracture risk and self-drilling efficacy. *Am. J. Orthod. Dentofac. Orthop.* 140: e181–e192.

12 Park, H., Jeong, S., and Kwon, O. (2006). Factors affecting the clinical success of screw implants used as orthodontic anchorage. *Am. J. Orthod. Dentofac. Orthop.* 130: 18–25.

13 Mischkowski, R.A., Kneuertz, P., Florvaag, B. et al. (2008). Biomechanical comparison of four different miniscrew types for skeletal anchorage in the mandibulo-maxillary area. *Int. J. Oral Maxillofac. Surg.* 37: 948–954.

14 Wilmes, B., Panayotidis, A., and Drescher, D. (2011). Fracture resistance of orthodontic mini-implants: a biomechanical in vitro study. *Eur. J. Orthod.* 33: 396–401.

15 Chen, C.H., Chang, C.S., Hsieh, C.H., and Tseng, Y.C. (2006). The use of microimplants in orthodontic anchorage. *J. Oral Maxillofac. Surg.* 64: 1209–1213.

16 Wilmes, B., Rademacher, C., Olthoff, G., and Drescher, D. (2006). Parameters affecting primary stability of orthodontic mini-implants. *J. Orofac. Orthop.* 67: 162–174.

17 Wu, T., Kuang, S., and Wu, C. (2009). Factors associated with the stability of mini-implants for orthodontic anchorage: a study of 414 samples in Taiwan. *J. Oral Maxillofac. Surg.* 67: 1595–1599.

18 Lim, S., Cha, J., and Hwang, C. (2008). Insertion torque of orthodontic miniscrews according to changes in shape, diameter and length. *Angle Orthod.* 78: 234–240.

19 Pithon, M.M., Nojima, M.G., and Nojima, L.I. (2011). In vitro evaluation of insertion and removal torques of orthodontic mini-implants. *Int. J. Oral Maxillofac. Surg.* 40: 80–85.

20 Chen, Y., Shin, H., and Kyung, H.M. (2008). Biomechanical and histological comparison of self-drilling and self-tapping orthodontic microimplants in dogs. *Am. J. Orthod. Dentofac. Orthop.* 133: 44–50.

21 Chen, Y., Lee, J.W., Cho, W.H., and Kyung, H.M. (2010). Potential of self-drilling orthodontic microimplants under immediate loading. *Am. J. Orthod. Dentofac. Orthop.* 137: 496–502.

22 Cha, J., Yoon, T., and Hwang, C. (2008). Insertion and removal torques according to orthodontic mini-screw design. *Korean J. Orthod.* 38: 5–12.

23 Heidemann, W., Terheyden, H., and Gerlach, K.L. (2001). Analysis of the osseous/metal interface of drill free screws and self-tapping screws. *J. Craniomaxillofac. Surg.* 29: 69–74.

24 Kim, J., Ahn, S., and Chang, Y. (2005). Histomorphometric and mechanical analyses of the drill-free screw as orthodontic anchorage. *Am. J. Orthod. Dentofac. Orthop.* 128: 190–194.

25 Shank, S.B., Beck, F.B., d'Atri, A.M., and Huja, S.S. (2012). Bone damage associated with orthodontic placement of miniscrew implants in an animal model. *Am. J. Orthod. Dentofac. Orthop.* 141: 412–418.

26 Su, Y.Y., Wilmes, B., Honscheid, R., and Drescher, D. (2009). Comparison of self-tapping and self-drilling orthodontic mini-implants: an animal study of insertion torque and displacement under lateral loading. *Int. J. Oral Maxillofac. Implants* 24: 404–411.

27 Buchter, A., Wiechmann, D., Koerdt, S. et al. (2005). Load-related implant reaction of mini-implants used for orthodontic anchorage. *Clin. Oral Implants Res.* 16: 473–479.

28 Berens, A., Wiechmann, D., and Dempf, R. (2006). Mini- and microscrews for temporary skeletal anchorage in orthodontic therapy. *J. Orofac. Orthop.* 67: 450–458.

29 Kim, Y.H., Yang, S., Kim, S. et al. (2010). Midpalatal miniscrews for orthodontic anchorage: factors affecting clinical success. *Am. J. Orthod. Dentofac. Orthop.* 137: 66–72.

30 Kuroda, S., Nishii, Y., Okano, S., and Sueishi, K. (2014). Stress distribution in the mini screw and alveolar bone during orthodontic treatment: a finite element study analysis. *J. Orthod.* 41: 275–284.

31 Lin, T., Tsai, F., Chen, C., and Lin, D. (2013). Factorial analysis of variables affecting bone stress adjacent to the orthodontic anchorage mini-implant with finite element analysis. *Am. J. Orthod. Dentofac. Orthop.* 143: 182–189.

32 Shantavasinkul, P., Akkus, O., Palomo, J.M., and Baumgaertel, S. (2016). Surface strain distribution of orthodontic miniscrews under load. *Am. J. Orthod. Dentofac. Orthop.* 150: 444–450.

33 Cousley, R.R.J. (2009). A stent-guided mini-implant system. *J. Clin. Orthod.* 43: 403–407.

34 Buchter, A., Wiechmann, D., Koerdt, S. et al. (2005). Load-related implant reaction of mini-implants used for orthodontic anchorage. *Clin. Oral Implants Res.* 16: 473–479.

35 Cha, B., Lee, Y., Lee, N. et al. (2008). Soft tissue thickness for placement of an orthodontic miniscrew using an ultrasonic device. *Angle Orthod.* 78: 403–408.

36 Cha, J., Yoon, T., and Hwang, C. (2008). Insertion and removal torques according to orthodontic mini-screw design. *Korean J. Orthod.* 38: 5–12.

37 Chang, J.Z., Chen, Y., and Tung, Y. (2012). Effects of thread depth, taper shape, and taper length on the mechanical properties of mini-implants. *Am. J. Orthod. Dentofac. Orthop.* 141: 279–288.

38 Carano, A., Lonardo, P., Velo, S., and Incorvati, C. (2005). Mechanical properties of three different commercially available miniscrews for skeletal anchorage. *Prog. Orthod.* 6: 82–97.

39 Barros, S.E., Janson, G., Chiqueto, K. et al. (2011). Effect of mini-implant diameter on fracture risk and self-drilling efficacy. *Am. J. Orthod. Dentofac. Orthop.* 140: e181–e192.

40 Wilmes, B., Panayotidis, A., and Drescher, D. (2011). Fracture resistance of orthodontic mini-implants: a biomechanical in vitro study. *Eur. J. Orthod.* 33: 396–401.

41 Deguchi, T., Nasu, M., Murakami, K. et al. (2006). Quantitative evaluation of cortical bone thickness with computed tomographic scanning for orthodontic implants. *Am. J. Orthod. Dentofac. Orthop.* 129: 721.e–e12.

42 Motoyoshi, M., Hirabayashi, M., Uemura, M., and Shimizu, N. (2006). Recommended placement torque when tightening an orthodontic mini-implant. *Clin. Oral Implants Res.* 17: 109–114.

43 Wilmes, B., Rademacher, C., Olthoff, G., and Drescher, D. (2006). Parameters affecting primary stability of orthodontic mini-implants. *J. Orofac. Orthop.* 67: 162–174.

44 Wilmes, B., Ottenstreuer, S., Su, Y., and Drescher, D. (2008). Impact of implant design on primary stability of orthodontic mini-implants. *J. Orofac. Orthop.* 69: 42–50.

45 Lim, S., Cha, J., and Hwang, C. (2008). Insertion torque of orthodontic miniscrews according to changes in shape, diameter and length. *Angle Orthod.* 78: 234–240.

46 Cho, K. and Baek, S. (2012). Effects of predrilling depth and implant shape on the mechanical properties of orthodontic mini-implants during the insertion procedure. *Angle Orthod.* 82: 618–624.

47 An, J.H., Kim, Y.I., Kim, S.S. et al. (2019). Root proximity of miniscrews at a variety of maxillary and mandibular buccal sites: reliability of panoramic radiography. *Angle Orthod.* 89: 611–616.

48 Garfinkle, J.S., Cunningham, L.L., Beeman, C.S. et al. (2008). Evaluation of orthodontic mini-implant anchorage in premolar extraction therapy in adolescents. *Am. J. Orthod. Dentofac. Orthop.* 133: 642–653.

49 Cho, U., Yu, W., and Kyung, H. (2010). Root contact during drilling for microimplant placement. *Angle Orthod.* 81: 130–136.

50 Suzuki, E.Y. and Suzuki, B. (2007). A simple three-dimensional guide for safe miniscrew placement. *J. Clin. Orthod.* 41: 342–346.

51 Liu, H., Liu, D., Wang, G. et al. (2010). Accuracy of surgical positioning of orthodontic miniscrews with a computer-aided design and manufacturing template. *Am. J. Orthod. Dentofac. Orthop.* 137: 728.e1–728.e10.

52 Bae, M., Kim, J., Park, J. et al. (2013). Accuracy of miniscrew surgical guides assessed from cone-beam computed tomography and digital models. *Am. J. Orthod. Dentofac. Orthop.* 143: 893–901.

4

Maximising Mini-implant Success
Clinical Factors

4.1 Clinical Technique Factors

4.1.1 Insertion Technique

As with all clinical techniques, it's an unfortunate truth that mini-implant success rates increase with clinical experience [1–4]. Therefore, if you're gaining experience in mini-implant techniques, it's advisable to preplan the insertion steps and biomechanics (as outlined in Chapter 5), and consider the use of a guidance stent to reduce root proximity risks. In addition, there is some evidence that 3D (cone beam computed tomography – CBCT) imaging may reduce the risks of root contact and hence improve success rates. For example, an *in vitro* study of mini-implant insertions in skulls showed a 5% risk of root contact with the use of small-volume CBCT compared to a 55–60% rate when no radiograph or a 2D radiograph was used for planning [5]. While CBCT may not be justifiable where it is clinically apparent that there is plenty of interproximal space, arguably it would help orthodontists with little experience of mini-implants. Ideally, a guidance stent (refer to Chapters 3 and 4) would then be used to replicate this 3D planning in the clinical environment.

Mini-implants may be inserted manually with a customised screwdriver or using a contra-angle handpiece. This technique choice is a practical one depending on the ease of intraoral access and hence screwdriver directional control and handling. The other difference is that it is easier to appreciate and control the insertion torque with a manual screwdriver, whereas tactile sensation is lost with the handpiece.

The key technique variations which have been studied by researchers are whether a pilot hole is drilled prior to mini-implant insertion and whether the insertion should be made perpendicular to the cortex or angled obliquely. Unlike restorative dental implant techniques, predrilling for orthodontic mini-implants does not involve drilling a full-depth pilot hole. The aim of predrilling is to reduce the insertion torque to an acceptable level by perforation of the cortical plate, since the greatest effect of drilling occurs within the most superficial 2 mm of drilling depth [6–8]. This is consistent with the clinical observation of a drop in drilling resistance once the cortex has been perforated. However, predrilling has been associated with an increased mini-implant failure rate in adolescents [9]. This makes sense given that growing patients have lower maximum insertion torque statistics than adults. Therefore, it is ideal to avoid predrilling in adolescent patients and also in maxillary buccal and anterior mandibular sites, where the cortex is relatively thin and less dense anyway. Conversely, self-drilling mini-implants benefit from perforation of the cortex in areas of dense/thick cortex (specifically the posterior mandible and palate) in order to avoid excessive insertion torque and the associated generation of microcracks and bone damage [10–16]. This can be achieved with a cortical punch which only perforates the cortex rather than a pilot drill which readily drills beyond 2 mm depth [17].

> Self-drilling mini-implants benefit from perforation of the cortex in areas of dense/thick cortex in order to avoid excessive insertion torque.

The design features of some mini-implants essentially limit their insertion to being perpendicular (90°) to the surface. However, several animal studies have recorded the highest insertion torque values and increased secondary stability with a 20–30° apically directed insertion angle rather than it being perpendicular to the bone surface [18–21]. This is due to enhanced engagement of the cortex and appears to be especially favourable in the maxilla (where the cortex is less robust). Oblique insertions are also favourable in terms of reducing labiolingual insertion depth and hence proximity to the roots [22,23].

4.1.2 Root Proximity

Close proximity of the mini-implant body and adjacent roots (Figure 4.1) should be avoided in order to avoid

The Orthodontic Mini-Implant Clinical Handbook, Second Edition. Richard Cousley.
© 2020 John Wiley & Sons Ltd. Published 2020 by John Wiley & Sons Ltd.

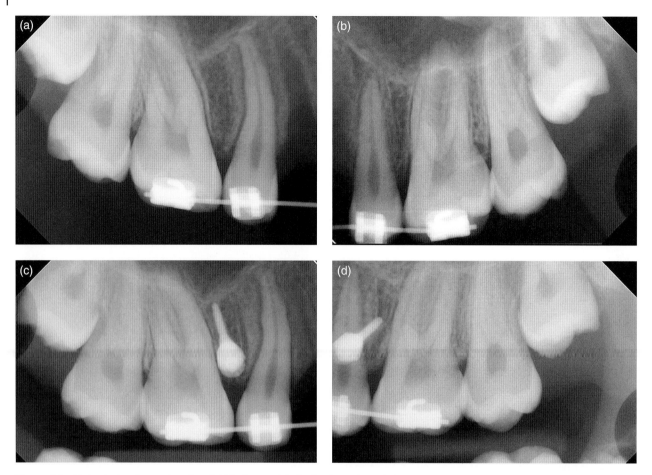

Figure 4.1 Periapical radiographs taken (a,b) before and (c,d) after insertion of bilateral maxillary mini-implants. There is a large interproximal space on the right side (a,c), but a smaller distance on the left side (b,d), with the consequence of radiographic overlap and likely close root proximity on the left side (d).

periodontal and root damage, although histological studies show that complete cellular cementum repair usually occurs after root trauma [23–32]. In effect, the major problem with close implant–root proximity is that it provides inadequate bone coverage for the threads, destabilises the mini-implant (rather than the tooth) and increases failure rates [33–40]. For example, a CBCT study of 228 mini-implants (inserted in buccal sites mesial to the maxillary first molar) demonstrated a statistically significant link between root proximity and success rates, and indicated that 0.5 mm separation between mini-implants and adjacent root surfaces is required [39]. In contrast, higher success rates with increasing cortex thickness appeared to be a less significant influence. Therefore, root proximity is a greater risk factor than modest reductions in cortical thickness [38,39]. This appears to be because of the transfer of unfavourable masticatory forces to the mini-implant via the adjacent tooth [41].

In clinical terms, root contact, or even close proximity, may be detected during mini-implant insertion by a sharp increase in insertion resistance [27,28,42], although an increase in insertion torque does not always occur on root contact [43]. This is also likely to result in blunting of the mini-implant tip, patient discomfort (provided that only superficial anaesthesia has been used), and a dull note on percussion of the affected tooth. Consequently, these signs should be taken as indicators of close proximity and the mini-implant withdrawn and reinserted at a different location or angle.

On the other hand, if signs of root contact are missed and the mini-implant is left *in situ*, then it is not inevitable that it will fail. For example, a retrospective CBCT study of 147 buccal mini-implants showed that 20% had some degree of root contact, particularly with the root on the distal side of the insertion site [44]. This is because there was probably a strong tendency for freehand insertions to be angulated (aimed) towards the more distal tooth. Since the failure rate of these mini-implants was 21% (compared to 2% for the non-contact mini-implants), this means that 80% of the mini-implants in root contact were still successful. In other words, root contact strongly predisposes to failure but does not guarantee it.

The major problem with close implant–root proximity is that this provides inadequate bone coverage for the threads, destabilises the mini-implant and increases failure rates.

4.1.3 Force Application

Mini-implant loading stimulates a favourable physiological response in the adjacent bone provided that the force level is tolerable for this tissue. This has been demonstrated in terms of increasing bone–implant contact, relatively more bone formation (than resorption), increases in cortical thickness and alveolar density and removal torque [45–55]. In turn, these bone changes contribute to secondary stability of the mini-implant. However, there is no clear evidence currently available regarding the optimum force levels tolerated by mini-implants. Therefore, it is sensible to be cautious and only apply a light initial force, for instance 50 g during the first 4–6 weeks, and thereafter limit forces to the normal orthodontic range, which is 150–200 g.

It is helpful to understand some relevant concepts of basic bone biology, especially that peri-implant bone is dynamic and undergoes a series of bone healing phases following mini-implant insertion. These phases involve:

1) inflammatory acceleration
2) active bone resorption
3) a latency or transition period
4) predominantly new bone formation.

Crucially, mini-implant stability is at its lowest level at the end of the resorptive phase, during the third week in humans, in both alveolar and midpalate sites [56–58]. However, buccal sites with a thin cortical bone layer may be most susceptible to this reduction in bone support since the primary stability at such sites is relatively low, even before the effects of bone resorption manifest after several weeks. Hence, this three-week postinsertion stage represents the pivotal point between reliance on the diminishing effects of primary and increasing effects of secondary stability. Whilst immediate loading is feasible, especially in adults [17,46,59,60], the results of a prospective clinical study suggest that delayed loading may be beneficial for adolescent patients [60]. This may be judged clinically by having a tactile feeling for the maximum insertion torque; if this is felt to be low when manually rotating the screwdriver during the final insertion stage then consider a loading delay of 6–12 weeks.

Only apply a light initial force, for instance 50 g, during the first four weeks in adults and six weeks in adolescents, before applying normal forces, of 150 g.

4.2 Introducing Mini-implants to your Clinical Practice

We're often told that it's easier to learn new things (e.g. techniques) at a young age, and this maxim appears to hold true for orthodontic anchorage. Therefore, many colleagues have benefited by integrating bone anchorage into their clinical practice within their specialist training programme. However, adopting mini-implant anchorage may be a daunting proposition for many orthodontists, especially if working outside the potentially supportive environment of a specialist training establishment.

From my observations, this has led some orthodontists to argue that they can readily treat most cases without the need for bone anchorage, irrespective of the biomechanical and outcome advantages which may be gained with the latter. Alternatively, I would suggest that a more balanced approach involves the gradual introduction of mini-implant anchorage after attending a professional training course. A suitable course, with both academic and hands-on instruction, should empower the orthodontist to select appropriate cases, understand the essential clinical steps and learn key practical skills. Notably, this book is intended as an aid to this type of learning and not a replacement for it. A formal, structured course will also satisfy typical regulatory and medical indemnity requirements. For example, in the UK, all the major indemnity organisations have recognised mini-implants as a standard part of orthodontics since before 2010, and consequently do not require additional insurance cover for their use. However, (osseointegrating) palatal implants and mini-plates are excluded from this standard cover.

Following structured training, each orthodontist should consider whether to commence their mini-implant usage in a relatively routine orthodontic case, or by selecting a difficult case where conventional anchorage success is likely to be limited. A routine case (e.g. an adult requiring anchorage reinforcement for anterior teeth retraction purposes) has the advantage of allowing the orthodontist to focus on predictable mini-implant biomechanics, and to differentiate these effects from conventional fixed appliance treatment. Alternatively, a more complex case will appear to be more difficult on many levels, but it may be easier to justify the use of a new technique when other options are limited, especially in consent terms.

4.3 Patient Consent

It is important that you feel both confident and comfortable with your proposed treatment plan and that there is favourable risk/benefit ratio for mini-implants. It is also very helpful to use patient-friendly terms during the consent process and to use some physical or virtual model props. For example, I inform and educate patients and their parents by using a fixed appliance typodont model with several mini-implants *in situ*, and possibly clinical photographs of the proposed treatment scenario. Lay persons will appreciate this as a means to understanding complex clinical details. When you are starting to use mini-implants in your clinical practice, it's also worth preparing an explanatory sentence or two which can 'roll off your tongue', such as: "We wish to move your teeth in this direction and need an anchor point to help achieve this. This little anchor, known as a mini-implant, may sound a bit weird, but it's fitted within minutes after numbing just a small patch of your gum. It's even easier to remove later in your treatment, but since it's not permanent it means that about one in ten anchors doesn't achieve full stability and comes loose. This isn't painful or harmful, but it's a nuisance since the mini-implant then needs to be replaced after a few months".

> It is also very helpful to use patient-friendly terms, and to help educate patients by using a fixed appliance typodont model.

For clarity and medicolegal cover, it is important to document that the treatment details, mini-implant application and potential problems have been fully discussed, including whether a mini-implant information sheet has been given to the patient (which in itself is a very useful routine step). Informed consent also requires that valid, alternative treatment options are discussed. For example, bone anchorage can be compared to headgear wear and efficacy, with the knowledge that a randomised controlled trial comparing headgear and mini-implants has demonstrated that patients prefer mini-implant treatment [61]. In addition, the limitations of conventional anchorage should be explained. For example, if a Nance palatal arch is an option then one may cite a study that showed 29% anchorage loss in a Nance group compared to 46% in a control, dental unit-only, group [62].

Anchorage consent does not necessarily require a separate mini-implant consent process and form, in the same way that other adjunctive types of orthodontic appliances may be included within a single treatment plan description. Instead, mini-implant usage should be included as an integral part of the overall treatment options, plan and consent process. In the same vein, where relevant, it may be appropriate to charge private patients in terms of their whole treatment plan, rather than having a separate add-on fee for mini-implant anchorage. The exception to this may be if you are planning for a colleague to insert the mini-implant(s) on your behalf, in which case fees and liabilities will need to be agreed beforehand by the clinicians involved.

The main points to cover in written and verbal formats are listed in the next section. It may not be appropriate to highlight all these details to every patient, especially once you have experience and are able to discern the risks which are realistic or recurrent possibilities in your own clinical practice. A clinical audit of your caseload will provide valuable information and indicators of possible areas to focus on in this respect [63,64]. This will also assist with clinical governance assurance. Such an audit is easy to conduct if you keep an up-to-date database of your mini-implant cases. A sample database spreadsheet, used for case compilation and audit, is shown in Table 4.1. Alternatively, one may adapt national audits, such as the one run by the British Orthodontic Society since 2008 [65]. Interestingly, this reports lower success rates than the published studies, probably because it reflects the 'real world' where orthodontists with a wide range of skills were starting their mini-implant use and at a time when mini-implant knowledge and advice were much less refined. Large-scale audits may also be difficult due to incomplete data returns, where insertions are submitted but not removal data.

Table 4.1 A clinical database for mini-implant audit purposes

	Patient ID	Patient name	DOB	Malocclusion/ mini-implant use	Insertion site(s)	Number inserted	Insertion date	Removal date	Design/ size	Comments
1										
2										
3										
4										
5										
6										
7										
8										

4.4 Key Points to Consider for Valid Consent

4.4.1 Rationale for Mini-implant Anchorage

What are the benefits for this patient's treatment and what are the alternatives?

4.4.2 Patient Discomfort

Reassure the patient that this typically feels like a dull pressure ache and that it is self-limiting (usually resolving within one day of insertion). I often describe the pain as being due to a pressure wave within a confined space, and that it peaks within one hour before gradually resolving. However, it is also worth mentioning that the pressure discomfort may come and go during the first 24 hours.

4.4.3 Mini-implant Instability

Explain that there is an 80–90% success rate, and that mini-implant failure does not cause any permanent harm or infection problems. In the case of a failing mini-implant, premature mobility will be detected by the orthodontist and only leads to patient discomfort if there is gross mobility causing an irritation to surrounding soft tissues.

4.4.4 Periodontal/Root Contact

If close root proximity occurs during insertion then it is usually indicated by an uncomfortable sensation felt in the nearest tooth, and the orthodontist can then alter the mini-implant's position. Even in the event of tooth contact, the root tissues heal uneventfully and there is no risk of clinically detectable or long-term tooth damage. The major problem with close root proximity or contact is that it is likely to lead to mini-implant failure.

4.4.5 Mini-implant Fracture

This occurs in only a small percentage of cases, especially when correct planning and technique steps are followed (e.g. predrilling or perforating sites with dense cortical bone prior to insertion). Surgical removal of a fractured piece may only be required if it is likely to interfere with subsequent tooth movements or in the unlikely event that inflammation occurs (when the mini-implant is not sealed over by the adjacent soft tissues). On such rare occasions, it may be appropriate for the removal of a fractured part to be undertaken by an oral surgeon. This involves gaining access via a small mucoperiosteal flap and trephination of a narrow collar of bone around the mini-implant end, to enable the fractured fragment to be gripped and derotated out of the bone.

4.4.6 Mini-implant Displacement

This is not usually an issue from the patient's perspective since it may only be noticed by them if it interferes with oral hygiene and gingival hyperplasia occurs. Migratory movements do not cause pain *per se*. However, mini-implant displacement is more likely to occur in areas with thin cortical bone and occasionally warrants mini-implant replacement.

4.4.7 Written Information

This is best supplied in the form of a patient information sheet such as those produced by individual mini-implant distributors and professional bodies, such as the American or British Orthodontic Societies (www.bos.org.uk/Public-Patients/Orthodontics-for-Children-Teens/Treatment-brace-types/Orthodontic-mini-implants-TADs). An example of a distributor's patient leaflet is given in Figure 4.2.

4.5 Staff Training

This is straightforward, especially for any mini-implant system with a relatively small number of instruments and inventory (which makes it easy for staff to keep control of the stock). It is essential that your staff are familiar with the mini-implant kit and also understand the requirements for its sterilisation, cross-infection control and the aseptic nature of the insertion procedure. This may be easier if presterilised mini-implants are used (inserted directly from their sterile packaging). Notably, sterile gloves are not essential provided that only the untouched ends of sterile instruments are used to directly handle the mini-implant.

Orthodontic nurses and therapists readily understand the concept of anchorage reinforcement and may be able to relate this to their experiences of trying to encourage headgear wear. Once they have seen mini-implants being used, and the results achieved, they are often enthusiastic advocates for this treatment adjunct.

4.6 Patient Selection

Broadly speaking, when it comes to case selection, there are two categories in terms of anchorage requirements and treatment options: routine and complex cases. On one

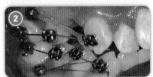

Photograph shows before treatment.

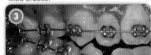

Upper and lower implants connected by
fixed braces.

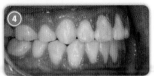

Immediately after removal of the upper implant.

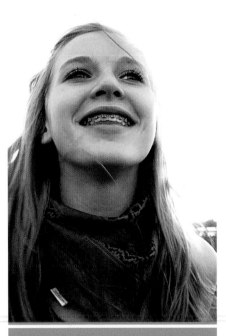

After treatment.

DB Orthodontics Ltd.
Ryefield Way,
Silsden,
West Yorkshire
BD20 0EF
United Kingdom

Tel: +44 1535 656 999
Fax: +44 1535 656 969
Email: sales@dbortho.com
Web: www.infinitas-miniimplant.co.uk

Cover photograph © lanuiop

DBO018

infinitas
mini implant system

Congratulations! You and your orthodontist are benefiting from a revolutionary new and research based orthodontic treatment. Your orthodontist has received specialist training in this technique in order to make your brace treatment as efficient and effective as possible.

What is a mini implant?

It's a very small (diameter 1.5 - 2mm) specially engineered titanium alloy screw which is placed into your gum and jaw bone thereby acting as an anchor point and greatly assisting with the precise movement of your teeth.

Actual size of 6mm mini implant

Will it be painful?

Local anaesthesia is used to numb a small area of your gum, and the mini implant is then gently inserted. You may experience an odd pressure sensation as this occurs. Once the numbness wears off you may feel some discomfort within the first 24 hours and approximately 50% of patients report taking simple painkillers (e.g. ibuprofen or acetaminophen) to resolve this.

Will it hurt when it is removed?

Mini Implants are simply removed when no longer needed, usually without the need for any anaesthesia - it's that easy! The mini implant site heals painlessly within several days after removal.

How long will the mini implant be in place?

Your orthodontist will determine how long the mini implant will be required, but in most cases you can expect to have it in place for a few months, however, it can be left in longer as necessary for individual patient requirements.

Should I expect any problems?

Research indicates that mini implants do not damage your teeth or other mouth tissues. The vast majority of mini implants remain stable during brace treatment and cause little nuisance. However, on occasion they can become loose prematurely. This is rarely painful, but may warrant replacement. If you have any questions or concerns about mini implants speak to your orthodontist.

What do I need to do?

Rinse this area with a anti-bacterial mouthwash, e.g. chlorhexidine, twice a day for the first five days.

During treatment, dip a small toothbrush in chlorhexidine mouthwash and use it to gently clean around the top of the mini implant.

Avoid using an electric toothbrush on the mini implant itself.

Don't fiddle with it!!

What if the implant causes irritation?

Place a small amount of orthodontic wax over the head of the mini implant. If the irritation persists contact your orthodontist.

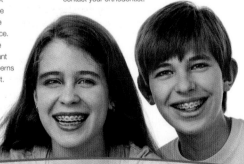

Figure 4.2 The two sides of a mini-implant patient information leaflet, which highlights the salient points of mini-implant usage and patient instructions, as part of the consent process. *Source:* Reproduced with kind permission from DB Orthodontics Ltd, UK.

hand, it is easy to become familiar with mini-implant insertion and use in a routine case, such as a patient who needs posterior anchorage reinforcement during retraction of the labial segment. In this scenario, the mini-implants are inserted in buccal positions using a manual technique such that hands-on experience is gained, and the overall treatment plan and progress are readily understood, tangible and relatively predictable. Hence, the effects of mini-implant anchorage may be gauged in a controlled clinical scenario.

Alternatively, at the start of your mini-implant career, you may feel more comfortable justifying their use in a complex case, such as an adult with multiple absent (anchor) teeth where the treatment options are very limited. Again, it is advisable to select a patient where manual (buccal) insertions are indicated, rather than 'jumping in' with a case requiring handpiece insertion and biomechanics which markedly differ from conventional (anchorage) approaches, such as molar intrusion with palatal mini-implants and a modified transpalatal bar.

References

1 Wu, T., Kuang, S., and Wu, C. (2009). Factors associated with the stability of mini-implants for orthodontic anchorage: a study of 414 samples in Taiwan. *J. Oral Maxillofac. Surg.* 67: 1595–1599.

2 Kim, Y.H., Yang, S., Kim, S. et al. (2010). Midpalatal miniscrews for orthodontic anchorage: factors affecting clinical success. *Am. J. Orthod. Dentofac. Orthop.* 137: 66–72.

3 Garfinkle, J.S., Cunningham, L.L., Beeman, C.S. et al. (2008). Evaluation of orthodontic mini-implant anchorage in premolar extraction therapy in adolescents. *Am. J. Orthod. Dentofac. Orthop.* 133: 642–653.

4 Cho, U., Yu, W., and Kyung, H. (2010). Root contact during drilling for microimplant placement. *Angle Orthod.* 81: 130–136.

5 Landin, M., Jadhav, A., Yadav, S., and Tadinada, A. (2015). A comparative study between currently used methods and small volume-cone beam tomography for surgical placement of mini implants. *Angle Orthod.* 85: 446–453.

6 Wilmes, B., Rademacher, C., Olthoff, G., and Drescher, D. (2006). Parameters affecting primary stability of orthodontic mini-implants. *J. Orofac. Orthop.* 67: 162–174.

7 Wilmes, B. and Drescher, D. (2009). Impact of insertion depth and predrilling diameter on primary stability of orthodontic mini-implants. *Angle Orthod.* 79: 609–614.

8 Cho, K. and Baek, S. (2012). Effects of predrilling depth and implant shape on the mechanical properties of orthodontic mini-implants during the insertion procedure. *Angle Orthod.* 82: 618–624.

9 Turkoz, C., Atac, M., Tuncer, C. et al. (2011). The effect of drill-free and drilling methods on the stability of mini-implants under early orthodontic loading in adolescent patients. *Eur. J. Orthod.* 33: 533–536.

10 Wilmes, B. and Drescher, D. (2011). Impact of bone quality, implant type, and implantation site preparation on insertion torques of mini-implants used for orthodontic anchorage. *Int. J. Oral Maxillofac. Surg.* 40: 697–703.

11 Miyawaki, S., Koyama, I., Inoue, M. et al. (2003). Factors associated with the stability of titanium screws placed in the posterior region for orthodontic anchorage. *Am. J. Orthod. Dentofac. Orthop.* 124: 373–378.

12 Yano, S., Motoyoshi, M., Uemura, M. et al. (2006). Tapered orthodontic miniscrews induce bone-screw cohesion following immediate loading. *Eur. J. Orthod.* 28: 541–546.

13 Morarend, C., Qian, F., Marshall, S.D. et al. (2009). Effect of screw diameter on orthodontic skeletal anchorage. *Am. J. Orthod. Dentofac. Orthop.* 136: 224–229.

14 Barros, S.E., Janson, G., Chiqueto, K. et al. (2011). Effect of mini-implant diameter on fracture risk and self-drilling efficacy. *Am. J. Orthod. Dentofac. Orthop.* 140: e181–e192.

15 Shank, S.B., Beck, F.B., d'Atri, A.M., and Huja, S.S. (2012). Bone damage associated with orthodontic placement of miniscrew implants in an animal model. *Am. J. Orthod. Dentofac. Orthop.* 141: 412–418.

16 Nguyen, M.V., Codrington, J., Fletcher, L. et al. (2017). Influence of cortical bone thickness on miniscrew microcrack formation. *Am. J. Orthod. Dentofac. Orthop.* 152: 301–311.

17 Buchter, A., Wiechmann, D., Koerdt, S. et al. (2005). Load-related implant reaction of mini-implants used for orthodontic anchorage. *Clin. Oral Implants Res.* 16: 473–479.

18 Wilmes, B., Su, Y., and Drescher, D. (2008). Insertion angle impact on primary stability of orthodontic mini-implants. *Angle Orthod.* 78: 1065–1070.

19 Inaba, M. (2009). Evaluation of primary stability of inclined orthodontic mini-implants. *J. Oral Sci.* 51: 347–353.

20 Zhao, L., Xu, Z., Wei, X. et al. (2011). Effect of placement angle on the stability of loaded titanium microscrews: a microcomputed tomographic and biomechanical analysis. *Am. J. Orthod. Dentofac. Orthop.* 139: 628–635.

21 Xu, Z., Wu, Y., Zhao, L. et al. (2013). Effect of placement angle on the stability of loaded titanium microscrews in beagle jaws. *Angle Orthod.* 83: 659–666.

22 Ono, A., Motoyoshi, M., and Shimizu, N. (2008). Cortical bone thickness in the buccal posterior region for orthodontic mini-implants. *Int. J. Oral Maxillofac. Surg.* 37: 334–340.

23 Lee, Y., Kim, J., Baek, S. et al. (2010). Root and bone response to the proximity of a mini-implant under orthodontic loading. *Angle Orthod.* 80: 452–458.

24 Chen, Y., Shin, H., and Kyung, H.M. (2008). Biomechanical and histological comparison of self-drilling and self-tapping orthodontic microimplants in dogs. *Am. J. Orthod. Dentofac. Orthop.* 133: 44–50.

25 Ahmed, K.S., Rooban, T., Krishnaswamy, N.R. et al. (2012). Root damage and repair in patients with temporary skeletal anchorage devices. *Am. J. Orthod. Dentofac. Orthop.* 141: 547–555.

26 Brisceno, C.E., Rossouw, P.E., Carrillo, R. et al. (2009). Healing of the roots and surrounding structures after intentional damage with miniscrew implants. *Am. J. Orthod. Dentofac. Orthop.* 135: 292–301.

27 Chen, Y.H., Chang, H.H., Huang, C.Y. et al. (2008). Root contact during insertion of miniscrews for orthodontic anchorage increases the failure rate: an animal study. *Clin. Oral Implants Res.* 19: 99–106.

28 Hembree, M., Buschang, P.H., Carrillo, R. et al. (2009). Effects of intentional damage of the roots and surrounding structures with miniscrew implants. *Am. J. Orthod. Dentofac. Orthop.* 135: 280e1–280e9.

29 Kadioglu, O., Buyukyilmaz, T., Zachrisson, B.U., and Maino, B.G. (2008). Contact damage to root surfaces of premolars touching miniscrews during orthodontic treatment. *Am. J. Orthod. Dentofac. Orthop.* 134: 353–360.

30 Maino, B.G., Weiland, F., Attanasi, A. et al. (2007). Root damage and repair after contact with miniscrews. *J. Clin. Orthod.* 41: 762–766.

31 Renjen, R., Maganzini, A.L., Rohrer, M.D. et al. (2009). Root and pulp response after intentional injury from miniscrew placement. *Am. J. Orthod. Dentofac. Orthop.* 136: 708–714.

32 Ghanbarzadeh, M., Heravi, F., Abrishamchi, R. et al. (2017). Cementum and dentin repair following root damage caused by the insertion of self-tapping and self-drilling miniscrews. *J. Orthod. Sci.* 6: 91–96.

33 Motoyoshi, M., Uemura, M., Ono, A. et al. (2010). Factors affecting the long-term stability of orthodontic mini-implants. *Am. J. Orthod. Dentofac. Orthop.* 137: 588.e1–e5.

34 Asscherickx, K., Vande Vannet, B., Wehrbein, H., and Sabzevar, M.M. (2008). Success rate of miniscrews relative to their position to adjacent roots. *Eur. J. Orthod.* 30: 330–335.

35 Dao, V., Renjen, R., Prasad, H.S. et al. (2009). Cementum, pulp, periodontal ligament, and bone response after direct injury with orthodontic anchorage screws: a histomorphologic study in an animal model. *J. Oral Maxillofac. Surg.* 67: 2440–2445.

36 Kang, Y., Kang, Y., Kim, J. et al. (2008). Stability of mini-screws invading the dental roots and their impact on the paradental tissues in beagles. *Angle Orthod.* 79: 248–255.

37 Kuroda, S., Yamada, K., Deguchi, T. et al. (2007). Root proximity is a major factor for screw failure in orthodontic anchorage. *Am. J. Orthod. Dentofac. Orthop.* 131: S68–S73.

38 Min, K., Kim, S., and Kang, S. (2012). Root proximity and cortical bone thickness effects on the success rate of orthodontic micro-implants using cone-beam computed tomography. *Angle Orthod.* 82: 1014–1021.

39 Jung, Y., Kim, S., and Kang, K. (2013). Placement angle effects on the success rate of orthodontic microimplants and other factors with cone-beam computed tomography. *Am. J. Orthod. Dentofac. Orthop.* 143: 173–181.

40 Watanabe, H., Deguchi, T., Hasegawa, M. et al. (2013). Orthodontic miniscrew failure rate and root proximity, insertion angle, bone contact length, and bone density. *Orthod. Craniofacial Res.* 16: 44–55.

41 Zhou, G., Zhang, X., Qie, H. et al. (2018). Three-dimensional finite element analysis of the stability of mini-implants close to the roots of adjacent teeth upon application of bite force. *Dent. Mater. J.* 37: 851–857.

42 Wilmes, B., Su, Y.Y., Sadigh, L., and Drescher, D. (2008). Pre-drilling force and insertion torques during orthodontic mini-implant insertion in relation to root contact. *J. Orofac. Orthop.* 69: 51–58.

43 Motoyoshi, M., Uchida, Y., Matsuoka, M. et al. (2014). Assessment of damping capacity as an index of root proximity in self-drilling orthodontic mini-implants. *Clin. Oral Investig.* 18: 321–326.

44 Shinohara, A., Motoyoshi, M., Uchida, Y., and Shimizu, N. (2013). Root proximity and inclination of orthodontic mini-implants after placement: cone-beam computed tomography evaluation. *Am. J. Orthod. Dentofac. Orthop.* 144: 50–56.

45 Gracco, A., Cirignaco, A., Cozzani, M. et al. (2009). Numerical/experimental analysis of the stress field around miniscrews for orthodontic anchorage. *Eur. J. Orthod.* 31: 12–20.

46 Buchter, A., Wiechmann, D., Gaertner, C. et al. (2006). Load-related bone modelling at the interface of orthodontic microimplants. *Clin. Oral Implants Res.* 17: 714–722.

47 Cha, J.Y., Lim, K.J., Song, J.W. et al. (2009). Influence of the length of the loading period after placement of

orthodontic mini-implants on changes in bone histomorphology: microcomputed tomographic and histologic analysis. *Int. J. Oral Maxillofac. Implants* 24: 842–849.

48 Deguchi, T., Takano-Yamamoto, T., Kanomi, R. et al. (2003). The use of small titanium screws for orthodontic anchorage. *J. Dent. Res.* 82: 377–381.

49 Luzi, C., Verna, C., and Melsen, B. (2009). Immediate loading of orthodontic mini-implants: a histomorphometric evaluation of tissue reaction. *Eur. J. Orthod.* 31: 21–29.

50 Serra, G., Morais, L.S., Elias, C.N. et al. (2010). Sequential bone healing of immediately loaded mini-implants: histomorphometric and fluorescence analysis. *Am. J. Orthod. Dentofac. Orthop.* 137: 80–90.

51 Woods, P.W., Buschang, P.H., Owens, S.E. et al. (2009). The effect of force, timing, and location on bone-to-implant contact of miniscrew implants. *Eur. J. Orthod.* 31: 232–240.

52 Zhang, L., Zhao, Z., Li, Y. et al. (2010). Osseointegration of orthodontic micro-screws after immediate and early loading. *Angle Orthod.* 80: 354–360.

53 Al Maaitah, E.F., Safi, A.A.M., and Abdelhafez, R.S. (2012). Alveolar bone density changes around miniscrews: a prospective clinical study. *Am. J. Orthod. Dentofac. Orthop.* 142: 758–767.

54 Migliorati, M., Drago, S., Gallo, F. et al. (2016). Immediate versus delayed loading: comparison of primary stability loss after miniscrews placement in orthodontic patients – a single centre blinded randomized clinical trial. *Eur. J. Orthod.* 38: 652–659.

55 Iijima, M., Nakagaki, S., Yasuda, Y. et al. (2013). Effect of immediate loading on the biomechanical properties of bone surrounding the miniscrew implants. *Eur. J. Orthod.* 35: 577–582.

56 Ure, D.S., Oliver, D.R., Kim, K.B. et al. (2011). Stability changes of miniscrew implants over time. A pilot resonance frequency analysis. *Angle Orthod.* 81: 994–1000.

57 Wei, X., Zhao, L., Xu, Z. et al. (2011). Effects of cortical bone thickness at different healing times on microscrew stability. *Angle Orthod.* 81: 754–759.

58 Nienkemper, M., Wilmes, B., Pauls, A., and Drescher, D. (2014). Mini-implant stability at the initial healing period. A clinical pilot study. *Angle Orthod.* 84: 127–133.

59 Moon, C., Lee, D., Lee, H. et al. (2008). Factors associated with the success rate of orthodontic miniscrews placed in the upper and lower posterior buccal region. *Angle Orthod.* 78: 101–106.

60 Motoyoshi, M., Matsuoka, M., and Shimizu, N. (2007). Application of orthodontic mini-implants in adolescents. *Int. J. Oral Maxillofac. Surg.* 36: 695–699.

61 Sandler, J., Murray, A., Thiruvenkatachari, B. et al. (2014). Effectiveness of 3 methods of anchorage reinforcement for maximum anchorage in adolescents: a 3-arm multicenter randomized clinical trial. *Am. J. Orthod. Dentofac. Orthop.* 146: 10–20.

62 Al-Awadhi, E.A., Garvey, T.M., Alhag, M. et al. (2015). Efficacy of the Nance appliance as an anchorage-reinforcement method. *Am. J. Orthod. Dentofac. Orthop.* 147: 330–338.

63 Mistry, P.M. and Cousley, R.R.J. (2009). An audit of mini-implant success rates. *Br. Orthod. Soc. Clin. Effect Bull.* 22: 13–15.

64 Cousley, R.R.J. (2011). A re-audit of orthodontic mini-implant success rates. *Br. Orthod. Soc. Clin. Effect Bull.* 26: 7–9.

65 Bearn, D.R. and Alharbi, F. (2015). British Orthodontic Society national audit of temporary anchorage devices (TADs): report of the first thousand TADs placed. *J. Orthod.* 42: 214–219.

5

Mini-implant Planning

As with all orthodontic treatments, it's important to properly plan each mini-implant case from the outset and the principles outlined in this chapter will help to inform this diagnostic and treatment planning process. These are summarised in the flowchart in Figure 5.1 which highlights the considerations according to whether direct and indirect anchorage is planned. In a sense, this chapter provides a comprehensive *aide-memoire* on mini-implant planning, and at first glance suggests that there's a lot of information to analyse and remember. However, not all points apply to every case and experience will quickly lead you to discern the relevant steps for specific types of cases. In addition, common clinical scenarios are described in a sequential manner in the remaining book chapters and while this entails some degree of repetition, it ensures that nothing relevant is left out for each clinical scenario.

5.1 Mini-implant Planning

5.1.1 Treatment Goals and Anchorage Requirements

It may be a cliché but every successful treatment outcome begins with a plan. Therefore, it's essential that as the first step, one determines the aims of treatment following a comprehensive orthodontic assessment. The treatment options and details will then flow from this, and lead to the planning process. The only differences may be that your treatment options and expectations may be greater with mini-implant usage than with conventional treatment, for example achieving full overjet reduction in a Class II camouflage case or non-surgical correction of an anterior openbite.

5.2 Mini-implant Location

Determine the ideal anteroposterior and buccal/palatal location(s) for mini-implant(s) according to the anchorage requirements, anatomical features and biomechanical

perspectives for each clinical scenario. For example, since incisor retraction requires posterior anchorage, the typical mini-implant insertion site is on the buccal side of the alveolus between the second premolar and first molar teeth. This is because this site is easily accessible and provides adequate cortical bone support plus interproximal space. It is also easier to attach buccal mini-implants (than palatal ones) to a labial fixed appliance. In contrast, more anterior insertion sites may not provide sufficient distance for effective traction aver a period of time, and may increase vertical side-effects due to a steeper vector of traction (if auxiliaries known as powerarms are not added to the fixed appliance). The optimum insertion sites will be described in detail in each specific clinical scenario chapter.

> Consider the ideal anteroposterior and buccal/palatal site(s) according to anchorage requirements, anatomical features and biomechanical perspectives.

5.3 Hard Tissue Anatomy and Radiographic Imaging

The starting point for detailed mini-implant planning begins with a physical examination of the patient's topographical (surface) detail, including the soft tissue features. Two-dimensional and/or three-dimensional radiographs then supplement this clinical assessment by providing information on the underlying available bone volume and adjacent anatomical structures. Either physical (dental) or 3D virtual model records provide the final tier of planning information and may also be used for stent fabrication whereby the insertion plan is transferred to the patient's mouth. The process of model examination is also a useful exercise for the orthodontist in being methodical about planning, and free from patient contact. This ought to reduce potential operator error and enable the observation of small details. For example, it's often easier to observe alveolar surface undulations on a

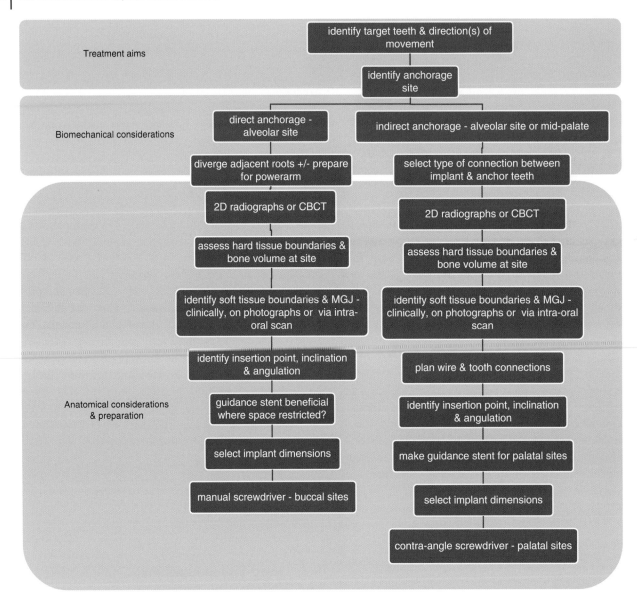

Figure 5.1 Flowchart highlighting the most common insertion site planning considerations.

physical model than in the patient's mouth, where a surface concavity indicates the interproximal area between the prominences of adjacent roots.

Given dentistry's historical reliance on 2D radiography, many orthodontists are still accustomed to thinking of both dentoalveolar and palatal areas as 2D structures. However, we should really consider dentate (interproximal) and palatal areas of the jaws as 3D spaces or volumes, and plan each potential insertion site in terms of its boundaries and bone volume in all three planes:

- the mesiodistal (anteroposterior) distance, as bordered by dental roots in dentate alveolar sites. In turn, the positions (e.g. tip) and morphology of adjacent tooth roots are important considerations

- alveolar (transverse) width
- the vertical limit in terms of the most coronal or superficial cortical bone surface, for example the alveolar crestal bone or palatal surface
- the vertical limit in terms of proximity to the most apical surface or structure, for example the maxillary sinus, nasal floor and midpalatal suture
- the bone morphology (in particular, whether there is alveolar necking or conversely a convex alveolar shape).

Mesiodistal and vertical anatomical information can still be derived from 2D radiographs, such as panoramic (orthopantomograph – OPG) and intraoral periapical views (Figure 5.2a,b). Panoramic radiographs are readily available as part of the patient's diagnostic stage, and should be used for preliminary evaluation of insertion sites. However, periapical radiographs (Figure 5.2b,c) are preferable to panoramic views immediately prior to mini-implant insertion since they enable more detailed analysis of the shape, position and angulation of dental roots. For example, the unfavourable mesial bowing of the upper left first molar's

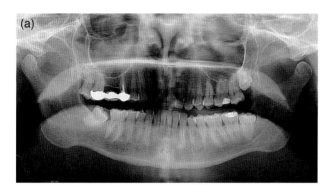

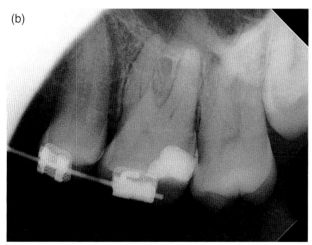

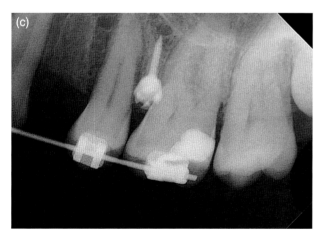

Figure 5.2 (a) Panoramic and (b) intraoral pretreatment radiographs of the dentition as used to visualise the interproximal area between the left maxillary second premolar and first molar teeth. (c) The intraoral radiograph is repeated to confirm the position of a mini-implant in this site.

mesiobuccal molar root may be missed on the OPG seen in Figure 5.2a (since it is outside the focal trough), but is visible in the periapical view (Figure 5.2b). However, periapical radiographs are prone to parallax errors if a film or sensor holder is not used for positional standardisation. This is demonstrated by the apparent differences in upper left first molar root morphology in the pre- and postinsertion periapicals taken with the x-ray tube in different mesiodistal positions in Figure 5.2b,c.

There is some evidence that 3D (cone beam computed tomography – CBCT) imaging may reduce the risks of root contact and hence improve success rates. For example, an *in vitro* study of mini-implant insertions in skulls showed a 5% risk of root contact with the use of small-volume CBCT compared to a 55–60% rate when no radiograph or a 2D radiograph was used for planning [1]. Whilst a CBCT may not be justifiable where it is clinically apparent that there is plenty of interproximal space, arguably it would help those orthodontists with little experience of mini-implants. This will increasingly be the norm with ongoing reductions in CBCT dosage (especially for small fields of view) and availability. Ideally, a 3D guidance stent (described in Chapter 3) would then be used to replicate this 3D planning in the clinical environment.

Cone beam CT now provides the fullest amount of 3D radiographic information and is increasingly justifiable in mini-implant scenarios given the relatively low radiation dose levels associated with modern radiography machines and the limited (small) fields of view. It is also worth remembering that CBCT images may already be available for some patients with clinical problems such as ectopic teeth or jaw deformity, without the need for further imaging specifically for mini-implant planning (Figure 5.3). CBCT scans also provide a means of estimating the cortical bone thickness and density, although density measurements are less accurate than the use of Hounsfield units in medical CT systems.

For midpalatal insertion sites, the main considerations are the depth of the palatal bone (including the nasal spine in the midline), the patency of the midpalatal suture and the proximity of the incisive canal and nasopalatine vessels. The palate depth can be assessed on a lateral cephalogram, but the bone depth tends to be underestimated on this radiograph, by as much as 2 mm [2]. Therefore, if this is a critical detail then a CBCT may be justified to provide coronal and sagittal CBCT views (Figure 5.3c,d). CBCT images also provide useful information on the midpalatal suture width and integrity (Figure 5.4).

Several authors have described the midpalate areas which are likely to provide sufficient bone depth for mini-implants as either the 'T zone' [3] or bilateral 'footprint'-like areas [4]. The latter, based on a systematic review of

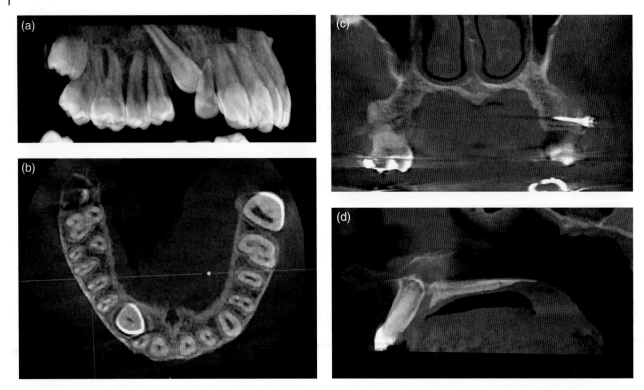

Figure 5.3 (a) A reformatted CBCT image of the right maxilla taken to assess the position of the ectopic right maxillary tooth and resorption of adjacent roots. This view also readily shows the available interproximal space mesial to the upper right first molar, partly due to the favourable curvature of the adjacent second premolar root. (b) The alveolar width, root positions and cortical depth are seen in this axial sectional view taken at the midroot level. The interproximal bone volume is appreciable in terms of the sizes and positions of all three first molar roots. (c) A coronal CBCT view showing midface and alveolar anatomy, plus the normal inclination of a buccally inserted maxillary mini-implant. (d) A sagittal CBCT view of midpalate morphology and (oronasal) depth, highlighting the relative positions of the incisor root and nasopalatine canal. This view is helpful for midpalate insertion site planning.

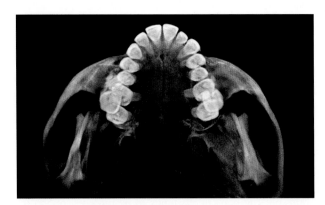

Figure 5.4 A reformatted CBCT image of the maxilla in a 19-year-old female, as viewed from the inferior aspect. The hard palate anatomy, incisive canal and midpalatal suture are easily seen. The palatal root positions, sizes and morphologies are also evident, especially on rotation of the image.

vertical bone measurements, describes a paramedian area situated distal to both maxillary incisors and palatal to both premolars. The T zone concept relates to the adequate availability of anterior bone depth across much of the hard palate between the premolars, but this increasingly becomes limited to the midpalate area in more distal sites of the palate (Figure 5.5).

Whilst there is wide patient variation in terms of palatal bone depth and density, a CBCT scan may not be justifiable in every case, especially where a short (e.g. 6mm body length) mini-implant is to be inserted in a paramedian site at the mesiodistal level of the premolar teeth. A simple rule of thumb has been described by Ludwig and colleagues which assists with midpalate planning [5]. They related the anterior palate bone and cortical depths to superficial landmarks and found that insertion on or distal to the third palatal rugae consistently places mini-implants within adequate bone and clear of the incisive canal. This soft tissue landmark is stable and clinically identifiable, hence negating the need for elaborate bone assessment whilst planning for midpalate insertions. This approach has been corroborated by their reported success rate of an amazing 99% for midpalate insertions performed in 40 consecutive adolescent and adult patients [6].

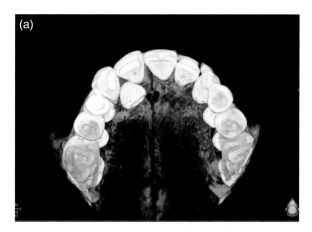
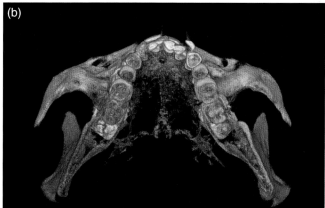

Figure 5.5 Reformatted CBCT image of the maxilla in (a) adolescent and (b) adult subjects. The midpalatal suture is patent in (a), but seen as obliterated in (b). The T zone is seen as the relatively opaque area of palate running transversely between the premolars and then extending posteriorly as either (a) parasagittal strips bordering the suture or (b) a single sagittal strip (without the suture radiolucency).

5.4 Soft Tissue Anatomy

Ideally, mini-implants should be inserted through the attached gingiva (not loose mucosa) for two key reasons: to prevent either the cheek or lip soft tissues wrapping around the mini-implant threads during insertion, and to minimise the risk of destabilisation of the mini-implant from plaque accumulation, peri-implant inflammation, and (mobile) soft tissue movements. The occlusal boundary of the attached tissue is superficially indicated by the gingival margin. However, remember that the correct limit, set by the alveolar bone crest level, is approximately 2 mm more occlusal than the soft tissue margin. The apical boundary (on the buccal aspect) is formed by the mucogingival junction (MGJ) and any adjacent frenal attachments (Figure 5.6). Insertion close to the MGJ tends to provide access to the largest interproximal alveolar space because the adjacent tooth roots are more narrow and tapered at this more apical level. Therefore, it is often recommended that the buccal insertion site is close to this margin because of this desire to gain access to the greatest bone volume.

This has been eloquently advocated by Dr Sebastian Baumgaertel who has described a shift from 'mechanics-driven' to 'anatomy-driven' insertion site determination [7,8]. In effect, this means that the orthodontist should choose the insertion site first, based on anatomical criteria, then match the biomechanical configuration to this. This has been made possible by the introduction of two separate treatment adjuncts: wire struts for indirect anchorage and powerarms for direct traction. Powerarms are my preferred option in many clinical scenarios, in both arches since they are simple to connect with direct traction auxiliaries (Figure 5.7). This newer focus subtly but clearly differs

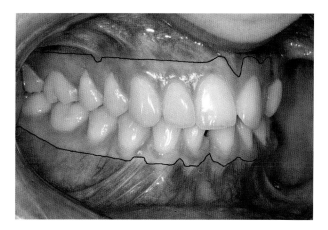

Figure 5.6 The upper and lower mucogingival junctions are highlighted as black lines between the attached and free mucosal tissues.

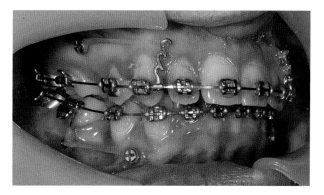

Figure 5.7 Two different versions of powerarms being used in the upper arch for incisor retraction and for molar protraction in the lower arch. The mini-implants have been inserted close to the MGJ and the powerarms create a horizontal vector of traction.

from 'early' insertion protocols for direct anchorage, used prior to the introduction of powerarms, where the insertion site was more coronal in an effort to reduce the vertical vector of traction (and hence rotational side-effects). Fortunately, it is now feasible and desirable for the decision on the vertical insertion level to be primarily dictated by anatomical and root proximity factors rather than biomechanical considerations.

It is worth remembering that the apparent height of the buccal attached gingiva is artificially exaggerated on a dental model because the sulcular tissues are easily stretched during the impression process. Therefore, if you are using a dental model to plan a buccal alveolar insertion, first record the clinical height of the attached gingiva (distance from the gingival margin) at the impression appointment, or verify it from clinical photographs. The apical insertion limit on the palatal side of the maxillary alveolus is best determined by palpation of the tissues to determine areas of firm attachment. Palatal alveolar insertions should be planned in areas where the mucosa displays little sign of mobility and compressibility.

> The apparent height of buccal attached gingiva is artificially exaggerated on a dental model because the sulcus is easily stretched during the impression process.

5.5 Vertical Location and Inclination

The vertical level and angle of a mini-implant insertion are affected by two factors: the interproximal bone space and the height of attached gingiva. It is now generally accepted that the vertical insertion position should be close to the MGJ rather than at a coronal level (where I originally placed mini-implants in order to reduce the side-effects of oblique traction). This principle has been supported by recent evidence from a retrospective study of 260 buccal mini-implants where the success rate increased with greater distance from the alveolar crest [9]. Therefore, the authors recommended relatively apical insertion levels, but if this was not feasible because of an insufficient height of attached gingiva then the mini-implant should be inserted with a 30° apical angulation.

An ideal mini-implant insertion site should provide at least a 0.5 mm margin of bone around the threads, with it generally being the case that greater interproximal space is available at more apical levels, due to the tapering shape of the adjacent roots. However, greater interproximal space (between roots) does not always equate to increased bone volume. The two exceptions to this rule,

limiting mini-implant insertion to a relatively coronal level in maxillary posterior alveolar sites, occur when the sinus floor has migrated in an inferior/occlusal direction. This may be due to the long-standing absence of a maxillary molar (Figure 5.8a,b) or occasionally it is solely due to anatomical variation (Figure 5.8c,d). Whilst root divergence may be used to increase the available interproximal width, it is not feasible to alter the level of the sinus floor. Therefore, if this is particularly problematic, it will be necessary to consider a different insertion site (Figure 5.9).

The overlying soft tissue is relevant since this dictates the range of vertical levels available for the insertion to be sited within the attached gingiva. However, this choice may be limited in patients with only a narrow band (height) of attached gingiva, such that the mini-implant often needs to be inserted at an oblique angle, for example 20–30° in the maxilla and 10–20° in the mandible, in order to keep its neck (and head) within the attached gingiva, while directing its body apically between the roots (Figure 5.10). As a rule of thumb, the wider the band of attached gingiva then the more apical the insertion point and the more 'horizontal' the insertion angle (i.e. perpendicular to the buccal alveolar bone surface). Conversely, the narrower the band of attached gingiva then the more coronal the insertion point and the greater the need for an oblique insertion angle.

Vertically angled (oblique) insertion of mini-implants is also favourable in terms of increasing the engagement of the alveolar cortex. This is especially relevant in sites with thin cortex, such as the buccal side of the maxilla and anterior alveolar sites [10].

Hence, a mini-implant's vertical level and angle of insertion influence its head position, emergence profile and ease of attachment. In particular, the head of an obliquely angled mini-implant, when inserted in an area of restricted attached gingival height, emerges at a relatively coronal level and its lateral (buccal) edge will be more prominent than the medial (palatal) aspect. This may irritate the opposing buccal (cheek) mucosa. In addition, the vertical position of the head affects the vector of force application such that an apical head position potentially produces an oblique traction vector (Figure 5.11a) compared to a position closer to the fixed appliance level (Figure 5.11b) if a powerarm is not used. This aspect will be discussed further in the chapters on clinical biomechanics.

5.6 Insertion Timing

In my early years of mini-implant usage, and especially prior to the introduction of powerarms, I tended to add the bone anchorage at the start of treatment, that is, at the fixed appliance bond-up. However, nowadays the ideal

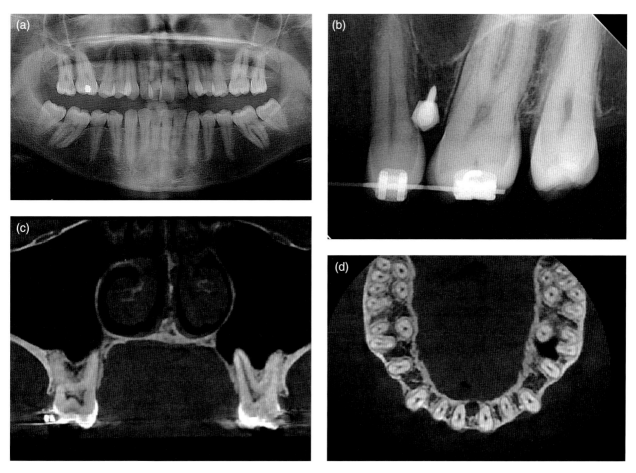

Figure 5.8 (a) Pretreatment panoramic and (b) intraoral postinsertion radiographs of an adult with early loss of all first molars. The maxillary sinus floor is at a relatively coronal level bilaterally, which limits the vertical (apical) level of mini-implant insertion. (c) A coronal CBCT sectional view of the maxilla in a young adult female, showing large maxillary sinuses and projection of the first molar roots into the sinuses, especially on the left side. (d) An axial sectional CBCT view of the patient shown in (c) shows the left sinus, rather than alveolar bone, in the interproximal space between the first molar and second premolar roots (the first premolars are absent).

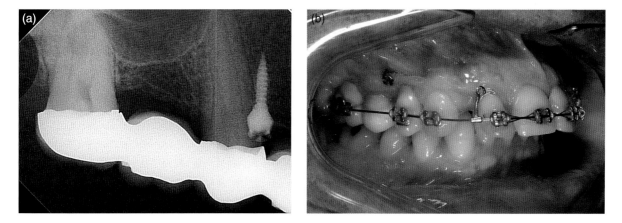

Figure 5.9 (a) Intraoral radiograph of an adult where early loss of a first molar and subsequent lowering of the sinus floor necessitated insertion of a mini-implant mesial rather than distal to the second premolar tooth. (b) This photograph shows immediate traction from this mini-implant to a powerarm, but the additional anatomical limitations posed by the soft tissues in this case are also seen.

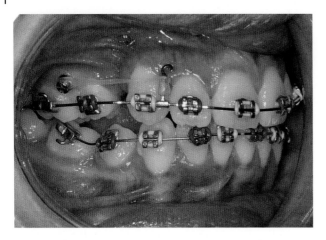

Figure 5.10 The clear elastomeric attachment provides horizontally orientated traction from the mini-implant head directly to a powerarm on the fixed appliance, for *en masse* retraction of the anterior teeth.

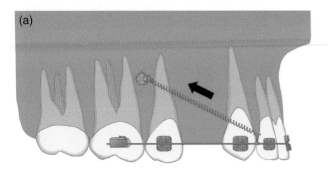

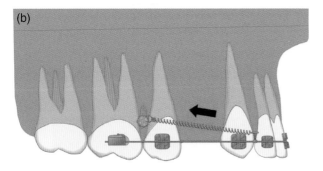

Figure 5.11 Diagrams of (a) oblique and (b) horizontal vectors of traction to the anterior teeth from a buccal mini-implant inserted at a relatively apical and coronal level, respectively.

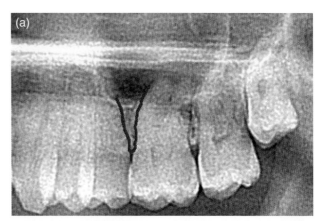

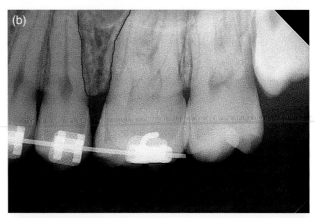

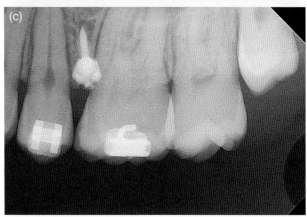

Figure 5.12 (a) Pretreatment panoramic, (b) preinsertion and (c) postinsertion intraoral radiographs. The insertion site between the left maxillary second premolar and first molar roots is highlighted in red in images (a) and (b). Root divergence has been performed to widen the interproximal space before radiograph (b) was taken.

stage for mini-implant anchorage is determined according to the extent of arch alignment (and root clearance) needed before mini-implant insertion. Crucially, if there is insufficient interproximal space at the planned insertion site then it is ideal to undertake a preliminary phase of fixed appliance treatment in order to diverge the roots and hence facilitate mini-implant insertion (Figure 5.12). This is achieved by bonding the bracket(s) with a modified tip, especially adding a mesial tip to the normal second premolar

bracket orientation (Figure 5.13). Notably, this preparatory step is both simple and reversible, yet it makes buccal mini-implant insertions much easier. My clinical impression is also that the increase in interproximal space provides more available bone volume for the insertion pressure (and pain) to dissipate through, before reaching the periodontal ligament (and pain receptors) of adjacent teeth.

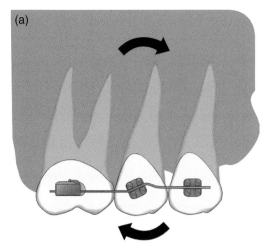

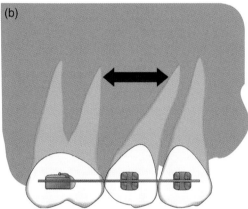

Figure 5.13 Diagrams of the premolar and first molar teeth where (a) the second premolar bracket has been bonded with the mesial tip to cause (b) mesial tipping of this root during the fixed appliance alignment phase and hence an increase in this interproximal space.

The bracket position is then corrected during the fixed appliance finishing stage (after explantation). Furthermore, it may be biomechanically beneficial to align the full arch such that it is ready to accommodate a rigid (e.g. 0.019×0.025 in. stainless steel) archwire and powerarm by the time of mini-implant insertion. This helps with sliding mechanics and the reduction of unfavourable vertical side-effects.

> If in doubt about the amount of interproximal space, then undertake a preliminary phase of fixed appliance treatment in order to diverge the roots and hence facilitate mini-implant insertion.

5.7 Guidance Stent

Fabricate a stent (as described in Chapter 3) if you think it will be helpful for the insertion stage. This depends on factors such as your level of experience and the ease of visual

and physical access to the insertion site. Mini-implant experience appears to provide more accurate and reproducible insertions, whereas inexperience has been shown to result in greater root proximity errors [11–13]. Hence, a stent may be invaluable for those with little or no mini-implant expertise, so that the mini-implant position is first determined *in vitro* for the majority of anchorage locations. However, even experienced orthodontists find a stent very useful in posterior areas which are difficult to see by direct vision and reach with a manual screwdriver and/or where the interproximal space is limited (requiring a high degree of insertion accuracy).

It is best that the treating orthodontist fully plans the insertion site and angles on a working or virtual model, rather than delegating this to a technician. Hence, the orthodontist is directly responsible for planning the case. Once planned, then the model and positional information are passed to the technician or nurse for physical fabrication of the stent. It is advisable to allow 1–2 weeks between impression/scanning and insertion appointments for this preparatory process to be undertaken.

5.8 Mini-Implant Dimensions

Determine the optimum body diameter and length primarily according to the insertion site, but by also considering general patient factors such as age and, to a lesser extent, the patient's body mass (Table 5.1, Figure 5.14). In general, narrow-diameter mini-implants (e.g. the Infinitas 1.5 mm version) are selected for interproximal sites, whereas a larger diameter (e.g. 2.0 mm) may be safely inserted in edentulous sites and the midpalate. A long (e.g. 9 mm) body length is ideal for posterior maxillary sites since this length gains additional stability (from cancellous bone engagement) in such areas with potentially suboptimal cortical bone depth. However, short (e.g. 6 mm) mini-implants are likely to have sufficient stability in adult patients in areas of thick and dense cortex, such as the posterior mandible and midpalate.

A short body length is also preferred for horizontal (perpendicular) insertions in sites with limited buccolingual alveolar width or palatal bone depth, such as anterior maxillary and mandibular alveolar sites, and the midpalate. The anterior alveolar bone depth may be assessed on a lateral cephalogram (Figure 5.15) or a CBCT (Figure 5.3d). If the depth is too shallow then the mini-implant tip may perforate the palatal/lingual side of the alveolus or nasal floor, respectively. This is less likely when mini-implants are inserted obliquely, hence enabling the safe use of 9 mm body length versions in the anterior alveolus. This is particularly relevant if the insertion site is restricted to a

Table 5.1 Clinical scenarios where additional details dictate that a wide diameter or long length mini-implant may be advantageous (compared to standard adult conditions)

Secondary clinical consideration	Diameter variation	Length variation
Adolescent patient with reduced cortical support (compared to an adult)	2.0 rather than 1.5 mm: increases bone engagement, more feasible in palatal alveolar (wide interproximal space) and midpalate sites	9 rather than 6 mm: increases secondary stability, e.g. in a posterior mandibular site
Elderly patient, especially postmenopausal female	2.0 rather than 1.5 mm: increases bone engagement	9 rather than 6 mm: increases secondary stability
Patient with a low body mass index where cortical thickness may be reduced	2.0 rather than 1.5 mm: increases bone engagement, e.g. in palatal sites	9 rather than 6 mm: increases secondary stability
Thicker than average or spongy palatal soft tissues	2.0 rather than 1.5 mm: allows for incomplete body insertion	9 rather than 6 mm reduces tipping moment effect (due to higher profile head projection)

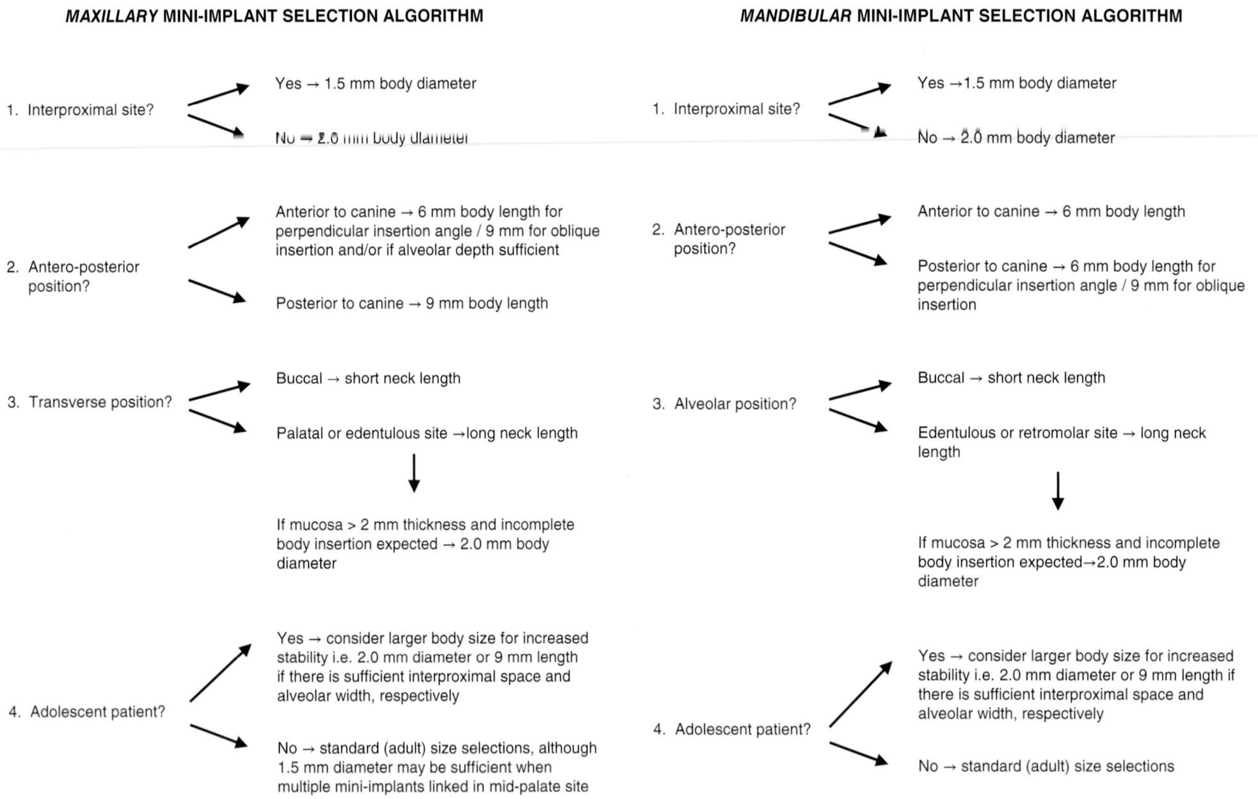

MAXILLARY MINI-IMPLANT SELECTION ALGORITHM

1. Interproximal site?
   - Yes → 1.5 mm body diameter
   - No → 2.0 mm body diameter

2. Antero-posterior position?
   - Anterior to canine → 6 mm body length for perpendicular insertion angle / 9 mm for oblique insertion and/or if alveolar depth sufficient
   - Posterior to canine → 9 mm body length

3. Transverse position?
   - Buccal → short neck length
   - Palatal or edentulous site → long neck length

   If mucosa > 2 mm thickness and incomplete body insertion expected → 2.0 mm body diameter

4. Adolescent patient?
   - Yes → consider larger body size for increased stability i.e. 2.0 mm diameter or 9 mm length if there is sufficient interproximal space and alveolar width, respectively
   - No → standard (adult) size selections, although 1.5 mm diameter may be sufficient when multiple mini-implants linked in mid-palate site

MANDIBULAR MINI-IMPLANT SELECTION ALGORITHM

1. Interproximal site?
   - Yes → 1.5 mm body diameter
   - No → 2.0 mm body diameter

2. Antero-posterior position?
   - Anterior to canine → 6 mm body length
   - Posterior to canine → 6 mm body length for perpendicular insertion angle / 9 mm for oblique insertion

3. Alveolar position?
   - Buccal → short neck length
   - Edentulous or retromolar site → long neck length

   If mucosa > 2 mm thickness and incomplete body insertion expected → 2.0 mm body diameter

4. Adolescent patient?
   - Yes → consider larger body size for increased stability i.e. 2.0 mm diameter or 9 mm length if there is sufficient interproximal space and alveolar width, respectively
   - No → standard (adult) size selections

Figure 5.14 Algorithms (flowcharts) highlighting the most common considerations in the selection of optimum mini-implant body and neck dimensions according to the planned insertion site and directions.

coronal level by the narrowness of the band of attached gingiva (Figure 5.6).

Variations also occur in the length of mini-implant necks. In general, a short (e.g. 1.5 mm) neck is appropriate for most buccal insertion sites where the mucosa is thin. However, a long (e.g. 2.5 mm) neck version is used in areas with thick or loose mucosa, such as palatal and edentulous sites. This is a very useful rule of thumb but if necessary, the tissue thickness may be double checked, once the tissue has been anaesthe-

tised, by directly measuring the depth of the mucosa using a dental probe with an endodontic stopper on the end.

Determine the optimum body diameter and length primarily according to the insertion site, but also considering general patient factors such as age and, to a lesser extent, body mass.

Figure 5.15 Lateral cephalogram showing the midline palatal bone thickness and depth of the maxillary and mandibular alveolar processes. A 6 mm length midpalate mini-implant has been inserted, angled towards the anterior nasal spine. An indirect anchorage wire was shaped to follow the anterior palate's contour.

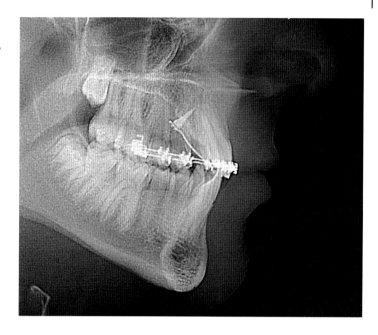

References

1 Landin, M., Jadhav, A., Yadav, S., and Tadinada, A. (2015). A comparative study between currently used methods and small volume-cone beam tomography for surgical placement of mini implants. *Angle Orthod.* 85: 446–453.

2 Wehrbein, H., Merz, B.R., and Diedrich, P. (1999). Palatal bone support for orthodontic implant anchorage – a clinical and radiological study. *Eur. J. Orthod.* 21: 65–70.

3 Wilmes, B., Ludwig, B., Vasudavan, S. et al. (2016). The T-Zone: median vs. paramedian insertion of palatal mini-implants. *J. Clin. Orthod.* 50: 543–551.

4 Winsauer, H., Vlachojannis, C., Bumann, Λ. et al. (2014). Paramedian vertical bone height for mini-implant insertion: a systematic review. *Eur. J. Orthod.* 36: 541–549.

5 Houfar, J., Kanavakis, G., Bister, D. et al. (2015). Three dimensional anatomical exploration of the anterior hard palate at the level of the third ruga for the placement of mini-implants – a cone-beam CT study. *Eur. J. Orthod.* 37: 589–595.

6 Di Leonardo, B., Ludwig, B., Lisson, J.A. et al. (2018). Insertion torque values and success rates for paramedian insertion of orthodontic miniimplants. *J. Orofac. Orthop.* 79: 109–115.

7 Baumgaertel, S. and Tran, T.T. (2012). Buccal mini-implant site selection: the mucosal fallacy and zones of opportunity. *J. Clin. Orthod.* 46: 434–436.

8 Baumgaertel, S. (2014). Hard and soft tissue considerations at mini-implant insertion sites. *J. Orthod.* 41: S3–S7.

9 Haddad, R. and Saadeh, M. (2019). Distance to alveolar crestal bone: a critical factor in the success of orthodontic miniimplants. *Prog. Orthod.* 20: 19.

10 Laursen, M.G., Melsen, B., and Cattaneo, P.M. (2013). An evaluation of insertion sites for mini-implants: a micro-CT study of human autopsy material. *Angle Orthod.* 83: 222–229.

11 Kim, Y.H., Yang, S., Kim, S. et al. (2010). Midpalatal miniscrews for orthodontic anchorage: factors affecting clinical success. *Am. J. Orthod. Dentofac. Orthop.* 137: 66–72.

12 Garfinkle, J.S., Cunningham, L.L., Beeman, C.S. et al. (2008). Evaluation of orthodontic mini-implant anchorage in premolar extraction therapy in adolescents. *Am. J. Orthod. Dentofac. Orthop.* 133: 642–653.

13 Cho, U., Yu, W., and Kyung, H. (2010). Root contact during drilling for microimplant placement. *Angle Orthod.* 81: 130–136.

6

Mini-implant Insertion

This chapter describes the insertion process for various typical mini-implant placement scenarios in a step-by-step manner.

6.1 Mini-implant Kit Sterilisation

The manufacturer's recommended sterilisation regimen must be followed so that the mini-implant kit and mini-implants (if purchased non-sterile) are available in a sterile state ready for the scheduled appointment. Multiple sterilisation cycles do not cause problematic surface changes in mini-implants, so they may be resterilised if not used the first time [1]. Technically, sterile patient drapes and gloves are not required provided that the mini-implants and the free ends of the instruments (which contact the tissues) are untouched by the non-sterile gloves and instead only handled using sterile instruments such as the mini-implant screwdriver or an orthodontic instrument such as a Weingarts plier.

6.2 Superficial Anaesthesia

Either local (LA) or topical anaesthetic agents may be used to achieve superficial anaesthesia. Unfortunately, profound topical anaesthetics are not readily obtainable in many countries such as the UK and commercially available agents may provide insufficient anaesthesia [2,3]. Furthermore, LA is more effective in thick mucosa, and the appearance of soft tissue blanching indicates that the insertion may proceed immediately. In contrast, topical agents require at least three minutes of tissue contact, even for thin buccal tissue sites [2]. However, topical application is still beneficial at the start of the procedure to reduce the discomfort of the injection, especially if one is injecting directly into the mucosa at the insertion site. My preferred clinical regimen involves

rubbing topical gel onto the tissues, using a cotton wool roll, followed a minute later by LA delivery with the needle inserted *obliquely* (at a sloping angle to the surface) into the insertion site mucosa (Figure 6.1). Direct injection avoids more generalised infiltrations or blocks and hence patient discomfort. This often requires less than 0.2 mL of LA per site, and it provides both rapid anaesthesia and a vasoconstrictive effect (which is useful if soft tissue is to be removed).

> Local anaesthetic is more effective in thick mucosa, plus the appearance of soft tissue blanching indicates that the insertion may proceed immediately.

The key principle is that the mucosa and periosteum are anaesthetised (remember bone doesn't have feelings!), but the periodontal tissues of adjacent teeth remain responsive. This should alert the clinician if either the position or direction of the mini-implant needs to be altered during insertion because of close proximity to an adjacent dental root, or occasionally the opposite side of the alveolus. However, some anxious patients may give false-positive feedback, that is, they overinterpret the pressure sensation as pain when the mini-implant is not actually approximating adjacent roots. This is also more likely in posterior mandibular sites, due to less alveolar elasticity with the higher cortical density.

It is always helpful to percuss the adjacent teeth before the end of the insertion process: pain implies that the mini-implant is in close proximity to, or in contact with, the periodontal membrane. A dull percussion note indicates a limited width of alveolar bone between the mini-implant and tooth, but this is not an indication for reinsertion in the absence of percussion pain. Indeed, it is helpful to percuss the teeth before mini-implant insertion so that a baseline sound is noted. If in doubt, then a periapical radiograph, taken during the insertion process, should confirm whether the patient's sensation is accurate

The Orthodontic Mini-Implant Clinical Handbook, Second Edition. Richard Cousley.
© 2020 John Wiley & Sons Ltd. Published 2020 by John Wiley & Sons Ltd.

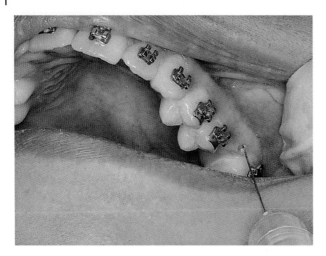

Figure 6.1 Local anaesthesia being injected directly into the insertion site soft tissues, with the needle at an oblique angle, on the mesial aspect of the maxillary second molar (where the first molar is absent).

or not. If necessary, the mini-implant can be reinserted at a different site or angle. If the insertion is clear of adjacent roots then further LA may be safely used to fully overcome any exaggerated patient discomfort.

> Percuss the adjacent teeth before the end of the insertion process: pain implies that the mini-implant is in close proximity to, or in contact with, the periodontal membrane.

6.3 Antibacterial Mouthwash

The patient should rinse the insertion site(s) for one minute using 0.2% chlorhexidine gluconate mouthwash. This helps to reduce the mucosal surface's bacterial levels immediately prior to insertion. It is also useful to give this bottle of mouthwash to the patient for postinsertion use, in order to optimise hygiene compliance. However, there is no benefit in widespread antibiotic prophylaxis [4]. The exception may be those patients at increased risk of infection, such as those with type 1 diabetes or a compromised immune response.

6.4 Stent Application (Optional)

'Freehand' insertion of a mini-implant is simple when there is ample interproximal space and the insertion site is easily accessible. In such cases, it may help to highlight the middle of the interproximal space by vertically indenting the gingival surface, using the side of a dental probe, in a line running apical to the contact point. Otherwise, a

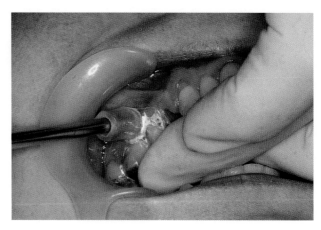

Figure 6.2 A manual screwdriver placed within the stent's buccal guidance cylinder. The stent's baseplate is being stabilised by finger pressure on its occlusal surface.

surgical stent helps to guide the insertion instruments, ideally in all three dimensions. This does not need to be sterile, but it must be disinfected prior to use. For example, it may be helpful to initially soak a stent in chlorhexidine mouthwash for 10 minutes immediately before it is fitted in the mouth. Also remember that care should be taken to minimise contact of the mini-implant threads with the stent material as the insertion instrument is lined up in the stent's guidance channel.

It is important to ensure that the stent is both rigid and adequately stabilised during usage, for example by finger pressure on the occlusal surfaces of a removable one (Figure 6.2). In addition, the screwdriver should not be leant on (pushed in one direction) whilst inside the guide cylinder. These precautions help to minimise flexing or movement of the stent and the subsequent risk of the screwdriver sticking in the stent when it is being released from the mini-implant. This arises because of a conflict between the paths of mini-implant insertion and screwdriver removal, when the stent has been moved or flexed.

> It is important to ensure that the stent is both rigid and adequately stabilised during usage.

6.5 Soft Tissue Removal

Use a soft tissue punch (mucotome) where the insertion is through either (thick) palatal attached tissue or through unattached/mobile buccal mucosa. The mucotome tip is positioned perpendicular to the tissue surface and simultaneously rotated and pressed through the soft tissue, using either a manual screwdriver handle or contra-angle handpiece. Once the bone surface has been contacted, the

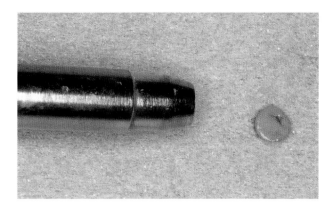

Figure 6.3 The circular piece of excised attached mucosa is seen adjacent to the Infinitas soft tissue punch (mucotome) used to remove it.

punch is rotated against it to cleanly incise the circle of soft tissue (Figure 6.3). The excision can be completed by removing the tissue plug with a curette or mosquitoes forceps. When a stent is used, it is best to provisionally indent the mucosa with the mucotome inserted in the guidance cylinder, and then temporarily remove the stent so that the mucotome can be applied perpendicular to the tissue surface and hence provide a consistent tissue cut.

Finally, it is important for an orthodontic assistant to hold a slow suction tip close to the tissue punch site since the cut tissue edge will bleed until the mini-implant neck seals the site.

6.6 Cortical Perforation

Full pilot drilling (of both cortical and cancellous bone layers) is required for non-drilling mini-implants but not for self-drilling designs. However, even self-drilling insertions benefit from perforation of the cortical plate where it is dense and thick, such as the posterior mandible and palate (both midpalate and alveolus) areas. Crucially, this involves making only a 1–2 mm perforation of the cortex (Figure 6.4) in contrast to an 8–10 mm pilot drilling depth. In effect, cortical perforation facilitates mini-implant insertion by reducing the risks of screw fracture and excessive insertion torque (which compromises secondary bone healing, as described in Chapter 2). In addition, some clinicians like to use a cortical punch to indent the cortex at many more insertion sites in order to provide a locating ('purchase') point for the mini-implant tip. This is especially useful to prevent slippage on the bone surface, where the alveolus has a convex contour and an oblique insertion is planned.

Cortical perforation may be performed with either a pilot drill, partially inserted into bone, or a customised bone punch. The latter has the advantage of a shoulder at the

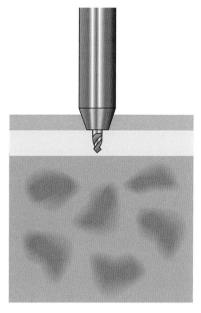

Figure 6.4 Diagram of the Infinitas cortical bone punch traversing the mucosa and inserting into a thick cortical layer.

end of the drill section, which limits the drilling depth (Figure 6.4). Such punches may be used either manually, in the manner of a screwdriver, or with a contra-angle handpiece. As with a mucotome, the cortical punch is rotated under axial pressure in order to penetrate the cortex. However, this can be a surprisingly quick and simple process since even manual perforation takes only a few seconds. Crucially, the punch should be directed at the planned insertion angles rather than at right angles to the surface (which differs from the mucotome application).

6.7 Mini-implant Insertion

The screwdriver should be fully engaged onto the mini-implant neck or head (depending on the type of implant design), but without excessive pressure since this may make it more difficult to subsequently detach the screwdriver. If there is doubt over whether the implant is securely engaged then shake the screwdriver over a sterile field to ensure that the mini-implant does not fall out.

A self-drilling mini-implant may be inserted directly through thin mucosa and into the bone (Figure 6.5), except in situations requiring preliminary perforations of the mucosa and/or cortex. Even when the cortex is initially perforated, insertion of a self-drilling mini-implant still continues in the normal manner. The insertion may be performed using a manual or handpiece-driven screwdriver. The former is recommended for buccal sites, since it gives the operator tactile feedback and fine motor control. However, it is crucial that the screwdriver rotations are

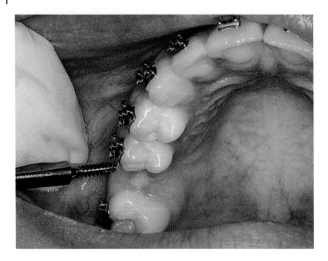

Figure 6.5 Freehand manual insertion of a 2.0 mm diameter mini-implant in the right maxillary edentulous molar site. The adjacent cheek and buccal sulcus are held taut (with finger pressure) to provide access and to prevent the loose mucosa from wrapping around the mini-implant threads.

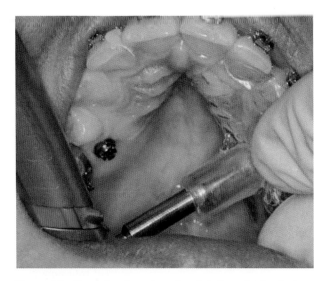

Figure 6.6 Handpiece insertion of an Infinitas mini-implant on the palatal aspect of the alveolus, where the end of the screwdriver insert fits within the 3D stent. The mini-implant's body can be seen through the plastic guidance cylinder.

limited to finger turns only, since any rotation of the wrist could readily exceed the maximum insertion torque for many clinical sites and result in secondary failure [5].

A contra-angle slow handpiece is used where direct access is limited, such as palatal or posterior buccal sites (Figure 6.6). I prefer using a customised cordless mini-implant handpiece which is capable of precise slow speed control (e.g. 25 rpm, to control the insertion depth and heat generation), providing a digital reading of the maximum insertion torque (in lieu of a tactile indication of this) and presetting the maximum torque below 30 Ncm (in order to avoid root injury and excessive bone strain).

Alternatively, one may use a speed reduction handpiece (with at least a 128:1 ratio) coupled with reduction of the dental unit's motor speed (e.g. from 40 000 to 10 000 rpm). This limits the maximum screwdriver speed to below 100 rpm while still delivering adequate insertion torque. Unfortunately, if insertion is attempted by solely reducing the dental chair/motor speed (and using a normal 1:1 or 4:1 ratio speed reduction handpiece) then there is a strong risk of inadequate torque delivery and the handpiece may stall mid-insertion.

> Even when the cortex is initially perforated, insertion of a self-drilling mini-implant still continues in the normal manner.

The mini-implant is inserted slowly by rotating the screwdriver handle clockwise with one's fingers and with firm seating pressure at the base of the handle. It is essential that one's wrist is stabilised and that the rotations are produced by digit movements alone. Remember it is a gentle procedure for both the patient and their bone. Care should also be taken not to alter the insertion angle during this process. Firm pressure is used initially to penetrate the cortical plate, applied by pressing the palm on the end of the manual screwdriver at the same time as rotating it. The insertional resistance tends to reduce once the first few threads appear to be submerging, and then the insertion process should continue solely by rotational means. As the mini-implant is gradually advanced into bone, the torque (resistance to screwdriver rotation) tends to increase, especially in posterior mandible sites and with a tapered body design, such as the 1.5 mm diameter Infinitas version (as the wider section of body engages the cortex). Excessive resistance, usually felt as difficulty in turning a manual screwdriver by finger pressure alone (without resorting to rotation of the wrist), may result in either implant fracture or delayed bone necrosis. In such circumstances, the insertion should either be paused for 10–20 seconds (giving time for the viscoelastic nature of bone to allow its expansion around the mini-implant) or the mini-implant should be unscrewed by one to two anticlockwise turns before inserting it further with clockwise rotations. These measures may be repeated as necessary until the desired final insertion depth is approached (but do not derotate at the final insertion stage).

> As the mini-implant is gradually advanced into bone, the torque (resistance to screwdriver rotation) tends to increase.

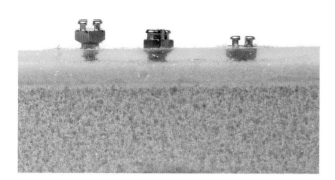

Figure 6.7 A photograph of Infinitas (short neck) mini-implants at three different stages of insertion in an artificial bone block (covered by a relatively thick soft tissue layer). The left mini-implant is underinserted since its neck is completely exposed. The tapered section of the middle mini-implant's neck is within the mucosa and the head is clear of the tissues. This mini-implant could be inserted by a maximum of one further turn (0.7 mm). The right mini-implant has been overinserted since its neck is submerged.

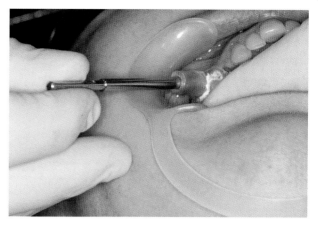

Figure 6.8 The long (manual) screwdriver insert is being detached from the mini-implant head after removal of the screwdriver handle. The end of the insert is held by two fingers in order to avoid lateral displacement and facilitate detachment in line with the mini-implant's long axis.

It is crucial to avoid overinserting a mini-implant, either by leaving an insufficient amount of the head exposed (for orthodontic attachment purposes) or by rotating it beyond the point of continued engagement in the bone (when it continues to rotate freely but without inserting more deeply). Equally, a mini-implant should never be partially unscrewed in an attempt to increase its emergence profile, since this will inevitably result in loss of stability. Therefore, it is best to control the final insertion stage by slowly rotating the screwdriver clockwise until the desired body insertion depth or head emergence profile is reached (Figure 6.7). This is a balance such that the tapered section of the neck is submerged but the whole head is readily accessible.

It is often helpful to detach the screwdriver at this stage in order to visually inspect the remaining exposed mini-implant threads and head–mucosa distance. When detaching the screwdriver, care should be taken to avoid excessive lateral or pull-out movements. In particular, if substantial pressure was required to penetrate the cortex then this may result in noticeable resistance to the first detachment attempt. Whilst it is very tempting to tug the screwdriver laterally, this must be avoided since it may conflict with the mini-implant's path of release from within the screwdriver, resulting in the widening of the mini-implant bed or even its fracture. Therefore, it is advisable to reduce the chances of lateral 'tugging' by first detaching the screwdriver handle (or handpiece). It is then easier to pull the screwdriver component off the mini-implant in a straight line, along the long axis of the implant-screwdriver, by grasping the insert's end with a forefinger and thumb grip (Figure 6.8).

> It is best to control the final insertion stage by slowly rotating the screwdriver clockwise until the desired body insertion depth or head emergence profile is reached.

If primary stability, as indicated by the final insertion torque, is unsatisfactory then the mini-implant should be removed and the insertion process repeated at a different site. Conversely, if a sudden increase in insertion torque is experienced then this is probably due to root contact (and the insertion should be stopped). However, when only superficial anaesthesia has been used, it is more likely that the patient will report pain in an adjacent tooth if the mini-implant approximates a root.

A simple test for root proximity, which I routinely perform, is to percuss the adjacent teeth during an alveolar site insertion. An alteration in tone indicates a reduction in the amount of bone separation between the mini-implant and root. This is a particularly useful warning sign if there is a distinct difference in percussion tone between the two adjacent teeth, indicating closer proximity to one tooth in particular. If a tooth is painful to percuss then this suggests actual root contact. If close root proximity is suspected then an intraoral radiograph will help to check the mini-implant position in relation to adjacent structures during the insertion process (Figure 6.9a). If this shows a radiographic overlap of the mini-implant and a tooth root then reinsertion in either a new position or angle is indicated. For example, if the mini-implant position is much closer to one tooth in the mesiodistal direction, then the mini-implant should be removed and reinserted in a more

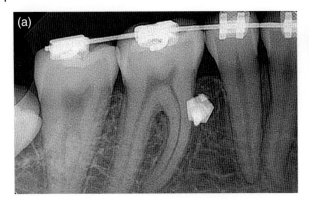 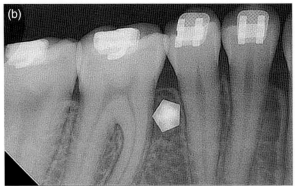

Figure 6.9 Periapical radiographs taken (a) during and (b) after insertion of a buccal mini-implant between the mandibular second premolar and first molar teeth. The patient complained of pain during the initial insertion and the first radiograph confirmed excessively close proximity to the first molar root. The mini-implant was then reinserted by choosing a more mesial surface point (apical to the contact point), as shown in (b).

neutral insertion point, ideally apical to the contact point (Figure 6.9b). However, if the insertion point looks reasonably neutral but the tip of the mini-implant is angled towards a tooth, then the mini-implant may be reinserted in the same insertion site but at a corrected angle (aimed to follow under the contact point).

The same mini-implant may be reused if it is fully removed and then immediately reinserted without touching other oral tissues. However, the mini-implant tip may have been blunted during the original insertion, especially if there was high initial insertion torque or root contact [6]. In that case, a cortical punch should be used to help penetrate the cortex at a new insertion site. If an adjacent suitable site is not available at the same clinical appointment, for example where more root divergence is required, then allow a minimum of three months before repeating the insertion in the same site. This will allow time for bone infill, as demonstrated in a recent animal study of bone healing after explantation [7]. Even then, it is often helpful to diverge the adjacent tooth roots, to provide a greater range of insertion site positions, before attempting reinsertion. This may be done by either adding a second-order bend to the archwire or rebonding one of the adjacent brackets at a different tip, as described in Chapter 5 (see Figure 5.8).

6.8 Mini-implant Fracture

Fortunately, this is an infrequent occurrence, typically associated with excessive torque due to insertion in high-density bone, contact of the mini-implant with a tooth root or deviation of the insertion path (when the mini-implant is already partially inserted). In the case of root contact, one would expect the patient to feel pain, but this may not

occur if the level of anaesthesia has affected the periodontal membrane as well as superficial tissues.

Most mini-implant fractures occur flush with the cortical surface, leaving the retained fragment submerged and difficult to retrieve. Provided that the mini-implant is manufactured from a titanium or titanium alloy material then it can be left *in situ*, to be covered over by soft tissue healing, if the orthodontist is confident that it will not interfere with any remaining tooth movement or cause root trauma (Figure 1.4). However, if it is necessary to remove the retained fragment so that a new mini-implant can be inserted, or if an adjacent tooth needs to move towards this site, then a small surgical procedure is required. This involves elevation of a mucoperiosteal flap and trephination of a narrow trough of bone around the fragment so that an instrument, such as a Weingarts plier, can be used to unscrew it. Given that a surgical flap is required, many orthodontists will prefer to advise the patient of the problem immediately after the fracture and then refer the patient to a surgical colleague for this procedure at a later date.

6.9 Postoperative Instructions

It is advisable to provide the patient with both verbal and written instructions on postinsertion analgesics (usually only taken in the first 24 hours), chlorhexidine usage and advice not to fiddle with the mini-implant or touch it with an electric toothbrush. 'Traditional' oral hygiene advice was that chlorhexidine mouthwash should be used twice daily for five days. However, in order to prevent tooth staining, a better long-term option is for the patient to dip a small manual toothbrush into the chlorhexidine and brush daily and gently around the mini-implant head in order to inhibit peri-implant tissue inflammation or hyperplasia.

6.10 Force Application

Most mini-implant types can and should be loaded immediately, unless the final insertion torque was very low, that is, there was minimal screwdriver resistance on final seating. As a rule of thumb, it is advisable that only a light (approximately 50 g) force is applied for the first four and six weeks in adults and adolescents, respectively. This is easily applied by a gently stretched elastomeric chain, and it allows time for the bone healing response to stabilise the mini-implant. Indeed, it is favourable that the elastomeric force decays within the first few weeks at the same time that the mini-implant's primary stability is reducing. This has been shown by resonance frequency studies to result in the minimum total bone stability at three weeks after insertion [8–10]. Subsequently, various kinds of attachments, such as preformed nickel titanium coil springs and elastomeric chains, can be placed for direct loading with conventional continuous orthodontic force levels, for example 200 g.

Care should be taken to avoid derotational effects on both directly and indirectly loaded mini-implants since an anticlockwise movement may result in a reduction in secondary stability [11,12]. This affects mini-implants with a bracket-like head design, such as the Infinitas, but is readily avoided in direct traction scenarios by placing an elastomeric chain around the external circumference to be rotationally neutral. When a NiTi coil spring is used, it should be fitted on the wing (corner) which is either in the line of traction (Figure 6.10a) or most likely to cause subtle clockwise rotation of the head (Figure 6.10b).

> As a rule of thumb, it is advisable that only a light (approximately 50 g) force is applied for the first four and six weeks in adults and adolescents, respectively.

Indirect anchorage loading may also be applied immediately via an auxiliary wire (ligature or rigid wire) either connected to the fixed appliance or simply bonded to an adjacent tooth. The latter scenario may utilise a cross-tube on the main archwire and intermediary rectangular steel wire, as illustrated in Chapter 1.

6.11 Biomechanics

It is now clear that fixed appliances can exert more profound three-dimensional effects, especially in the vertical direction, when mini-implants are utilised. Therefore, customised mechanics are required in order to maximise the desired effects and minimise side-effects. These details are discussed in relation to specific clinical scenarios in the following chapters.

6.12 Explantation

Mini-implants are removed once the need for anchorage reinforcement has abated, although if there is any doubt over future anchorage requirements, they can easily be left *in situ* and unloaded for several months. This gives the orthodontist the option of turning anchorage on and off. In contrast, can you imagine trying to convince a patient to recommence wearing headgear after you had given them

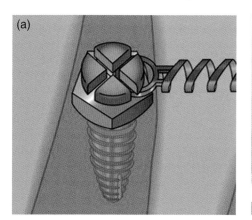
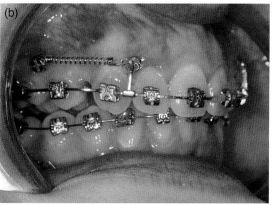

Figure 6.10 (a) Illustration of a mini-implant where the traction spring has been attached to the wing in line with the direction of traction. (b) Photograph of a mini-implant loaded by direct connection of a closing coil spring on the mesiogingival wing of its head. This will produce a small clockwise moment. The other end of the spring is ligated to a fixed appliance powerarm to retract the anterior teeth.

the 'all clear'! Since mini-implants do not osseointegrate in terms of clinical ankylosis, they are easily removed, usually without the need for local anaesthesia. The exception to this occurs in cases with submerged mini-implant heads or in the upper labial area where soft tissue sensation may be heightened.

Explantation is performed by fully engaging the screwdriver (both manual and handpiece versions) onto the mini-implant and rotating it anticlockwise. Rotate the implant fully out of its socket, without pulling it out since this causes pain due to the threads catching on the peri-implant soft tissue. No special postremoval precautions (e.g. suturing or analgesics) are required, and both the soft tissues and bone heal uneventfully (the former within several days).

6.13 Summary of Mini-implant Insertion Steps

1) Case selection: identify the anchorage requirements.
2) Records and planning.
   - Obtain records (+/− a working model for stent fabrication)
   - Obtain informed consent
   - Determine the insertion site and timing
   - Fabricate a stent as required
   - Select optimum mini-implant dimensions
3) Mini-implant insertion.
   - Superficial anaesthesia (blanch the mucosa)
   - Chlorhexidine mouthwash for one minute
   - Fit stent (if applicable, presoaked in chlorhexidine)
   - Soft tissue removal – if site is in thick or loose mucosa
   - Perforate cortex – for posterior mandible and palate sites in adults
   - Insert mini-implant with slow steady screwdriver rotations
   - If torque is high then pause for 10–20 seconds or partially derotate
   - Percuss adjacent teeth to gauge implant–root proximity
   - If root proximity apparent then take a radiograph or reinsert implant
4) Postinsertion.
   - Apply light (e.g. 50 g) traction for the first six weeks
   - Provide verbal and written patient instructions and mouthwash

5) Explantation: rotate mini-implant anticlockwise until fully removed.

6.14 Maximising Mini-implant Success: Ten Clinical Tips

1) Gain experience with manually performed buccal insertions before attempting palatal insertions (with a contra-angle handpiece). This helps develop a feel for manual control and insertion torque.
2) Direct or indirect anchorage: identify the ideal insertion site (in terms of anatomical and biomechanical considerations) and the type of attachment to the fixed appliance at the treatment planning stage.
3) 'Develop' the insertion site (interproximal space) by diverging the adjacent roots during initial fixed appliance alignment. This is achieved by altering the tip of adjacent brackets, for example adding a mesial bracket tip in order to mesially tip an upper second premolar crown.
4) Use a guidance stent, especially if you are inexperienced with mini-implants or not the treating orthodontist, but also for difficult-to-access (e.g. palatal) insertion sites.
5) Use superficial anaesthesia, at least until the risk of root proximity has been discounted, so that live patient feedback from adjacent periodontal membranes is available.
6) Do not overinsert the mini-implant: it will be prone to tissue overgrowth and/or will loosen if subsequent partial derotation is attempted.
7) Always apply light (circa 50 g) traction for the first six weeks, or even leave unloaded in adolescents where the insertion torque has been low.
8) Correct minor secondary (delayed) mobility of a mini-implant by simple further clockwise rotation by one to two turns (without the need for anaesthesia).
9) Apply anteroposterior traction to a powerarm on a rigid stainless steel archwire. This will reduce intrusive side-effects and maximise bodily movement of the target teeth.
10) Insert mini-implants in palatal and midpalatal sites for maximum intrusion and distalisation effects, respectively.

References

1 Akyalcin, S., McIver, H.P., English, J.D. et al. (2013). Effects of repeated sterilization cycles on primary stability of orthodontic mini-screws. *Angle Orthod.* 83: 674–679.

2 Kwong, T.S., Kusnoto, B., Viana, G. et al. (2011). The effectiveness of Oraqix versus TAC$_{(a)}$ for placement of orthodontic temporary anchorage devices. *Angle Orthod.* 81: 754–759.

3 Valieri, M.M., Salvatore de Freitas, K.M., Valarelli, F.P., and Cançado, R.H. (2014). Comparison of topical and infiltration anesthesia for orthodontic mini-implant placement. *Dental Press J. Orthod.* 19: 76–83.

4 Łyczek, J., Kawala, B., and Antoszewska-Smith, J. (2018). Influence of antibiotic prophylaxis on the stability of orthodontic microimplants: a pilot randomized controlled trial. *Am. J. Orthod. Dentofac. Orthop.* 153: 621–631.

5 Estelita, S., Janson, G., Chiqueto, K. et al. (2012). Selective use of hand and forearm muscles during mini-implant insertion: a natural torquimeter. *J. Orthod.* 39: 270–278.

6 Chung, C.J., Jung, K., Choi, Y.J., and Kim, K. (2014). Biomechanical characteristics and reinsertion guidelines for retrieved orthodontic miniscrews. *Angle Orthod.* 84: 878–884.

7 Kim, S.J., Ha, Y.D., Kim, E. et al. (2019). Dynamics of alveolar bone healing after the removal of orthodontic temporary anchorage devices. *J. Periodontal Res.* 54 (4): 388–395.

8 Ure, D.S., Oliver, D.R., Kim, K.B. et al. (2011). Stability changes of miniscrew implants over time. A pilot resonance frequency analysis. *Angle Orthod.* 81: 994–1000.

9 Wei, X., Zhao, L., Xu, Z. et al. (2011). Effects of cortical bone thickness at different healing times on microscrew stability. *Angle Orthod.* 81: 754–759.

10 Nienkemper, M., Wilmes, B., Pauls, A., and Drescher, D. (2014). Mini-implant stability at the initial healing period. A clinical pilot study. *Angle Orthod.* 84: 127–133.

11 Cho, Y., Cha, J., and Hwang, C. (2010). The effect of rotation moment on the stability of immediately loaded orthodontic miniscrews: a pilot study. *Eur. J. Orthod.* 32: 614–619.

12 Park, K., Lee, E., Shin, S. et al. (2011). Evaluation of the effect of force direction on stationary anchorage success of mini-implant with a lever arm-shaped upper structure. *Angle Orthod.* 81: 776–782.

7

Retraction of Anterior Teeth

When most orthodontists think of anchorage, it's probably a scenario involving the use of an intraoral appliance or headgear to stabilise the maxillary molars in the anteroposterior (AP) dimension during retraction of the anterior teeth. Unsurprisingly, this was one of the first identified applications for mini-implants, with traction applied directly from the mini-implant (typically inserted buccally between first molar and second premolar roots), sparing molar involvement and hence anchorage loss. It's now clear, both from clinical experience and published studies, that mini-implant usage enables ideal orthodontic treatment goals to be much more reliably achieved than with the traditional gold standard of headgear anchorage [1–8]. In addition, unlike conventional anchorage options, mini-implant anchorage offers direct, maximum anchorage reinforcement in both the maxillary and mandibular arches. In effect, mini-implants represent the twenty-first century's gold standard for orthodontic anchorage because of their key benefits:

- complete anchorage control, with minimal patient compliance requirements
- controlled, bodily retraction of anterior teeth
- more efficient, quicker treatment through *en masse* retraction of the six anterior teeth (rather than two-stage retraction of the canines then incisor teeth).

Mini-implant anchorage enables full incisor retraction without posterior anchorage loss, even when the canine and incisor teeth are retracted *en masse*. In addition, anchorage *gain* has been observed such that the maxillary molars have been distalised by a small amount. This may occur by a combination of archwire binding in the molar tube which causes the retractive force to shunt the whole arch distally, and by the continuation of traction after closure of premolar spaces. It is probably ironic that if this occurs then it will be appropriate in some cases to close residual space by anchorage loss (after removal of the mini-implants).

The second key benefit of mini-implant anchorage, over conventional options, is the increased control of the target (anterior) teeth movements. However, this only occurs with direct traction and not with indirect mini-implant anchorage where conventional traction is applied between the anchor and target teeth (Figure 7.1). Therefore, only correctly executed direct traction biomechanics produce bodily control of the anterior teeth during their retraction and even some incisor intrusion (which is ideal in Class II cases with a deep overbite) [7,9–12]. This contrasts with the recognised side-effect of incisor retraction in conventional straight-wire mechanics where the retractive force causes incisor extrusion and retroclination. My original use of buccal mini-implant anchorage not only replicated this side-effect but unexpectedly increased its expression, because of the effect of obliquely directed traction (Figure 7.2). Fortunately, this side-effect is unlikely nowadays following the introduction of powerarms (elongated vertical hooks either crimped on the anterior part of the archwire or bonded to anterior teeth). These enable direct traction to be applied with a more 'horizontal' vector and the force delivered closer to the centre of resistance of either the entire block of anterior teeth (Figure 7.3) [3,8,13–15] or a single canine tooth [16]. If a commercial version is not available for purchase, then a single-tooth powerarm may be created by combining a crimpable one with a bondable base, or by soldering a rigid extension wire onto the hook of a canine bracket (Figure 7.4). As a result, powerarms have revolutionised the delivery and effects of mini-implant anchorage for controlled AP tooth movements.

On the other hand, vertical biomechanical side-effects may be advantageous in patients presenting with either a reduced overbite or small anterior openbite since they will benefit from some incisor extrusion (provided that this is acceptable in terms of upper incisor display), ideally coupled with modest molar intrusion. In this situation, the mini-implant biomechanics cause clockwise rotation of the entire maxillary arch, manifesting as incisor extrusion

The Orthodontic Mini-Implant Clinical Handbook, Second Edition. Richard Cousley.
© 2020 John Wiley & Sons Ltd. Published 2020 by John Wiley & Sons Ltd.

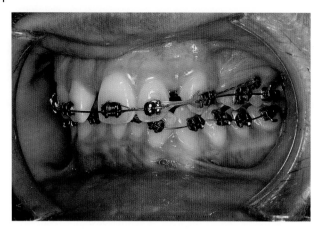

Figure 7.1 Indirect anchorage involving a stainless steel ligature from the posterior mini-implant to the canine bracket and elastomeric traction from this canine to retract the adjacent incisors. This avoids vertical side-effects, but equally does not provide bodily control of the incisor movements.

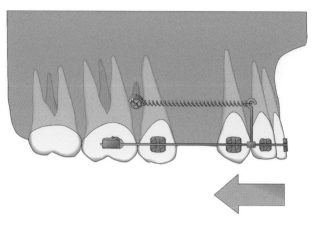

Figure 7.3 Diagram showing a horizontal vector of traction from the posterior mini-implant to an anterior powerarm, causing bodily retraction of the anterior teeth (without molar intrusion).

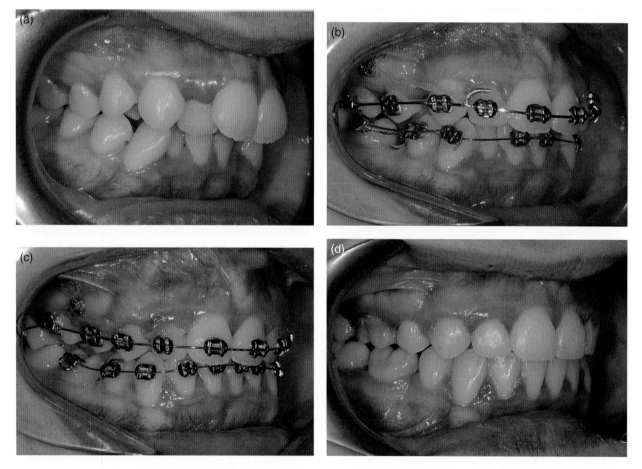

Figure 7.2 (a) This patient had extraction of the upper first premolar teeth for *en masse* canine and incisor retraction. (b) Oblique elastomeric traction was applied from the mini-implant to short hooks on the 0.019 × 0.025 in. steel archwire. (c) This traction vector caused intrusion of the upper first molars, as evidenced by the lateral openbite and vertical step between the first and second molar teeth. Cessation of oblique traction coupled with bonding of the second molar caused vertical settling of the buccal teeth prior to debond (d).

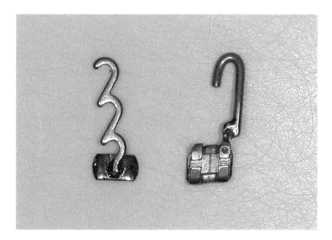

Figure 7.4 Photographs of single-tooth powerarms. The left one has been made by cutting off a crimpable powerarm's existing base and soldering it to a bondable base. The right powerarm was created by soldering a rigid round wire to the hook of a canine bracket.

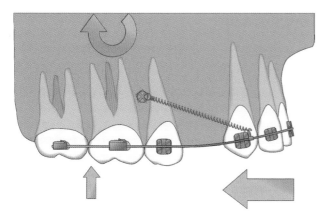

Figure 7.5 Diagram showing the effects of an oblique vector of traction where the mini-implant is apical to the anterior point of force application, causing rotation of the whole maxillary arch (manifesting as incisor retroclination and molar intrusion).

and molar intrusion (Figure 7.5). The molar intrusive side-effect indirectly assists with Class II correction, due to favourable mandibular counter-clockwise autorotation (measured as a reduction in the mandibular plane angle and an increase in the sella-nasion-B point [SNB] angle). In contrast to average or deep overbite cases, this biomechanical set-up deliberately requires the creation of a steep vector of traction where the mini-implant is inserted more apically than the point of traction application on the labial segment. In terms of the fixed appliance configuration, the terminal molars need to be included in the fixed appliance, and a rigid archwire should be in place. Otherwise, the application of direct traction with an oblique (vertically steep) vector to a flexible archwire causes pronounced distal tipping of the canine, incisor retroclination and a 'rollercoaster' buckling of the buccal segment (Figure 7.6).

In summary, the biomechanical configuration for incisor retraction ought to be decided at the treatment planning stage. The key considerations are the patient's age and overbite. Age is relevant since young adolescent patients may have insufficient alveolar bone support for mini-implant stability. Therefore, indirect, midpalate, anchorage is appropriate in these cases, accepting that the traction effects will mirror those of conventional straight-wire biomechanics. In terms of the overbite, patients with average and deep overbites should ideally have a direct anchorage configuration with the traction applied parallel to the occlusal plane from the mini-implant to a powerarm (Figure 7.3). This minimises the rotational effect on the whole arch and produces favourable bodily retraction of the anterior teeth. Patients with a reduced overbite or small openbite should have obliquely directed direct traction (Figure 7.5).

The final considerations are the anterior maxillary alveolar depth and nasopalatine size. There should be adequate cancellous alveolar bone depth to allow for the

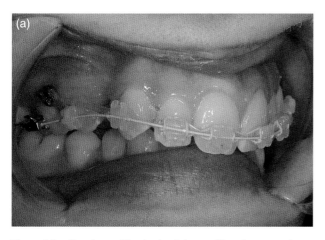

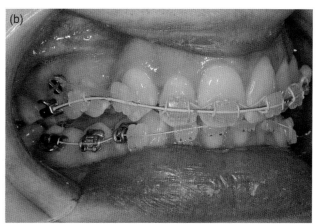

Figure 7.6 Alveolar necking in the right maxillary first premolar extraction site, resulted in very difficult distalisation of the adjacent canine in this adult patient. Consequently, elastomeric traction applied from the mini-implant to the upper canine bracket caused (a) distal tipping of the canine and a rollercoaster bowing of this 0.018 in. NiTi archwire, then (b) molar intrusion when traction continued on a rigid archwire.

Powerarms have revolutionized the effects of mini-implant anchorage for controlled AP tooth movements, but there needs to be sufficient anterior alveolar depth for the enhanced incisor root movement now possible.

enhanced range of palatal incisor root movement possible with powerarm (torque) control. If this is insufficient then limited use of powerarms is advisable, accepting that the incisors will retrocline as they are retracted. Otherwise, incisor root resorption may occur due to root contact with the palatal cortex (Figure 7.7) [17]. Given that the incisive canal may only be analysed fully via cone beam computed tomography (CBCT) (and not a lateral cephalogram), it may therefore be prudent (and justified) to take a CBCT of the anterior maxilla in patients who require substantial upper incisor retraction [18]. The various biomechanical scenarios will be illustrated in following sections of this chapter.

In average and deep overbite cases, mini-implant traction should be applied parallel to the occlusal plane by crimping a powerarm onto the anterior part of the archwire.

7.1 Clinical Objective

- Prevention of mesial movement (anchorage loss) of the upper or lower molar teeth during retraction of the anterior teeth for overjet reduction, relief of crowding and/or centreline correction.

7.2 Treatment Options

- Direct bone anchorage by the application of traction from a mini-implant inserted in a posterior alveolar site, in either jaw.
- Indirect alveolar bone anchorage using a mini-implant to stabilise the posterior teeth (the dental anchorage unit), for example by a ligature from the mini-implant to an anchor tooth (maxillary arch only) using midpalate mini-implants.
- Conventional anchorage, such as headgear, transpalatal arch (TPA), lingual arch.
- Intermaxillary elastics for indirect anchorage.
- Correction of the skeletal base (negating the anchorage requirements) using orthognathic surgery or orthopaedic (functional) appliance treatments.

7.3 Key Treatment Planning Considerations

- The anchorage requirements, as indicated by the overjet, incisor inclination, distance that the canines need to be retracted into Class I (allowing for any canine movements in the opposing arch), buccal segment relationships and extraction pattern.
- Overbite: this affects the ideal vertical level of the mini-implant and the vector of traction; that is, the more apical the position of the mini-implant head then the more potential for molar intrusion in a reduced overbite case.
- Centreline: is there a need for asymmetrical incisor retraction?

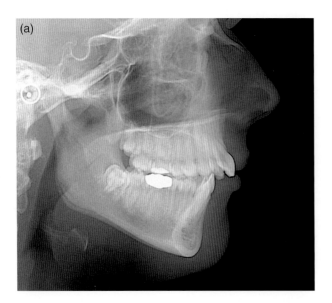
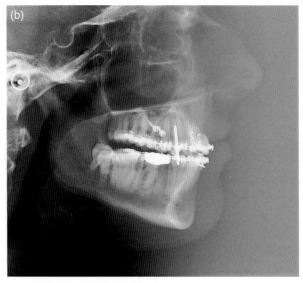

Figure 7.7 Lateral cephalograms of an adult patient (a) before treatment and (b) following mini-implant and powerarm incisor retraction mechanics. The anterior alveolar depth was limited and the incisor roots were short pretreatment, and the latter has worsened possibly due to the extent of palatal root movement.

- Morphological or prognostic differences between the posterior teeth which may influence the extraction pattern; for example, loss of a restored or macrodont/microdont second premolar may be indicated rather than a virgin first premolar even if this increases the anchorage demands.
- Is there sufficient interproximal space between the first molar and second premolar roots, or is preliminary root divergence required?
- The amount of incisor crowding: is there a need for preliminary canine retraction to enable incisor alignment/retraction?
- Age: there may be insufficient primary stability in alveolar sites in an adolescent patient because of their thin and less dense cortex. In such cases, consider using the midpalate as a source of indirect anchorage. For example, two mini-implants with a short body length and wide diameter (e.g. Infinitas 6 mm length, 2 mm diameter) may be inserted in parasagittal positions and used to anchor the Nance button of a TPA. This stabilises the upper molar anchor teeth, but there is still a risk of anchorage loss if the TPA distorts due to insufficient rigidity. There are also additional clinical time and (laboratory) cost implications due to the need for fabrication of a customised TPA or Nance arch, plus traction can only be applied in a conventional manner (at the coronal level from the molar hooks).

7.4 Biomechanical Principles

- Increased overbite case: apply direct traction to anterior powerarms on a rigid archwire and supplement the vertical control with a bite-opening curve in the archwire. One may also consider the adjunctive intrusion of the anterior teeth using additional anterior mini-implants.
- Reduced overbite case: bond the second molars (if fully erupted) during the alignment phase so that they can be actively intruded during space closure, by virtue of the rotational effect of oblique traction on the arch. The molars may be further intruded by direct vertical traction after the space closure phase.
- Determine the ideal mini-implant vertical position prior to insertion. For example, if there is sufficient height of attached gingiva then the mini-implant may be vertically sited at a relatively apical level, but with the potential effect of producing an oblique (steep) vector of traction and consequently molar intrusion if a powerarm is not added. Conversely, if there is only a narrow band of attached gingiva then the mini-implant is limited to a coronal insertion level, resulting in closer proximity to the archwire plane but little scope for intrusive effects.

- The force vector is best altered by application of the traction to a powerarm – an elongated hook attached to the archwire or a bracket (Figures 7.3 and 7.4). This has three effects/uses:
  - Elimination of the vertical component (vector) of the traction since the powerarm enables traction to be attached at the same vertical level as the mini-implant head. This minimises the risk of inadvertent molar intrusion, due to clockwise arch rotation.
  - The powerarm facilitates more bodily retraction of the incisors since the traction is applied closer to the centre of resistance of the anterior teeth.
  - A single tooth powerarm is also very useful for controlled canine retraction in cases requiring space for relief of incisor crowding (Figure 7.4). This greatly assists bodily canine distalisation and reduces the risk of the rollercoaster phenomenon (Figure 7.6) due to distal tipping of the canine. Indeed, a bondable powerarm even enables the application of traction when a flexible archwire is in place. Both patient comfort and rotational control of the target tooth are minimised if the powerarm has a relatively low profile (Figure 7.16i,j).
- Indirect anchorage, for example utilising a bone-anchored TPA, involves force application on the fixed appliance molar hooks. This means that biomechanical effects are similar to conventional straight wire approaches.

7.5 Midtreatment Problems and Solutions

- Vertical side-effects such as a lateral openbite and excessive incisor retroclination (Figures 7.2 and 7.6).
  - Avoid the application of traction with a flexible archwire *in situ* and when a working stainless steel archwire (e.g. 0.019 × 0.025 in.) has not fully levelled the arch.
  - Add a bite-opening curve to the working archwire.
  - Accept the openbite discrepancy until anchorage is no longer required, then remove the mini-implants, bond the second molars and use a flexible archwire to level the arch.
  - Vertical settling elastics may also be added, although most lateral openbites readily settle once traction has ceased and the archwire changes are expressed (Figures 7.2, 7.6 and 7.8).

7.6 Clinical Steps for a Posterior Mini-implant

7.6.1 Preinsertion

1) Increase the interproximal space available at the insertion site by bonding the second premolar bracket with the addition of approximately 30° of mesial tip. This

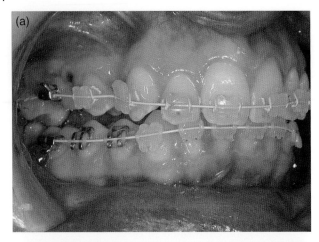

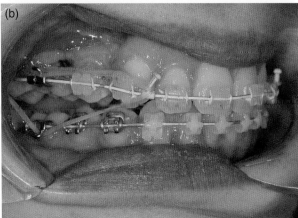

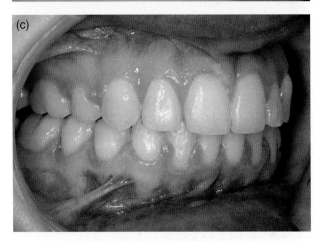

Figure 7.8 The patient shown in Figure 6.1 after (a) removal of the mini-implant and bonding of the upper second molar to assist with levelling. (b) An upper 0.019 × 0.025 in. NiTi archwire is combined with a triangular elastic to settle the lateral openbite. (c) Debond view.

causes the premolar root to move mesially during initial alignment.

2) If initial canine retraction is required, first align most of the arch to prepare for a 0.018 stainless steel working archwire. Then add a single-tooth powerarm to the canine crown or bracket. Otherwise, for *en masse* retraction, align and level the whole arch to prepare for a 0.019 × 0.025 steel archwire.

3) If desired, have a stent fabricated by taking an impression or intraoral scan of the arch two weeks before insertion. Avoid waxing out brackets and the buccal sulcus near the insertion site and record the clinical level of the mucogingival junction.

7.6.2 Mini-implant Selection

4) Maxilla: use a narrow long body, short neck mini-implant (e.g. the blue Infinitas version – 1.5 mm diameter, 9 mm length, short neck).

5) Mandible: use a narrow, short neck mini-implant (e.g. blue or pink Infinitas version – 1.5 mm diameter, 6 or 9 mm length, short neck). The body length selection depends on the anticipated cortical support such that a long length is selected in adolescent patients or if angulated insertion is indicated (because of limited attached gingival height).

7.6.3 Insertion

6) Identify the ideal buccal alveolar insertion point, through attached gingivae near the mucogingival junction (which does not require a soft tissue punch step), and between the second premolar and first molar roots.

7) Superficial anaesthesia of the insertion site.

8) Determine the angles of insertion. Interproximal mini-implants are generally inserted 'under' the adjacent teeth's contact points and perpendicular to the surface in the horizontal plane. Maxillary mini-implants may be inserted at either 90° (perpendicular to the surface) or angled obliquely by 20–30°, by inclining the screwdriver in an apical direction (Figure 7.9). Oblique insertion angles in the mandible tend to be less, for example 10–20°, because of the surface morphology and the thicker cortex.

9) Manual insertion is recommended where there is sufficient physical access (i.e. easy stretching of the cheek and buccal sulcus). Otherwise, handpiece insertion may be performed but with resultant loss of full tactile control.

10) Insert the mini-implant transmucosally, unless the site is in loose mucosa and requires a mucosal punch first.

11) A cortical bone punch is recommended as the first step for posterior mandibular sites in adult patients.

12) Complete the insertion to the point that the mini-implant neck is partially submerged but the head is fully accessible. This is best performed gradually and with intermittent release of the screwdriver during the final phase, so that overinsertion is avoided.

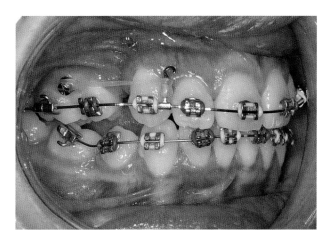

Figure 7.9 An adult patient with limited height of attached gingiva at the upper right buccal insertion site, requiring 20–30° oblique (apical) inclination of the mini-implant. Horizontal traction to the labial segment is achieved with a powerarm, featuring a composite resin stop to prevent coronal slippage of the traction auxiliary.

13) Percuss the adjacent teeth to gauge root proximity and take an intraoral radiograph if a problem is suspected.

7.6.4 Postinsertion

14) For initial canine retraction, apply traction directly from the mini-implant head to the canine bracket or powerarm.

15) For *en masse* labial retraction, crimp a powerarm to the archwire mesial to the canine bracket (Figure 7.3). Apply the traction at a level on the powerarm which creates a horizontal line of traction (parallel to the occlusal plane).

16) Immediately load the mini-implant with *light* traction for the first 5–6 weeks, for example with a lightly stretched powerchain. Subsequently apply normal levels of traction using a NiTi closing spring or elastomeric auxiliary.

17) If an increase in overbite is indicated then add posterior vertical traction from the mini-implant to the archwire, or to both molar and premolar attachments. This causes direct intrusion of the posterior teeth. This may require archwire contraction to avoid buccal crown flaring.

18) Discontinue the traction and consider explanting the mini-implant once the anchorage requirements have been met, for example Class I canines and incisors.

19) If a lateral openbite has developed then (after explantation) bond the upper second molars and level the arch using a flexible NiTi archwire (Figures 7.2 and 7.8). Vertical/box elastics may also be used to settle the buccal occlusion.

7.7 Biomechanical Options for Anterior Teeth Retraction

There are approximately eight different biomechanical set-ups involving mini-implant anchorage for canine and incisor teeth retraction purposes (Figures 7.10–7.17). These may involve both unilateral and bilateral bone anchorage, depending on the anchorage requirements. The different clinical scenarios are illustrated in the clinical cases shown in the remainder of this chapter and listed as follows.

1) **Indirect anchorage: midpalate anchorage of a TPA (Figure 7.10)**
   Perhaps the best option for adolescent patients with insufficient alveolar cortical maturity. However, it is limited to the maxillary arch and the use of conventional traction biomechanics.

2) *En masse* **(canine and incisor) retraction with a crimpable powerarm (Figure 7.11)**
   The most efficient option where the labial segment teeth are readily aligned prior to mini-implant insertions, in an average or deep overbite case.

3) **Incisor torque and intrusion, using a crimpable powerarm (Figure 7.12)**
   This is appropriate where the principal requirement is incisor torque, rather than substantial retraction with space closure, for example in non-extraction Class II division 2 patients.

4) **Incisor retraction and anterior openbite correction, using oblique traction (Figure 7.13)**
   This is suitable for Class II patients who primarily require retraction of anterior teeth plus correction of a reduced overbite or small anterior openbite (AOB). It utilises the vertical rotational side-effect caused by oblique traction and hence the use of powerarms is minimised.

5) **Single-tooth (canine) retraction, using a bondable powerarm (Figure 7.14)**
   This is used where initial canine retraction is required to alleviate incisor crowding. The anterior teeth may then be retracted *en masse* using the canine powerarm, or by switching to a crimpable powerarm.

6) **Canine retraction using sectional (buccal) fixed appliance (Figure 7.15)**
   An alternative approach where initial canine retraction is required to alleviate incisor crowding, and it is desirable to delay bonding of the incisor teeth (for aesthetics or pathology reasons) until space is readily available for their alignment.

7) **Single-tooth (canine) retraction in aligner cases (Figure 7.16)**
   This provides a means of maximum anchorage control during orthodontic aligner treatment and facilitates effective canine/incisor retraction.

8) **Lingual bondable powerarm and palatal alveolar anchorage (Figure 7.17)**

This is an alternative for canine/*en masse* retraction where a palatal alveolar mini-implant is preferable (rather than a buccal one).

7.8 Case Examples

1) **Indirect anchorage: midpalate anchorage of a TPA (Figure 7.10)**
   - A 13-year-old boy who presented with a Class II division 1 malocclusion on a mild skeletal II base, with bimaxillary proclination and associated bilabial protrusion (Figure 6.10a,b). He had a 9 mm overjet (OJ), a deep overbite (OB) and impacted lower second premolars, necessitating earlier extraction of the lower first premolars (Figure 7.10c–e).
   - The upper first premolars were extracted and an upper fixed appliance bonded. Exploratory insertion of a buccal alveolar mini-implant was abandoned due to the low insertion torque, so the midpalate was elected as the optimum anchorage site.
   - 1.5 mm diameter, 6 mm length, long neck Infinitas mini-implants were inserted in parasagittal sites, level with the upper premolars (Figure 7.10f). These were inclined by approximately 30° towards the anterior nasal spine and inserted with the assistance of a stent and contra-angle handpiece.
   - The working model, with mini-implant analogues, was also used to fabricate a modified Nance palatal arch. This featured two holes in the button which corresponded to the planned mini-implant head locations. Ideally, molar bands would have been used for the Nance arch, but this was not feasible due to the macrodont size of the molar teeth. Therefore, the Nance arch was bonded to the first molars, and the gaps between the mini-implant heads and the acrylic base were obturated with light-cured composite (Figure 7.10g).
   - Immediate elastomeric chain traction was applied from the molar tubes (of the indirectly anchored first molars) to the canine brackets (Figure 7.10h,i).
   - Class I canine and incisor positions were achieved after five months of traction, without the loss of anchorage (Figure 7.10j,k). The lower arch was bonded at this stage. There were residual upper arch spaces and Class III molar relationships, which provided scope for subsequent Class III traction (and hence lower incisor retroclination).
   - Residual upper arch spaces were closed with continued conventional traction after removal of the Nance palatal arch (Figure 7.10l–n). Mild palatal erythema

was present immediately after removal of the acrylic button (Figure 7.10o).
   - Debond facial and intraoral photographs showing a Class I profile and occlusion (Figure 7.10o–r).

2) ***En masse* (canine and incisor) retraction with a crimpable powerarm (Figure 7.11)**
   - An adult female presented with a Class II division 1 malocclusion on a moderate skeletal II base (Figure 7.11a–g), having declined orthognathic surgery. She had a 12 mm OJ, a deep overbite and asymmetric Class II buccal segment relationships including a full unit Class II right canine relationship. Both dental centrelines were displaced to the left side, especially the upper arch, and with absence of the upper left second premolar and lower left first molar teeth.
   - The upper right first premolar was extracted to provide space for correction of the anterior crowding, upper centreline displacement, and the right canine and incisor relationships. The upper arch was then aligned with a fixed appliance, up to insertion of a 0.019×0.025 in. steel archwire.
   - A 1.5 mm diameter, 9 mm length, short neck Infinitas mini-implant was inserted in a buccal position mesial to the upper right first molar and immediate traction was applied to powerarms (Figure 7.11h–k).
   - The mini-implant was explanted after 16 months when Class I right canine and incisor relationships had been achieved, and no anchorage loss had been incurred (Figure 7.11l–o).
   - Debond followed four months later, accepting some residual displacement of the lower dental centreline to the left side (Figure 7.11q,r).

3) **Incisor torque and intrusion, using a crimpable powerarm (Figure 7.12)**
   - An adult female presented with a Class II division 2 malocclusion on a mild skeletal II base with a low maxillomandibular planes angle (Figure 7.11a–f). She complained of 'flat' upper incisors, increased maxillary gingival display on smiling and hypodontia (absence of both lower second premolars).
   - The upper arch was aligned for seven months with fixed appliances, up to insertion of a 19×25 in. steel archwire. Small spaces opened, distal to the upper lateral incisors, during this alignment phase.
   - 1.5 mm diameter, 9 mm length, short neck Infinitas mini-implants were inserted in a buccal position mesial to the upper right first molar and immediate traction was applied to crimpable powerarms (Figure 7.12g,h).
   - The principal phase of powerarm traction was stopped after eight months to allow occlusal settling.

The mini-implants remained *in situ* for potential further traction (Figure 7.12i–k).

- The patient was debonded after 24 months of treatment, after establishment of the appropriate lower premolar spaces (Figure 7.12m–p). She was pleased with the improvements in the upper incisor level and torque, and declined crown lengthening gingival surgery.

4) **Incisor retraction and anterior openbite correction, using oblique (direct buccal) traction (Figure 7.13)**

- A 17-year-old male presented with a Class II division 1 malocclusion on a skeletal I base with increased maxillomandibular planes angle and lower anterior facial height (Figure 7.13a–e). He had a 7.5 mm OJ, a 4 mm AOB and a partial left lateral openbite. The upper incisor display was acceptable. There was severe maxillary arch crowding, with palatal exclusion of the upper right lateral incisor and severe displacement of the upper dental centreline to the right side. Conversely, the lower centreline was significantly displaced to the left side. The Class II buccal segment relationships were asymmetrical with half unit right and full unit left Class II canine relationships.
- The upper first premolars were extracted to provide space for correction of the anterior crowding, upper centreline displacement, and the canine and incisor relationships. Extraction of the lower right first premolar (for relief of crowding and centreline correction) was electively delayed until the vertical relationship had been improved.
- The upper arch, including the second molars but excluding the upper right lateral incisor, was aligned with a fixed appliance, up to insertion of a 018 in. steel archwire.
- Two 1.5 mm diameter, 9 mm length, short neck Infinitas mini-implants were inserted in a buccal position mesial to the first molars and immediate oblique elastomeric traction was applied to the canine brackets (Figure 7.13f–i). A NiTi spring was also inserted between the upper right central incisor and canine brackets.
- The upper right lateral incisor was bonded after five months of traction, and light oblique traction was continued with an initial 012 in. NiTi archwire in place (Figure 7.13k–m). At this stage, there was premature occlusal contact on the upper right central incisor and a rollercoaster effect was present, especially on the left side.
- The mini-implants were explanted after a total of 18 months when Class III incisor and canine relationships were present (Figure 7.13n–q). The upper sec-

ond premolar brackets were then rebonded to reverse the original root divergence effects.

- Superimposition of the lateral cephalograms taken at the start and end of the mini-implant phase showed upper first molar intrusion, without any AP anchorage loss, resulting in a small clockwise mandibular rotation (despite the patient's background vertical facial growth). The upper central incisors had moved palatally with extrusion yet bodily retraction, and there had been mild lower incisor proclination (Figure 7.13s).
- Active treatment was completed nine months later (Figure 7.13t–y), following lower arch space closure and limited use of elastics to close the left lateral openbite.

5) **Single-tooth (canine) retraction, using a bondable powerarm (Figure 7.14)**

- A 17-year-old male with a severe Class III malocclusion on a skeletal III base (Figure 7.14a–f) was planned for orthognathic surgery. He had severe upper arch crowding with buccal exclusion of the upper left canine and displacement of the upper centreline to the left side.
- The upper first premolars were extracted to provide space for correction of the anterior crowding, upper centreline displacement, and incisor retraction. The upper arch, excluding the lateral incisors, was then aligned with a fixed appliance, up to insertion of a 018 in. steel archwire.
- Two 1.5 mm diameter, 9 mm length, short neck Infinitas mini-implants were inserted in buccal positions mesial to the first molars. Immediate traction was applied to a powerarm bonded on the upper right canine and directly to the left canine bracket (Figure 7.14g–J).
- The upper lateral incisors were bonded, and the left mini-implant explanted nine weeks later. Standard elastomeric traction continued to the right canine powerarm, initially with a 012 in. NiTi archwire in place (Figure 7.14k–n). At this stage, there had been some distal tipping of the left canine, but not on the powerarm side.
- The patient was prepared for orthognathic surgery with the right mini-implant and powerarm still *in situ* (Figure 7.14o–t), to assist with the final centreline correction and incisor retraction postoperatively.
- The right mini-implant was explanted two months after and the patient debonded a further six months later, with final postoperative occlusal settling planned for the retention period (Figure 7.14u–x).

6) **Canine retraction using sectional (buccal) fixed appliance (Figure 7.15)**

- An adult female presented with a Class II division 1 malocclusion on a skeletal I base (Figure 7.15a–f). She had proclined upper central incisors, an increased OB and moderate upper anterior dental crowding. The canine relationship was three-quarter unit Class II bilaterally.
- Given the pre-existing tooth discolourations, it was agreed to delay bonding the upper incisors until space was available for their rapid alignment. Therefore, treatment commenced with extraction of both upper first premolar teeth (for space provision) and provision of temporary composite resin pontics bonded to the distal surfaces of the upper canine teeth.
- The upper arch was aligned with bilateral sectional fixed appliances bonded on the canine, second premolar and first molar teeth. The premolar brackets were bonded with additional mesial tip to aid root divergence and alignment progressed until insertion of 19×25 in. steel sectional archwires.
- Two 1.5mm diameter, 9mm length, short neck Infinitas mini-implants were inserted in buccal positions mesial to the first molars and immediate oblique elastomeric traction applied to the canine brackets (Figure 7.15g–j).
- The upper incisors were bonded after five months of oblique traction, yet with no discernible rotation of the dental plane (Figure 7.15k–n). The mini-implant traction was paused during the 11 weeks of rapid incisor alignment (Figure 7.15o–q).
- The mini-implants were explanted after a total of 11 months *in situ*. Class I canine positions had been established and there was scope for some loss of anchorage during final space closure (Figure 7.11r–t).
- Debond occurred after a total of 21 months treatment (Figure 7.15u–z).

7) **Single-tooth (canine) retraction in aligner cases (Figure 7.16)**
  - An adult male presented with a Class I malocclusion on a skeletal I base with a history of upper right first premolar extraction and fixed appliance treatment, He had residual upper right premolar space, distal tipping of the upper right canine and a Class II right canine relationship (Figure 7.16a–d). He required space provision for incisor alignment then replace-

ment of the central incisor crowns, but declined further fixed appliance treatment.
- A limited treatment plan was agreed, involving a series of upper arch aligners to distalise the upper right canine and reposition the anterior teeth. The canine movements would be supported by mini-implant anchorage on the right side. In effect, the aligners provided the 'road map' for tooth movements and the mini-implant traction was the engine for the canine retraction (Figure 7.16e–f).
- A prototype plastic powerarm was bonded to the right canine and the aligner edges adjusted to allow for this. This proved to be irritating to the patient's lip so it was replaced with a lower profile metal powerarm until the canine had been retracted without distal tipping or any worsening of its mild rotation (Figure 7.16g–j).
- The final incisor movements were planned after four months of treatment (Figure 7.16k,l). This involved a further series of aligners, after removal of the mini-implant and powerarm.

8) **Lingual bondable powerarm and palatal alveolar anchorage (Figure 7.17)**
  - A 16-year-old female patient presented with a Class III malocclusion on a Class III skeletal base with a small AOB due to her divergent vertical pattern (Figure 7.17a–c). She was planned for maxillary molar intrusion (using bilateral palatal alveolar mini-implants) to correct the vertical discrepancies (Figure 7.17d–f) followed by a mandibular setback osteotomy to correct the Class III problems.
  - The immediate postoperative occlusion was planned to be Class I overall, but maintaining the upper centreline shift to the right side and half unit Class II left canine relationship (Figure 7.14g–i). A powerarm was bonded to the palatal surface of the upper left canine two months after surgery and elastomeric traction applied from the ipsilateral mini-implant to close the arch space mesial to the upper left second premolar tooth.
  - The mini-implants were explanted after five months, once the left canine relationship was Class I and the upper centreline correct. The patient was then debonded one month later (Figure 7.17j–l).

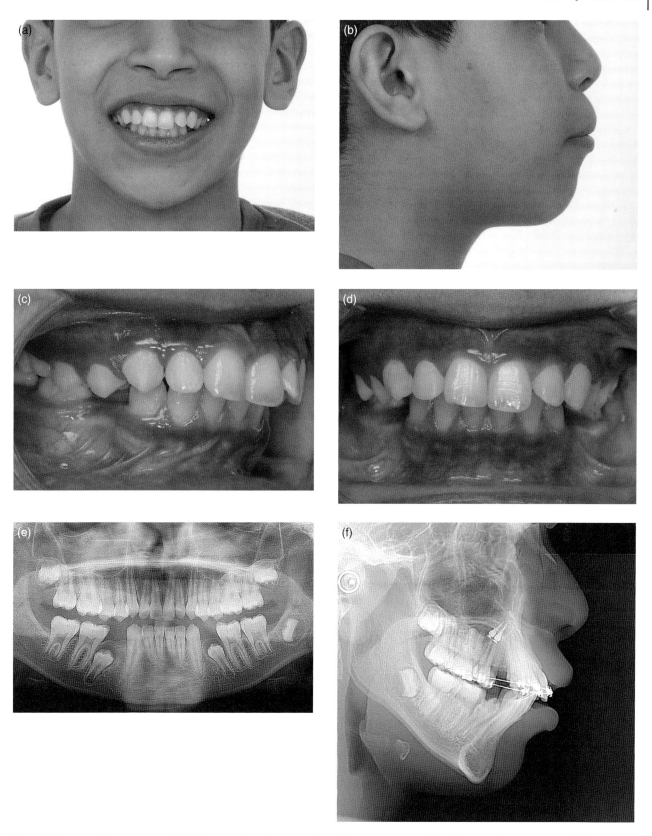

Figure 7.10 (a–e) Pretreatment. (f–i) Following insertion of palatal mini-implants, a modified Nance palatal arch and initial traction from the upper molar hooks to the canine brackets. (j,k) Labial segment retraction the canine relationships are Class I. (l–n) Continued traction following removal of the palatal arch. (o–r) Debond facial and intraoral photographs.

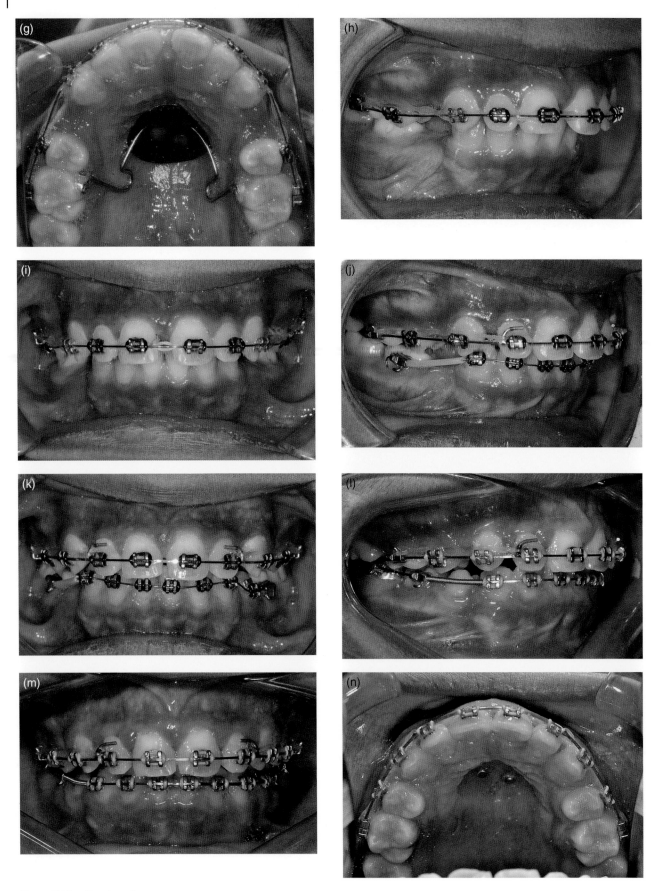

Figure 7.10 (Continued)

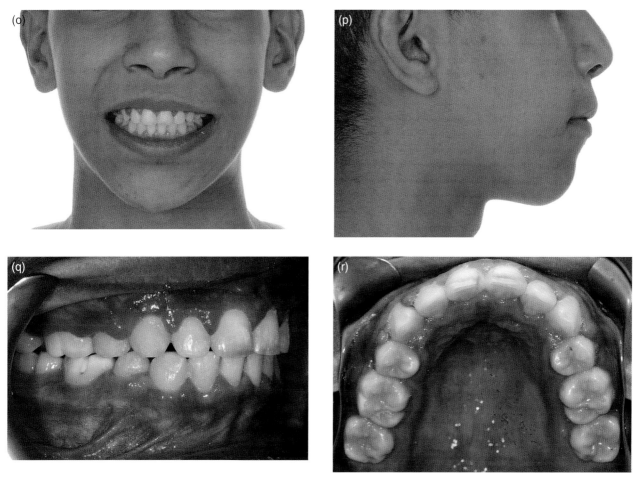

Figure 7.10 (Continued)

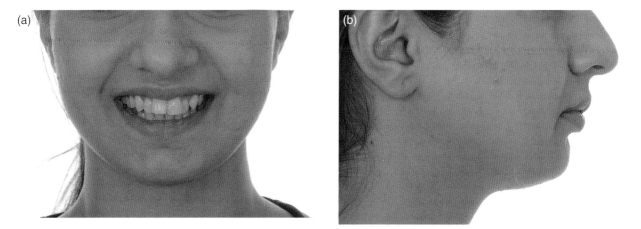

Figure 7.11 (a–g) Pretreatment views of the Class II division 1 malocclusion, with a Class II skeletal relationship and full unit Class II right canines. (h–k) Mini-implant traction to a crimpable powerarm commenced after extraction of the right maxillary first premolar and initial alignment. (l–o) Images taken immediately after *en masse* retraction of the labial segment, and at the time of the mini-implant removal. (p) Cephalometric superimposition of the cephalograms taken at the start and two months before the end of mini-implant traction (when a small anterior space was still present). (q,r) Debond views.

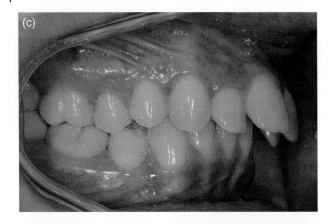

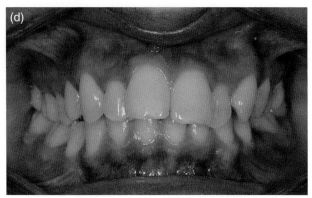

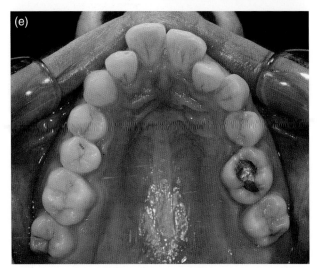

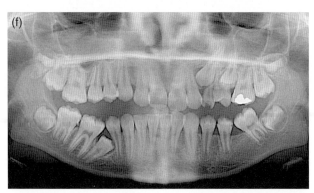

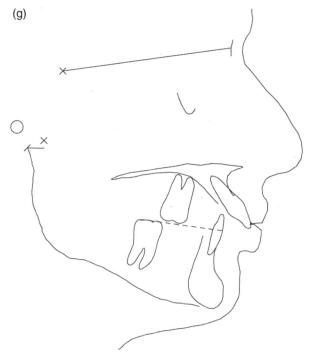

SKELETAL			SOFT TISSUES		
SNA	°	81.0	Lip Sep	mm	0.0
SNB	°	77.5	Exp UI	mm	1.5
ANB	°	3.0	LS-E	mm	-3.0
SN/MxP	°	2.5	LI-E	mm	-0.5
MxP/MnP	°	26.5	NLA	°	130.0
LAFH	mm	55.0	LLA	°	116.5
UAFH	mm	48.0	Holdaway	°	19.0
LAFH/TAFH	%	53.5			
LPFH	mm	36.0	NOSE PROMINENCE		
UPFH	mm	47.5			
PFH	mm	67.5	Nose tip	mm	24.5
Wits	mm	1.0	Nose angle	°	31.0
			CHIN PROMINENCE		
TEETH					
			Chin tip	mm	-2.5
Overjet	mm	11.5	B-NPo	mm	-4.0
Overbite	mm	4.0	LADH	mm	37.5
UI/MxP	°	122.5			
LI/MnP	°	89.0			
Iiangle	°	121.5			
LI-APo	mm	-1.5			
LI-NPo	mm	-1.5			

Figure 7.11   (Continued)

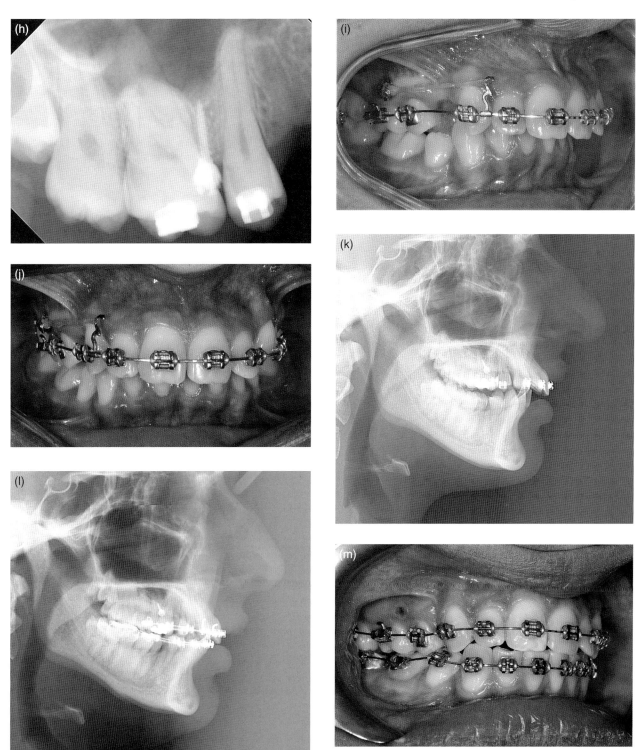

Figure 7.11 (Continued)

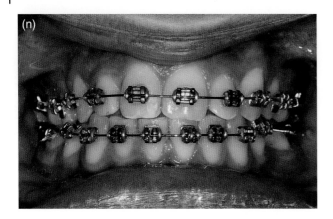

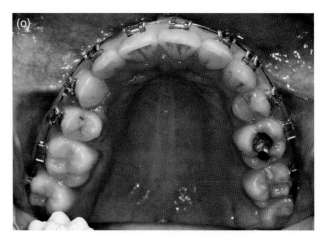

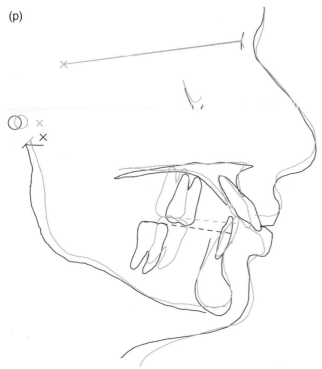

SKELETAL			SOFT TISSUES		
SNA	°	1.0	Lip Sep	mm	4.5
SNB	°	0.0	Exp UI	mm	2.5
ANB	°	0.5	LS-E	mm	-0.5
SN/MxP	°	2.0	LI-E	mm	-2.5
MxP/MnP	°	-2.5	NLA	°	19.5
LAFH	mm	-1.0	LLA	°	5.0
UAFH	mm	-1.0	Holdaway	°	-3.0
LAFH/TAFH	%	0.0			
LPFH	mm	1.0	NOSE PROMINENCE		
UPFH	mm	-2.0			
PFH	mm	0.5	Nose tip	mm	-1.0
Wits	mm	2.5	Nose angle	°	4.5

TEETH			CHIN PROMINENCE		
Overjet	mm	-7.0	Chin tip	mm	1.0
Overbite	mm	-0.5	B-NPo	mm	0.5
UI/MxP	°	-4.0	LADH	mm	-3.0
LI/MnP	°	10.0			
IIangle	°	-3.0			
LI-APo	mm	2.5			
LI-NPo	mm	3.0			

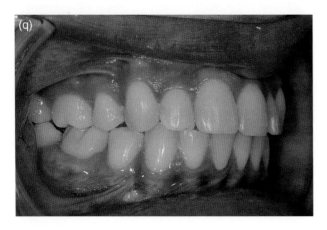

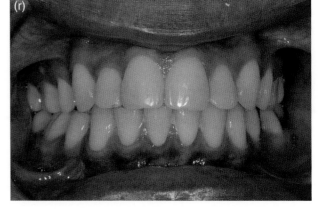

Figure 7.11   (Continued)

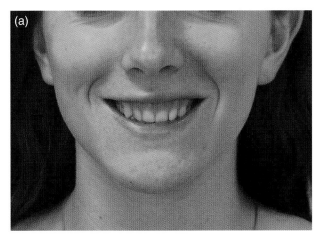

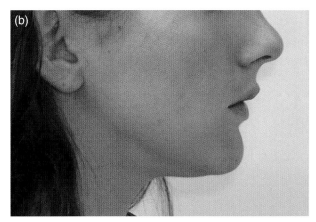

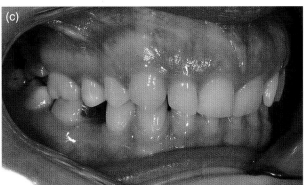

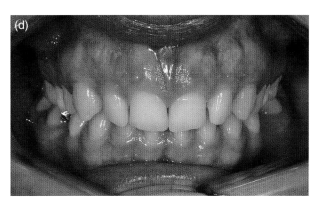

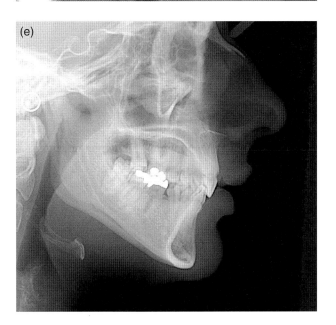

Figure 7.12 (a–d) Pretreatment views showing the Class II division 2 malocclusion, mild Class II skeletal base, asymmetrically increased incisor display, and lower edentulous site. (e,f) The cephalogram and measurements confirm the clinical findings and the severe upper incisor retroclination. (g,h) The start of traction from maxillary buccal mini-implants to crimpable powerarms. (i,j) End of the main traction phase. The mini-implants remained *in situ* whilst the upper second premolar brackets were repositioned (to reverse the original root divergent tip alteration. (k,l) A cephalogram taken at the end of the traction phase and superimposition of its measurements on the original one. These show that the upper central incisor root had moved palatally and superiorly, with a 19° increase in the incisor inclination, and significant reductions in both the overbite and upper incisor exposure. (m–p) Debond facial and intraoral views showing the OB reduction as a result of upper incisor intrusion.

(f)

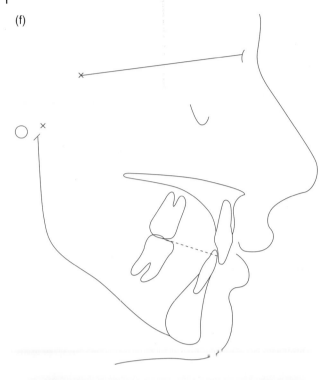

SKELETAL			SOFT TISSUES		
SNA	°	79.5	Lip Sep	mm	1.0
SNB	°	73.5	Exp UI	mm	5.0
ANB	°	6.0	LS-E	mm	−3 .0
SN/MxP	°	15.0	LI-E	mm	−3 .5
MxP/MnP	°	27.0	NLA	°	123.5
LAFH	mm	64.5	LLA	°	112.0
UAFH	mm	55.5	Holdaway	°	18.5
LAFH/TAFH	%	53.5			
LPFH	mm	41.0	NOSE PROMINENCE		
UPFH	mm	44.5	Nose tip	mm	28.0
PFH	mm	69.0	Nose angle	°	31.0
Wits	mm	1.5			
			CHIN PROMINENCE		
TEETH			Chin tip	mm	−11.5
Overjet	mm	3.0	B-NPo	mm	−0.5
Overbite	mm	5.0	LADH	mm	38.5
UI/MxP	°	92.0			
LI/MnP	°	84.0			
IIangle	°	157.0			
LI-APo	mm	−2.0			
LI-NPo	mm	2.0			

(g)

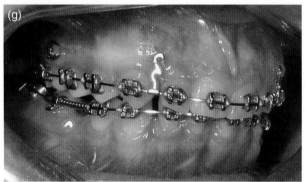

(h)

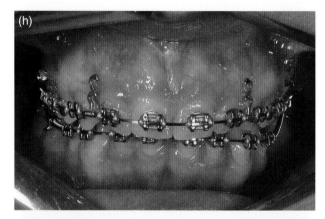

(i)

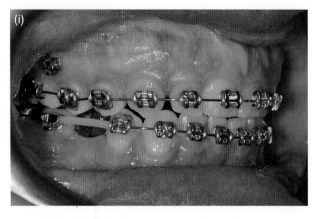

(j)

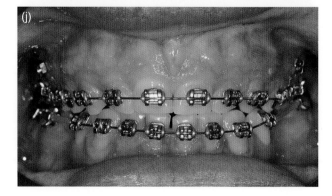

Figure 7.12 (Continued)

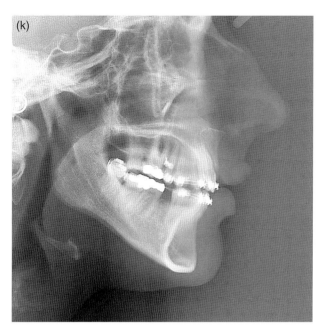

(k)

(l)

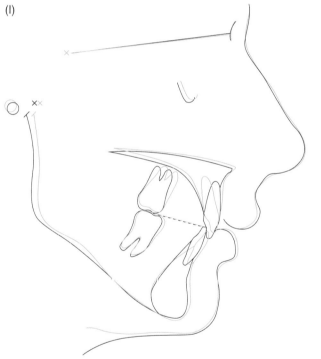

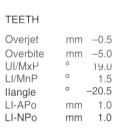

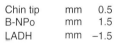

SKELETAL			SOFT TISSUES		
SNA	°	2.0	Lip Sep	mm	−0.0
SNB	°	1.5	Exp UI	mm	−2.5
ANB	°	1.0	LS-E	mm	−1.5
SN/MxP	°	1.5	LI-E	mm	1.5
MxP/MnP	°	−0.0	NLA	°	−7.0
LAFH	mm	1.5	LLA	°	−3.5
UAFH	mm	−1.0	Holdaway	°	0.0
LAFH/TAFH	%	1.0			
LPFH	mm	0.5	NOSE PROMINENCE		
UPFH	mm	−1.5			
PFH	mm	−0.0	Nose tip	mm	0.5
Wits	mm	−1.0	Nose angle	°	−1.5

TEETH			CHIN PROMINENCE		
			Chin tip	mm	0.5
Overjet	mm	−0.5	B-NPo	mm	1.5
Overbite	mm	−5.0	LADH	mm	−1.5
UI/MxP	°	19.0			
LI/MnP	°	1.5			
IIangle	°	−20.5			
LI-APo	mm	1.0			
LI-NPo	mm	1.0			

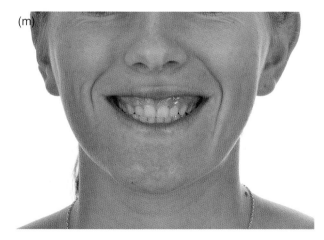

(m)

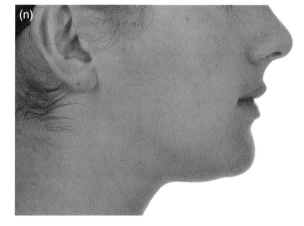

(n)

Figure 7.12 (Continued)

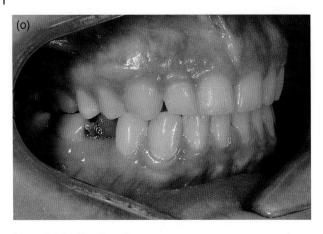

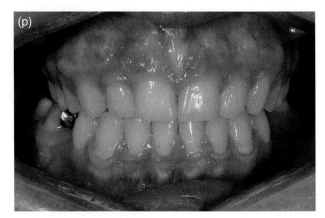

Figure 7.12 (Continued)

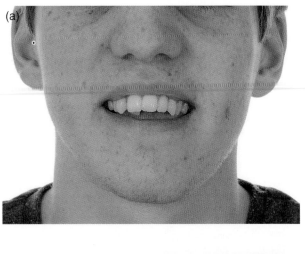

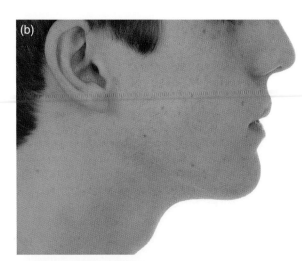

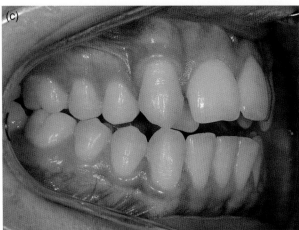

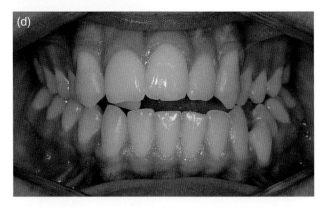

Figure 7.13 (a–e) Pretreatment photographs showing the Class II division 1 malocclusion, Class I skeletal base, increased lower anterior face height, acceptable upper incisor display, and severe maxillary crowding. (f–h) Photographs taken when oblique traction was applied from maxillary buccal mini-implants to the canine brackets. The overjet and AOB were 4 and 3 mm respectively at this stage. (i,j) Lateral cephalogram and measurements showing the key AP and vertical features at the start of the traction phase: skeletal I with a high mandibular plane angle, increased lower anterior face height, bimaxillary retroclination and an AOB. (k–m) Photographs taken when space had been opened for the upper right lateral incisor to be bonded. (n–p) Photographs taken on removal of the mini-implants, at the end of the traction phase. (q–s) A cephalogram taken at the end of the traction phase and superimposition of traction phase changes (prior to retraction of the lower incisors). These show that the upper first molars have been intruded with an associated modest reduction in the mandibular angle. The incisors have proclined a small amount with predominant bodily retraction of the upper incisors and some extrusion. (t–x) Debond facial and intraoral views.

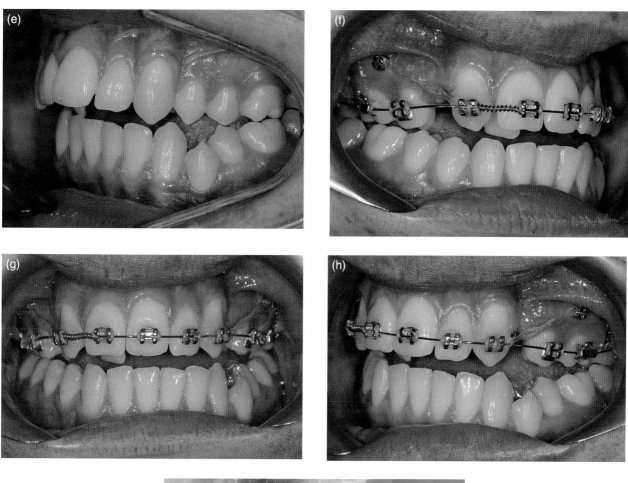

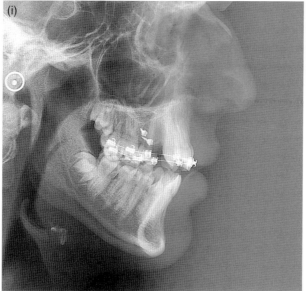

Figure 7.13 (Continued)

(j)

NAME | SEX | DOB | X-RAY DATE
LAW Samuel | | | 2015-06-19

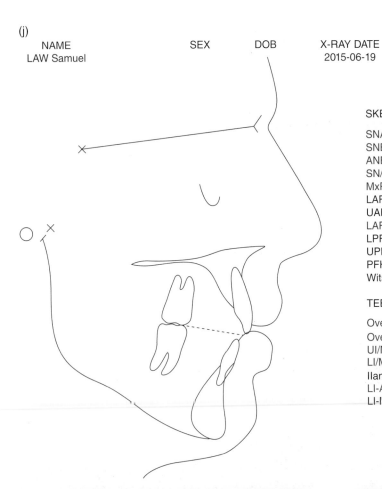

SKELETAL			SOFT TISSUES		
SNA	°	79.0	Lip Sep	mm	2.0
SNB	°	76.0	Exp UI	mm	3.0
ANB	°	3.0	LS-E	mm	−4.0
SN/MxP	°	−0.0	LI-E	mm	−1.5
MxP/MnP	°	35.0	NLA	°	132.5
LAFH	mm	71.5	LLA	°	130.0
UAFH	mm	47.5	Holdaway	°	12.5
LAFH/TAFH	%	60.5			
LPFH	mm	45.0	NOSE PROMINENCE		
UPFH	mm	49.0			
PFH	mm	80.0	Nose tip	mm	21.0
Wits	mm	2.5	Nose angle	°	29.0

TEETH			CHIN PROMINENCE		
			Chin tip	mm	−5.0
Overjet	mm	3.5	B-NPo	mm	−2.5
Overbite	mm	−2.5	LADH	mm	38.5
UI/MxP	°	94.0			
LI/MnP	°	88.0			
IIangle	°	142.0			
LI-APo	mm	1.0			
LI-NPo	mm	2.0			

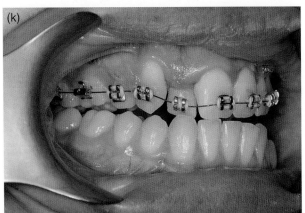

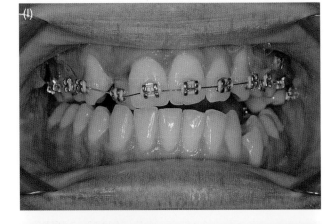

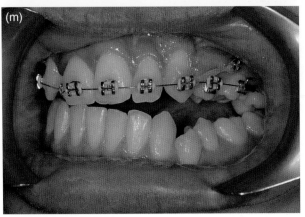

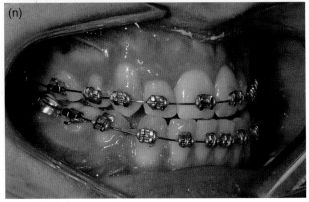

Figure 7.13 (Continued)

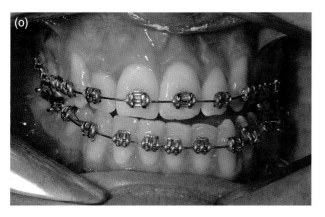

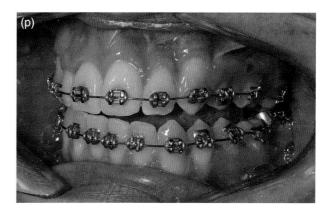

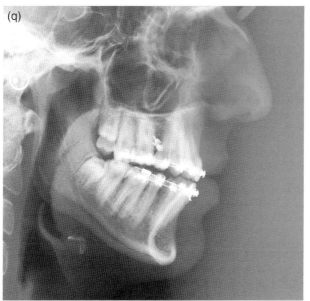

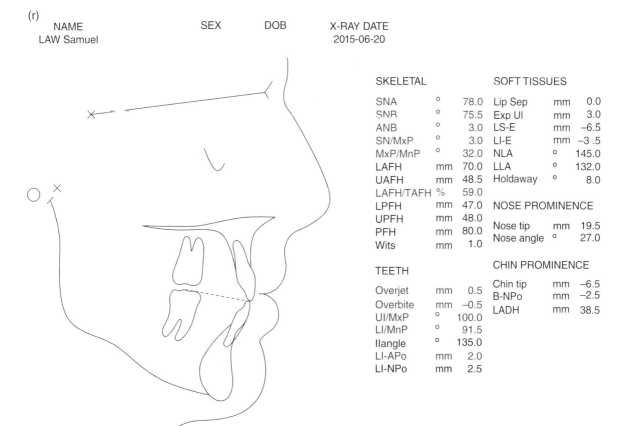

NAME
LAW Samuel

SEX

DOB

X-RAY DATE
2015-06-20

SKELETAL			SOFT TISSUES		
SNA	°	78.0	Lip Sep	mm	0.0
SNB	°	75.5	Exp UI	mm	3.0
ANB	°	3.0	LS-E	mm	−6.5
SN/MxP	°	3.0	LI-E	mm	−3.5
MxP/MnP	°	32.0	NLA	°	145.0
LAFH	mm	70.0	LLA	°	132.0
UAFH	mm	48.5	Holdaway	°	8.0
LAFH/TAFH	%	59.0			
LPFH	mm	47.0	NOSE PROMINENCE		
UPFH	mm	48.0			
PFH	mm	80.0	Nose tip	mm	19.5
Wits	mm	1.0	Nose angle	°	27.0

TEETH			CHIN PROMINENCE		
Overjet	mm	0.5	Chin tip	mm	−6.5
Overbite	mm	−0.5	B-NPo	mm	−2.5
UI/MxP	°	100.0	LADH	mm	38.5
LI/MnP	°	91.5			
IIangle	°	135.0			
LI-APo	mm	2.0			
LI-NPo	mm	2.5			

Figure 7.13 (Continued)

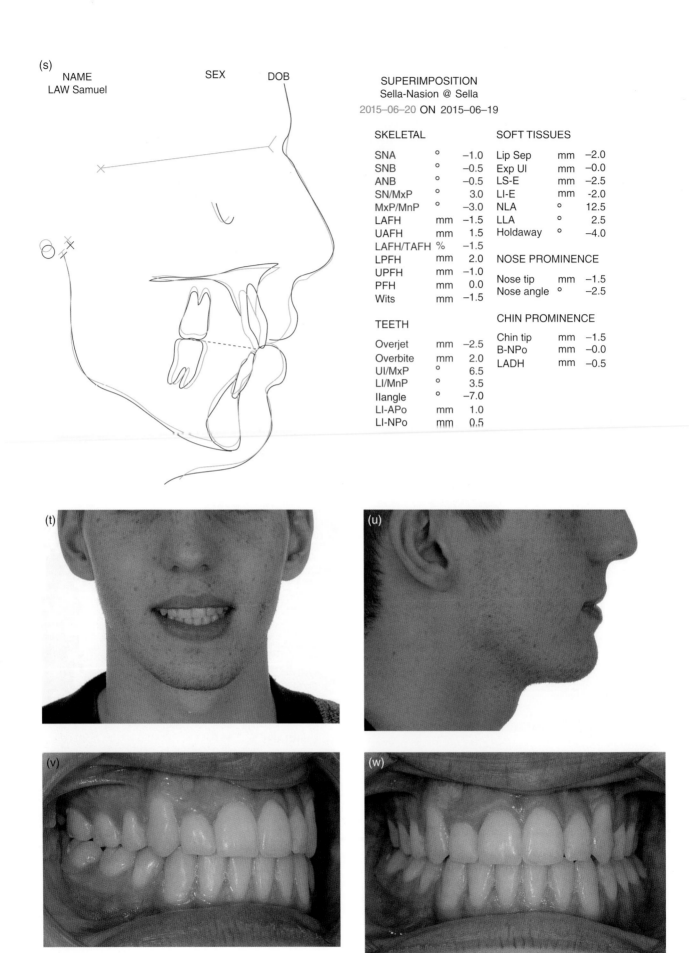

(s)

NAME
LAW Samuel

SEX

DOB

SUPERIMPOSITION
Sella-Nasion @ Sella
2015–06–20 ON 2015–06–19

SKELETAL			SOFT TISSUES		
SNA	°	−1.0	Lip Sep	mm	−2.0
SNB	°	−0.5	Exp UI	mm	−0.0
ANB	°	−0.5	LS-E	mm	−2.5
SN/MxP	°	3.0	LI-E	mm	−2.0
MxP/MnP	°	−3.0	NLA	°	12.5
LAFH	mm	−1.5	LLA	°	2.5
UAFH	mm	1.5	Holdaway	°	−4.0
LAFH/TAFH	%	−1.5			
LPFH	mm	2.0	NOSE PROMINENCE		
UPFH	mm	−1.0			
PFH	mm	0.0	Nose tip	mm	−1.5
Wits	mm	−1.5	Nose angle	°	−2.5

TEETH			CHIN PROMINENCE		
Overjet	mm	−2.5	Chin tip	mm	−1.5
Overbite	mm	2.0	B-NPo	mm	−0.0
UI/MxP	°	6.5	LADH	mm	−0.5
LI/MnP	°	3.5			
IIangle	°	−7.0			
LI-APo	mm	1.0			
LI-NPo	mm	0.5			

Figure 7.13 (Continued)

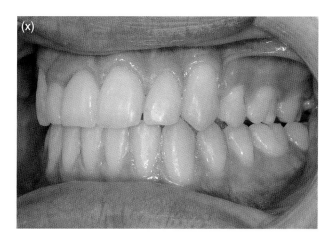

Figure 7.13 (Continued)

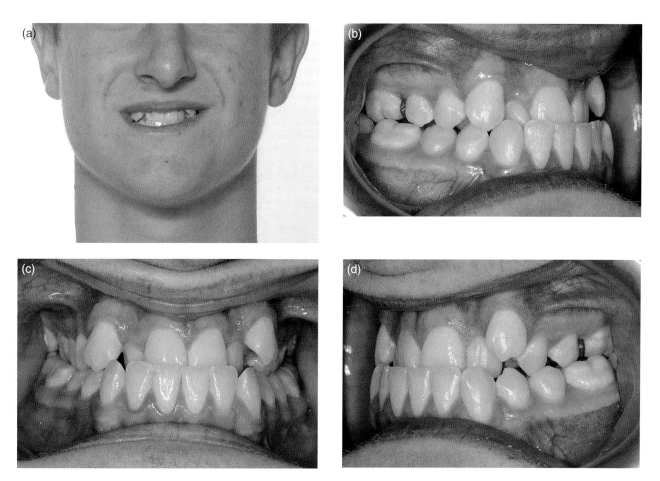

Figure 7.14 (a–e) Pretreatment photographs showing the Class III malocclusion and skeletal pattern, the severe maxillary arch crowding, and the upper centreline shift towards the left side. (f) The pretreatment lateral cephalometric measurements confirm the clinical findings. (g–j) Photographs taken on insertion of the maxillary buccal mini-implants and commencement of horizontal and oblique canine traction on the right and left sides respectively. (k–n) Photographs taken when the upper lateral incisors were bonded, a 012 in. NiTi archwire inserted and the left mini-implant explanted. (o–s) Preoperative photographs showing the passive elastomeric auxiliary connecting the mini-implant and powerarm, and the residual upper right premolar space and centreline discrepancy. (t) The preoperative cephalogram showing the skeletal discrepancy and the maintained upper incisor torque. (u–x) Debond facial and intraoral views showing the upper centreline correction and the need for longer term settling of the buccal occlusion and small space distal to the upper right lateral incisor.

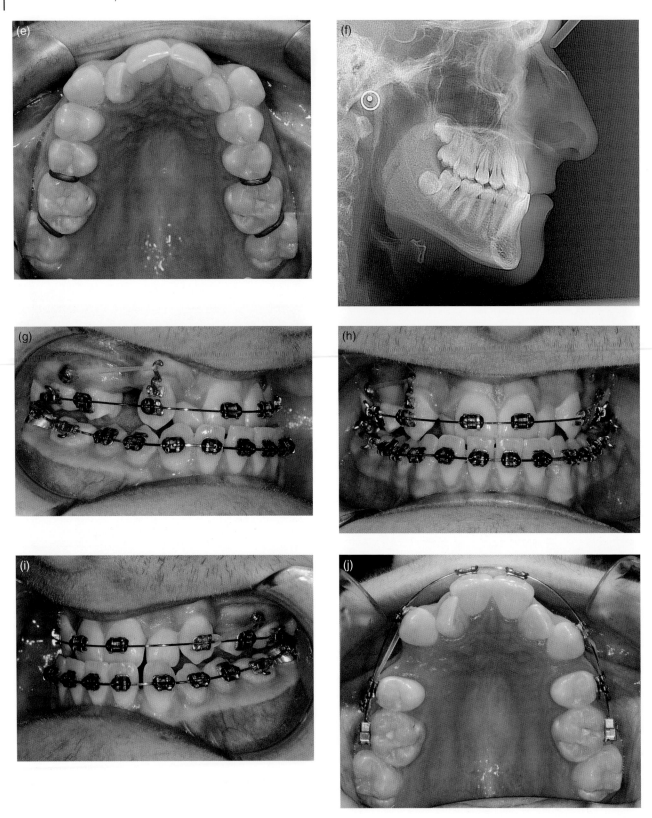

Figure 7.14 (Continued)

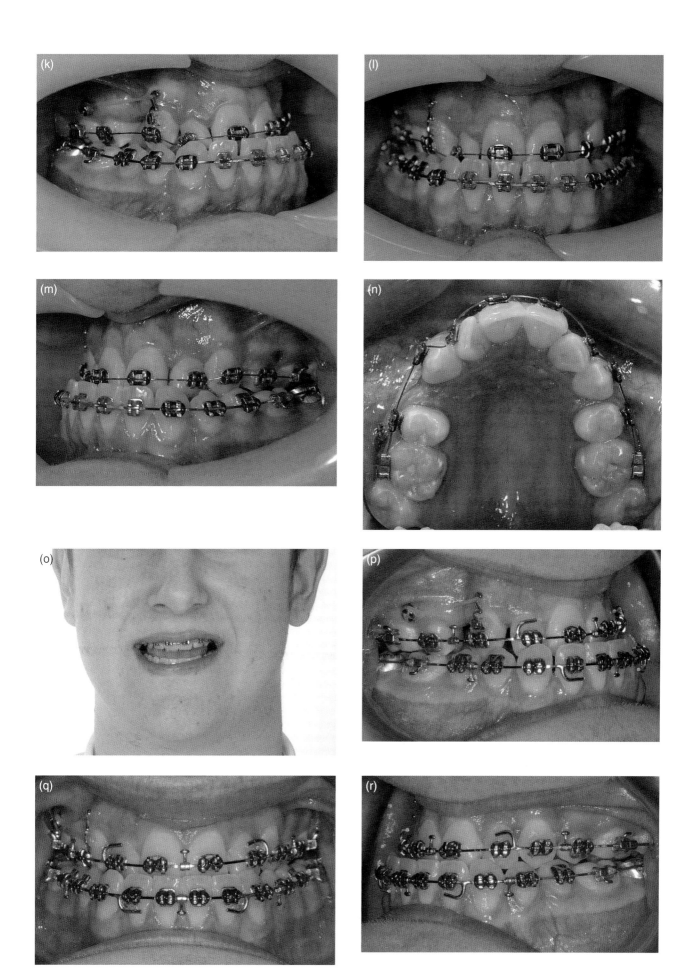

Figure 7.14 (Continued)

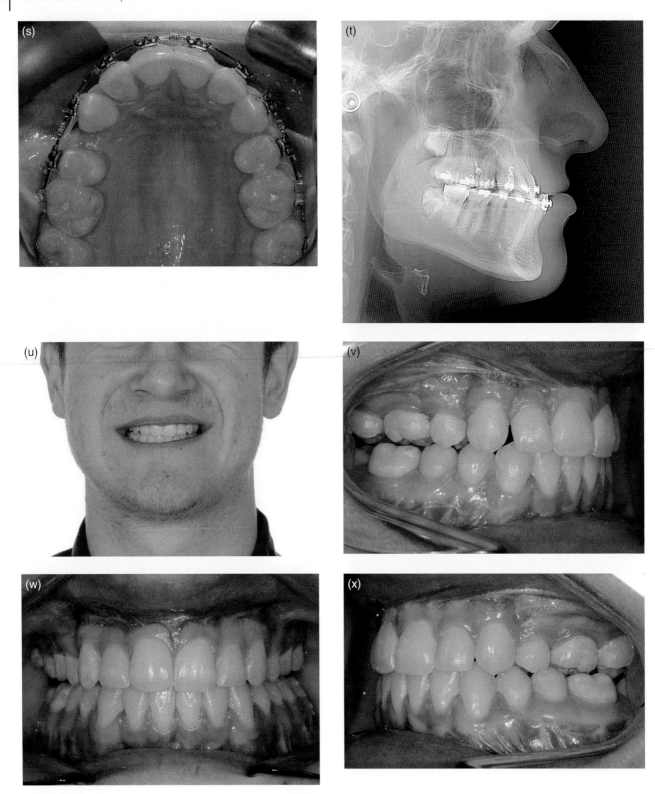

Figure 7.14 (Continued)

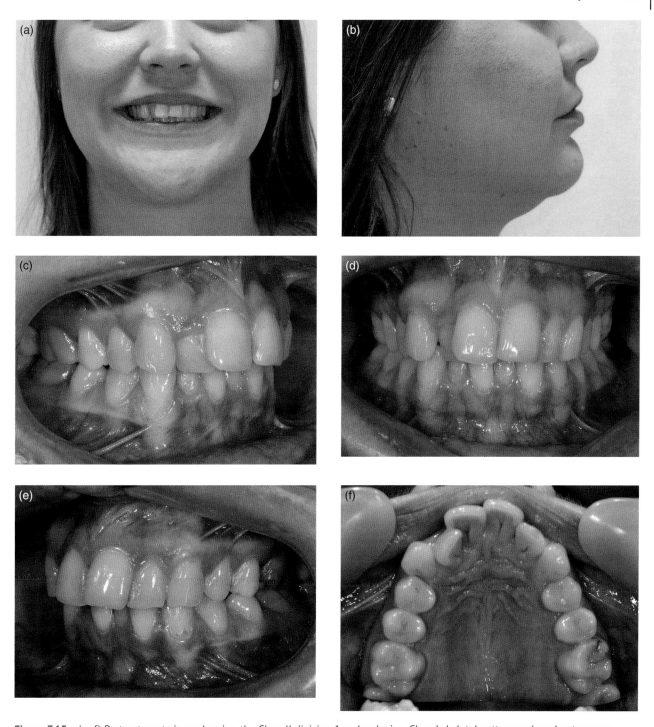

Figure 7.15 (a–f) Pretreatment views showing the Class II division 1 malocclusion, Class I skeletal pattern and moderate upper anterior crowding. (g–j) Photographs taken at the time of mini-implant insertion and placement of elastomeric traction to the upper canine brackets. (k–n) The mini-implants traction was paused at the time when the upper incisors were bonded. The multiple upper anterior spaces are evident and the residual extraction spaces camouflaged by the composite pontics. (o–q) The incisors were aligned sufficiently for insertion of a 19 × 25 in. NiTi archwire after 11 weeks. (r–t) Photographs taken after removal of the mini-implants, and when residual spaces were due to be closed with planned anchorage loss. (u–z) Debond facial and intraoral views, taken 21 months after the sectional appliances were bonded.

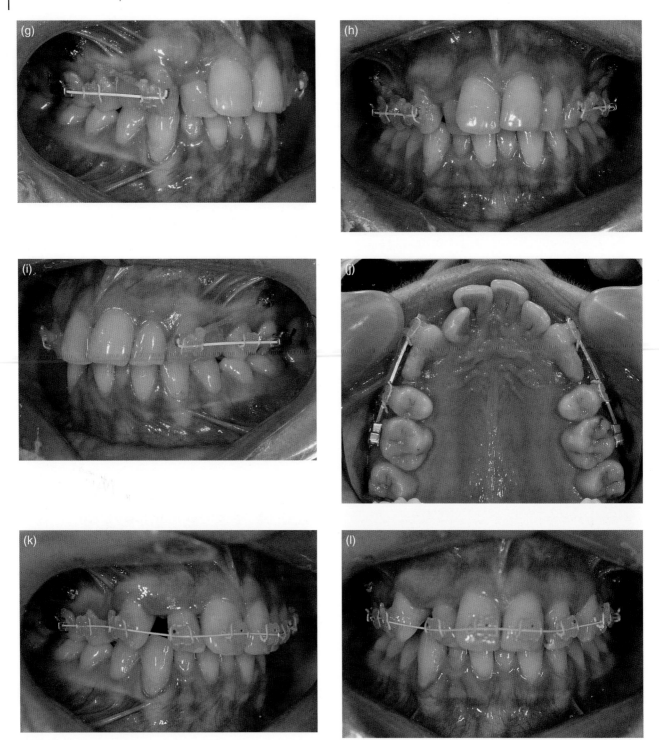

Figure 7.15 (Continued)

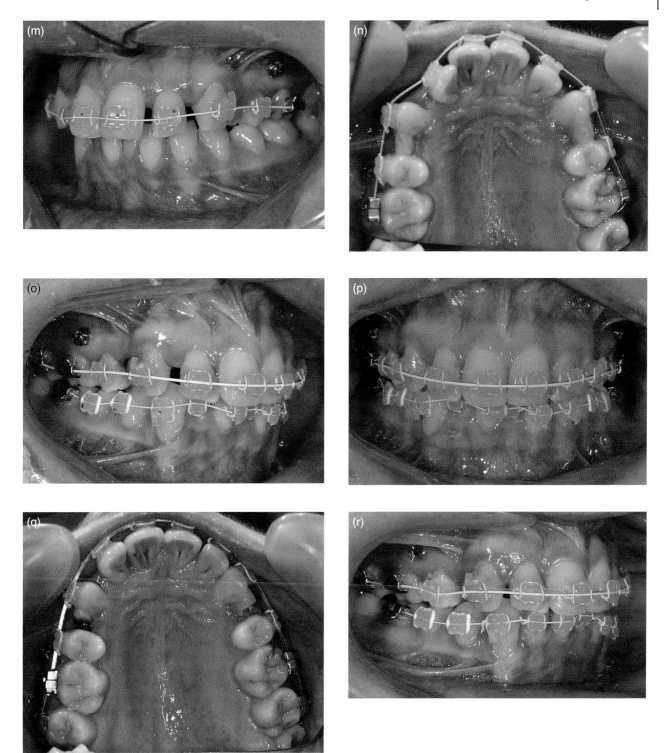

Figure 7.15 (Continued)

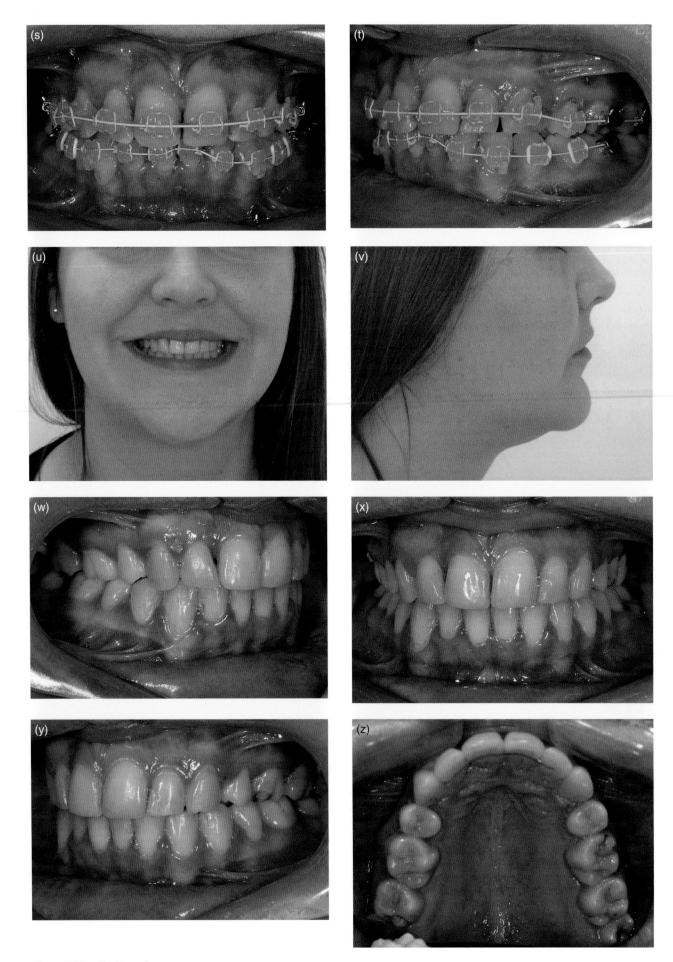

Figure 7.15 (Continued)

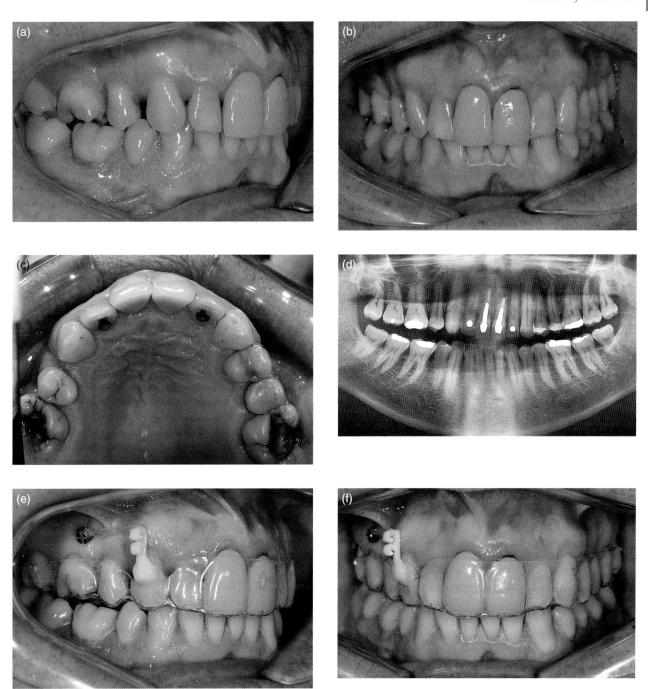

Figure 7.16 (a–c) Pretreatment photographs showing the Class I malocclusion, increased OB, Class II right canine position and residual upper right premolar space. (d) The panoramic radiograph shows absence of the upper right first premolar and mild distal angulation of the adjacent canine tooth. (e,f) Treatment starts with fitting of the first aligner and insertion of the buccal mini-implant, mesial to the right first molar. Elastomeric traction was applied to a plastic powerarm on the upper right canine. (g–j) Photographs showing the end of the traction phase, with (g,h) and without (i,j) the final aligner from the original planning phase *in situ*. (k,l) In the final aligner software planning process, the distalised upper right canine has the same small amount of distopalatal rotation as its pretreatment position (k). The canine distalisation enables planning of the final incisor alignment (l).

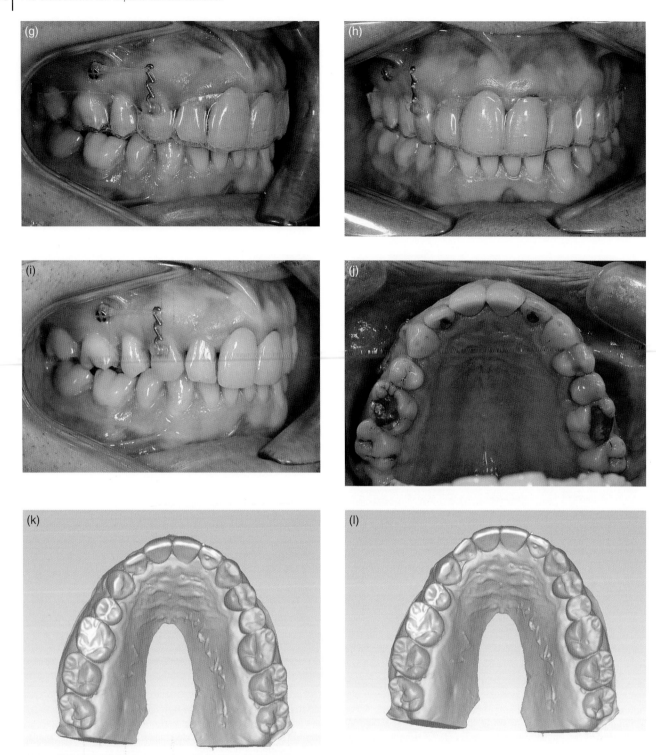

Figure 7.16 (Continued)

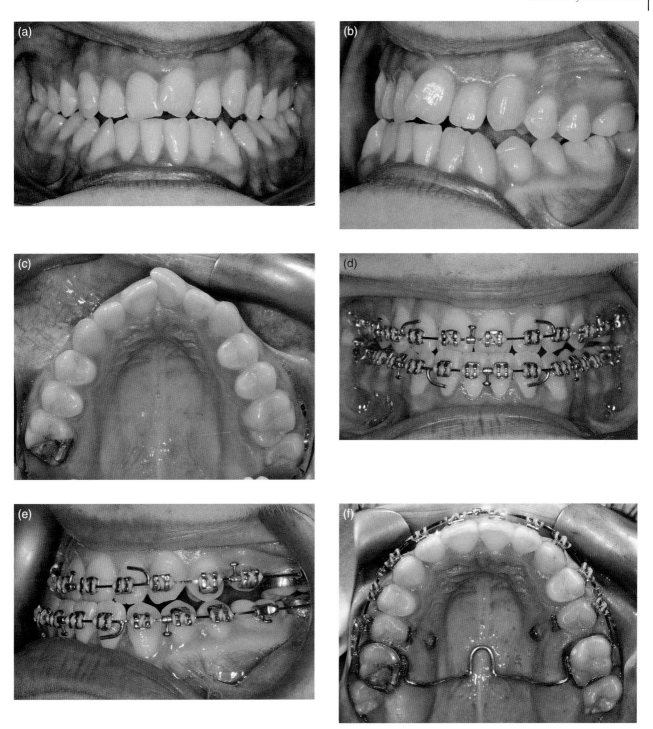

Figure 7.17 (a–c) Pretreatment intraoral photographs showing the Class III malocclusion, AOB, and upper centreline shift towards the right side. (d–f) The presurgical photographs show the improvements in alignment and overbite, but worsening of the Class III incisors and centreline mismatch. There is also space mesial to the distally tipped upper left second premolar crown. (g–i) Photographs taken after bonding of the metal powerarm on the palatal surface of the upper left canine crown and application of elastomeric traction from the ipsilateral palatal alveolar mini-implant. (j–l) Debond intraoral views showing the coincident centrelines and Class I canine relationship.

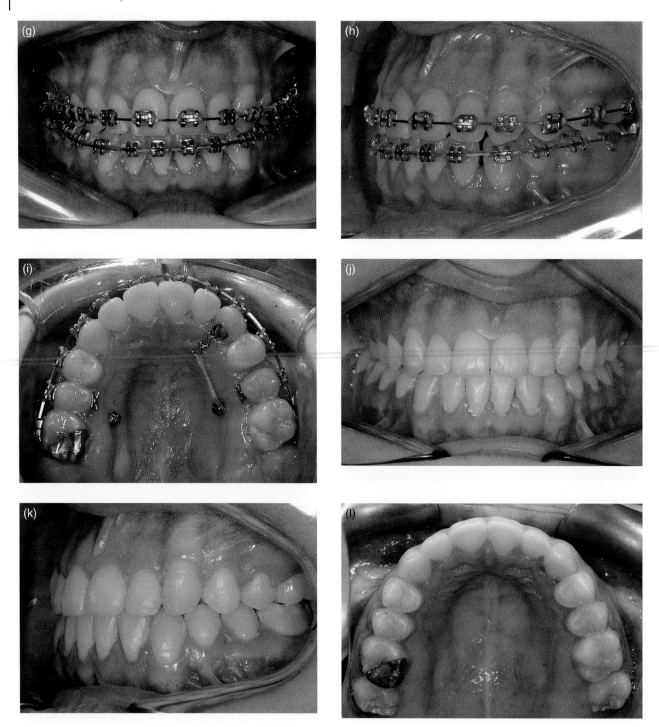

Figure 7.17 (Continued)

References

1 Koyama, I., Lino, S., Abe, Y. et al. (2011). Differences between sliding mechanics with implant anchorage and straight-pull headgear and intermaxillary elastics in adults with Bimaxillary protrusion. *Eur. J. Orthod.* 33: 126–131.

2 Kuroda, S., Yamada, K., Deguchi, T. et al. (2009). Class II malocclusion treated with miniscrew anchorage: comparison with traditional orthodontic mechanics outcomes. *Am. J. Orthod. Dentofac. Orthop.* 135: 302–309.

3 Lai, E.H., Yao, C.J., Chang, J.Z. et al. (2008). Three-dimensional dental model analysis of treatment outcomes for protrusive maxillary dentition: comparison of headgear, miniscrew, and miniplate skeletal anchorage. *Am. J. Orthod. Dentofac. Orthop.* 134: 636–645.

4 Lee, K., Park, Y., Hwang, C. et al. (2011). Displacement pattern of the maxillary arch depending on miniscrew position in sliding mechanics. *Am. J. Orthod. Dentofac. Orthop.* 140: 224–232.

5 Li, F., Hu, H.K., Chen, J.W. et al. (2011). Comparison of anchorage capacity between implant and headgear during anterior segment retraction. A systematic review. *Angle Orthod.* 81: 915–922.

6 Upadhyay, M., Yadav, S., Nagaraj, K., and Patil, S. (2008). Treatment effects of mini-implants for en-masse retraction of anterior teeth in bialveolar dental protrusion patients: a randomized controlled trial. *Am. J. Orthod. Dentofac. Orthop.* 134: 18–29.

7 Upadhyay, M., Yadav, S., Nagaraj, K., and Nanda, R. (2008). Dentoskeletal and soft tissue effects of mini-implants in class II division 1 patients. *Angle Orthod.* 79: 240–247.

8 Yao, C.J., Lai, E.H., Chang, J.Z. et al. (2008). Comparison of treatment outcomes between skeletal anchorage and extraoral anchorage in adults with maxillary dentoalveolar protrusion. *Am. J. Orthod. Dentofac. Orthop.* 134: 615–624.

9 Davoody, A.R., Posada, L., Utreja, A. et al. (2012). A prospective comparative study between differential moments and miniscrews in anchorage control. *Eur. J. Orthod.* 35: 568–576.

10 Upadhyay, M., Yadav, S., and Nanda, R. (2014). Biomechanics of incisor retraction with mini-implant anchorage. *J. Orthod.* 41: S15–S23.

11 Sibaie, S. and Hajeer, M.Y. (2014). Assessment of changes following en-masse retraction with mini-implants anchorage compared to two-step retraction with conventional anchorage in patients with class II division 1 malocclusion: a randomized controlled trial. *Eur. J. Orthod.* 36: 275–283.

12 Chen, M., Li, Z., Liu, X. et al. (2015). Differences of treatment outcomes between self-ligating brackets with microimplant and headgear anchorages in adults with bimaxillary protrusion. *Am. J. Orthod. Orthop.* 147: 465–471.

13 Sung, S.J., Jang, G.W., Chun, Y.S., and Moon, Y.S. (2010). Effective en-masse retraction design with orthodontic mini-implant anchorage: a finite element analysis. *Am. J. Orthod. Dentofac. Orthop.* 137: 648–657.

14 Ammar, H.H., Ngan, P., Crout, R.J. et al. (2011). Three-dimensional modelling and finite element analysis in treatment planning for orthodontic tooth movement. *Am. J. Orthod. Dentofac. Orthop.* 139: e59–e71.

15 Kojima, Y., Kawamura, J., and Fukui, H. (2012). Finite element analysis of the effect of force directions on tooth movement in extraction space closure with miniscrew sliding mechanics. *Am. J. Orthod. Dentofac. Orthop.* 142: 501–508.

16 RRJ, C. (2015). Controlled canine retraction using orthodontic mini-implants coupled with bondable powerarms. *J. Orthod.* 42: 315–323.

17 Chung, C.J., Choi, Y.J., and Kim, K. (2015). Approximation and contact of the maxillary central incisor roots with the incisive canal after maximum retraction with temporary anchorage devices: report of 2 patients. *Am. J. Orthod. Dentofac. Orthop.* 148: 493–502.

18 Pan, Y. and Chen, S. (2019). Contact of the incisive canal and upper central incisors causing root resorption after retraction with orthodontic mini-implants: a CBCT study. *Angle Orthod.* 89: 200–205.

8

Molar Distalisation

8.1 Alternatives to Mini-Implant Distalisation

Molar distalisation is an appropriate option in both the maxillary and mandibular arches to assist with Class II and Class III corrections, respectively. Contrary to advertising claims, all types of 'non-compliance' distalisation appliances lose anchorage, unless they are bone anchored [1].

What is more uncertain is when distalisation is the most appropriate treatment option. There appears to be wide geographic and individual variation amongst orthodontists in terms of the need for molar distalisation. The latter depends on the caseload in each clinic. For example, for many years, most of my clinical work has involved the treatment of severe malocclusions requiring either growth modification or orthognathic surgery, and not many 'simple' distalisation cases have crossed my threshold. For those who favour the logic of Class II orthopaedic correction by aiming to address the mandibular deficiency (rather than distalise maxillary molars) then mini-implants may be used to anchor either removable or fixed versions of orthopaedic appliance such as Twin Blocks (Figure 8.1) and Herbst/Forsus appliances, respectively [2–4]. The evidence to date indicates that this mandibular anchorage reduces the side-effects of the orthopaedic appliance, such as lower incisor proclination, and hence may increase the relative proportion of overjet reduction due to skeletal change. However, in the case of fixed-functional appliances this may still be limited by the maxillary arch headgear effect. Therefore, at present I think that this approach is mainly valid in patients who are past their pubertal growth peak and/or those with severe Class II malocclusions. In contrast, many of my patients have high-arched palates, which makes access to the hard palate difficult for palatal distaliser applications.

In terms of dentally focused camouflage treatments, there appears to be a 'cultural' shift in some countries such as the USA and Germany towards non-extraction Class II corrections involving molar distalisation, and in the Far East for Class III corrections. In the Class III scenarios, this typically involves mandibular prognathism cases (rather than predominantly maxillary hypoplastic ones), which is much more prevalent in this region of the world. However, it is worth considering the 'small print' when one sees or reads about the potential benefits of molar distalisation in many cases, since this tends to gloss over the need for second and/or third molar extractions, which in my mind renders the notion of *non-extraction* treatment void in such cases. When all the permanent teeth are present then the alternative of premolar extractions should not be overlooked as part of the informed consent process, since this often involves less morbidity.

Whilst *buccal* mini-implants are relatively easy to insert, their interproximal position, in close proximity to the buccal roots of adjacent molar teeth, limits the amount of nearby tooth movement which may occur. Consequently, buccal anchorage approaches provide only limited scope for molar distalisation and typically require a two-phase distalisation process: firstly for molar movement and secondly for retraction of the premolar and anterior teeth. Furthermore, the mini-implant anchorage needs to be relocated between these two phases, risking anchorage loss during this switch-over process. Fortunately, the availability of the hard palate for bone anchorage substantially increases the options for upper molar distalisation. Therefore, the choice of mini-implant site depends on the planned amount of maxillary molar movement and on whether the midpalate area is easily accessible (which may not be the case in high-arched palate cases). For example, up to half a unit of distalisation may readily be achieved using direct traction from mini-implants sited in the *palatal* alveolus. A greater range of distalisation and better bodily control of the molar movements are both achieved through indirect midpalatal anchorage of a customised distaliser appliance. Crucially, this differs from the use of 'non-compliance' distalisers since the incorporation of mini-implants avoids anchorage loss during both the

The Orthodontic Mini-Implant Clinical Handbook, Second Edition. Richard Cousley.
© 2020 John Wiley & Sons Ltd. Published 2020 by John Wiley & Sons Ltd.

distalisation and subsequent retraction phases, in the form of mesial movement/proclination of the anterior teeth and then molar anchorage loss [5,6]. The improved bodily control provided by a palatal distaliser occurs when the distalising force is applied at the level of the molar root furcation, rather than at the crown level [5,7,8]. This is readily achieved since the appliance sits at a relatively apical level in order to attach to the mini-implants and also for patient comfort.

Are patient age and stage of dental development relevant in distalisation cases? This question was addressed in a retrospective cephalometric study by Nienkemper et al. [8]. The sample of 51 patients was subdivided according to age and whether the upper second molars had erupted. It appears that these two variables did not affect the effectiveness of distalisation provided that higher forces (e.g. 500 g rather than 250 g per side) were used when the second molars were present intraorally and in adults.

> The improved bodily control provided by a palatal distaliser occurs when the distalising force is applied at the level of the molar root furcation, rather than at the crown level.

The options for distalisation of mandibular molars are limited to using anchorage sites in either the posterior alveolus (e.g. interproximally, just mesial to the first molar), the retromolar area, or the buccal shelf. However, the retromolar site may be complicated by the presence of the third molar, difficult physical access and a lack of attached gingiva (i.e. a shallow buccal sulcus). Therefore, the buccal shelf, as popularised by the Taiwanese orthodontist Dr Chris Chang, appears to offer the best anchorage site for any meaningful amount of lower molar distalisation [9]. This is because the mini-implant body can be inserted completely buccal to the molar roots (Figure 8.2). Dr Chang's recommended protocol describes that buccal shelf mini-implants should be inserted close to the mucogingival junction (MGJ) (with the sulcus tissues stretched), in a relatively vertical direction (perpendicular to the occlusal plane), leaving 5 mm of the screw head clear of the soft tissue surface [9]. He does not recommend predrilling in Far Eastern patients and probably because he uses relatively large-diameter stainless steel screws.

However, there appear to be anatomical differences between Caucasian and Far Eastern racial types. As such, the area immediately buccal to the lower first molar may not provide adequate bone volume in Caucasian patients [10,11].

Consequently, insertion sites distobuccal to the lower second molar have been recommended, with the additional recommendation of a planning cone beam computed tomography (CBCT) if the shelf dimensions are unclear. Unfortunately, this insertion site may have 4 mm depth of cortex, requiring predrilling, a wide (e.g. 2 mm diameter implant body), incomplete mini-implant insertion and also possible use of a (more fracture-resistant) stainless steel material.

Finally, given that there is no equivalent to the hard palate (for maxillary anchorage) for mandibular distalisation cases, an alternative source of skeletal anchorage there is the basal bone. However, this is not accessible without the elevation of a surgical flap and placement of a modified miniplate (Figure 8.3). Such miniplates feature a transmucosal neck extension for the application of traction at a distance from the anchorage site. The miniplate needs to be contoured to the bone surface and fixed with several bone screws. On balance, given the surgical nature of this procedure, it is likely that most orthodontists would refer to a surgical colleague for this form of anchorage insertion.

8.1.1 Class II Growth Modification Treatment, Involving Mini-implant Anchorage (Figure 8.1)

- This case illustrates enhanced growth modification treatment. I typically use a Twin Block type of orthopaedic appliance in early adolescent Class II cases. However, this male patient presented at the age of 15.5 years, after his peak pubertal growth phase (Figure 8.1a–c). Therefore, the effects of the orthopaedic appliance were augmented by the addition of mandibular mini-implant anchorage, with a view to reducing lower labial proclination side-effects and hence maximising the underlying skeletal changes.
- Bilateral mini-implants (1.5 mm diameter, 9 mm body length, short neck version) were inserted on the buccal aspect of the mandibular alveolus between the premolar roots. The sites were selected on the basis of those with sufficient pre-existing root separation (Figure 8.1d).
- The lower first premolars were anchored by the mini-implants via a 0.019 × 0.025 in. steel archwire connection (Figure 8.1d,e). A Twin Block appliance was worn for Class II corrections (Figure 8.1e).
- The Twin Block was discontinued and the mini-implants removed after 13 months of treatment (Figure 8.1h,i). This is a relatively prolonged time for this phase of treatment, in the author's experience, compared with younger adolescent patients.
- The patient progressed onto full upper and lower fixed appliances for 12 months, to achieve full alignment and occlusal consolidation (Figure 8.1j,k).

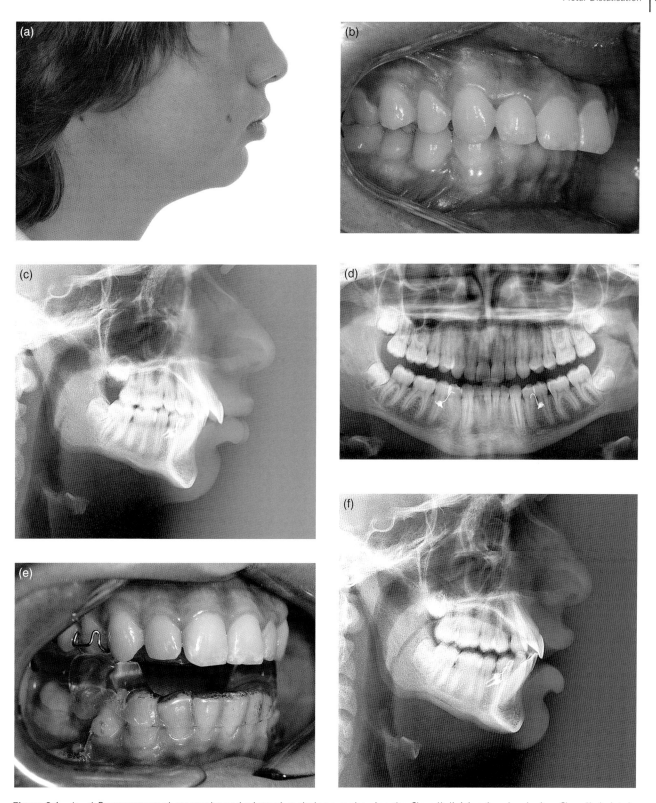

Figure 8.1 (a–c) Pretreatment photographs and a lateral cephalogram showing the Class II division 1 malocclusion, Class II skeletal base and reduced lower anterior face height. (d) A panoramic radiograph taken after insertion of bilateral mandibular mini-implants distal to the first premolars. (e) Photograph showing the Twin Block appliance *in situ* and a buccal mini-implant with sectional wire bonded to the adjacent first premolar crown. (f) Lateral cephalogram taken at the end of the orthopaedic phase. (g) Cephalometric superimpositions of the pretreatment and end of orthopaedic phase changes. This shows anterior and inferior movement of the chin, with minimal maxillary and incisor changes. (h,i) Photographs taken at the start of the fixed appliance phase, showing the overall Class I malocclusion and temporary lateral openbites. (j,k) Debond facial and intraoral photographs.

(g)

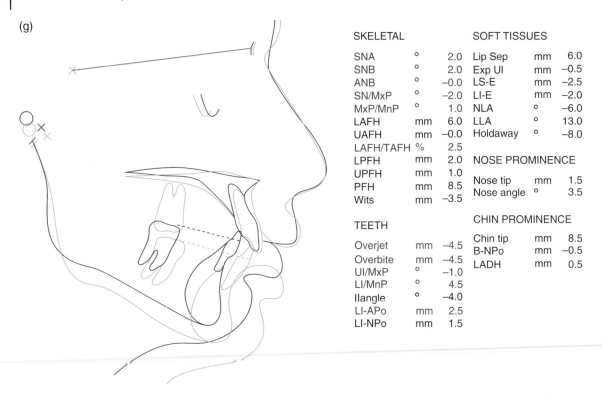

SKELETAL			SOFT TISSUES		
SNA	°	2.0	Lip Sep	mm	6.0
SNB	°	2.0	Exp UI	mm	−0.5
ANB	°	−0.0	LS-E	mm	−2.5
SN/MxP	°	−2.0	LI-E	mm	−2.0
MxP/MnP	°	1.0	NLA	°	−6.0
LAFH	mm	6.0	LLA	°	13.0
UAFH	mm	−0.0	Holdaway	°	−8.0
LAFH/TAFH	%	2.5			
LPFH	mm	2.0	NOSE PROMINENCE		
UPFH	mm	1.0			
PFH	mm	8.5	Nose tip	mm	1.5
Wits	mm	−3.5	Nose angle	°	3.5

TEETH			CHIN PROMINENCE		
Overjet	mm	−4.5	Chin tip	mm	8.5
Overbite	mm	−4.5	B-NPo	mm	−0.5
UI/MxP	°	−1.0	LADH	mm	0.5
LI/MnP	°	4.5			
Iiangle	°	−4.0			
LI-APo	mm	2.5			
LI-NPo	mm	1.5			

(h)

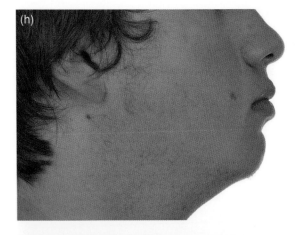

(i)

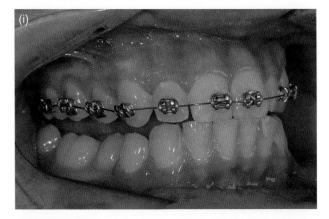

(j)

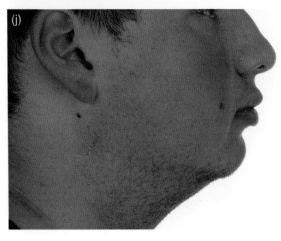

(k)

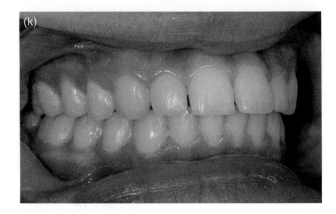

Figure 8.1 (Continued)

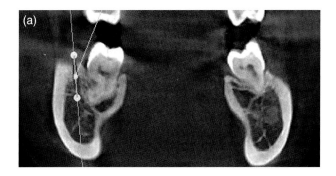

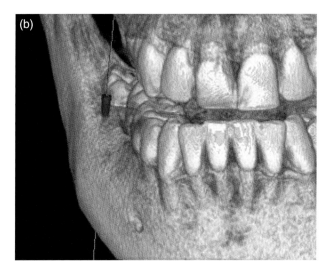

Figure 8.2 (a) A coronal view of a CBCT image showing the mandibular buccal shelf adjacent to the first molar tooth. A virtual implant (*red outline*) has been orientated for insertion in this buccal site. (b) The reformatted CBCT view shows the surface morphology of this right buccal shelf area and the top of a virtual implant projecting on the distobuccal aspect of the second molar crown.

8.1.2 Mandibular Distalisation Using Miniplate Anchorage (Figure 8.3)

- A 38-year-old male presented with a Class II division 1 malocclusion on a severe skeletal II base with a reduced maxillomandibular planes angle (Figure 8.3a–f). He required space provision for relief of his severe mandibular arch crowding, and for orthodontic decompensation. This was planned to be followed by a mandibular advancement osteotomy to correct his Class II discrepancies. Conventionally, lower premolar extractions would be warranted but management of the lower arch was greatly complicated by the absence of all lower second and third molars (Figure 8.3g). Consequently, it was agreed to avoid further loss of lower teeth by distalising the lower buccal teeth. However, this was complicated by the resorbed posterior alveolar ridges, meaning that mini-implant anchorage would not be feasible at these sites.
- Bilateral L-shaped maxillofacial surgical miniplates (Figure 8.3h) were fixed to the mandibular body by a sur-

geon under general anaesthesia, following elevation of surgical access flaps. The miniplates were modified by the surgeon cutting into the distal aspect of the most superior plate hole in order to form a hook.

- Bilateral sectional fixed appliances were bonded on the mandibular molar and premolar teeth, then elastomeric traction was applied from the miniplates to the molar tube hooks eight weeks after surgery (Figure 8.3i–k).
- The lower anterior teeth were bonded after six months of distalising traction, once initial spaces had been created for their alignment (Figure 8.3l–o).
- The patient was ready for a mandibular advancement osteotomy and advancement genioplasty after 16 months of presurgical orthodontics, once the arches had been aligned and the overjet increased to 10 mm by retraction of the lower incisor teeth (Figure 8.3p–s). The lower first molar had been distalised by a full unit, with some distal tipping and intrusive side-effect movements present at this stage.
- The miniplates were removed at this surgery and standard fixation plates inserted (Figure 8.3t).
- Active treatment was completed six months after orthognathic surgery (Figure 8.3u–z), accepting minor residual molar openbites.

8.2 Clinical Objectives of Molar Distalisation

- Distal movement of the molar teeth, without simultaneous mesial movement of the premolars and anterior teeth (anchorage loss).
- Retraction of the premolar and anterior teeth, following molar distalisation, without mesial movement (anchorage loss) of the distalised molars.

8.3 Treatment Options

- Buccal alveolar mini-implant anchorage (direct or indirect) in either arch.
- Palatal alveolar mini-implant anchorage.
- Midpalate mini-implant distaliser.
- Mandibular buccal shelf or retromolar mini-implant anchorage.
- Miniplate insertion on the infrazygomatic or mandibular body areas for maxillary and mandibular distalisation, respectively.
- Premolar extractions (where none have previously been undertaken), avoiding the need for molar distalisation.
- Headgear, possibly with an upper removable appliance (e.g. a 'Nudger'), for upper molar distalisation.
- Correction of the skeletal base (negating distalisation requirements) by orthognathic surgical or orthopaedic appliance treatments.

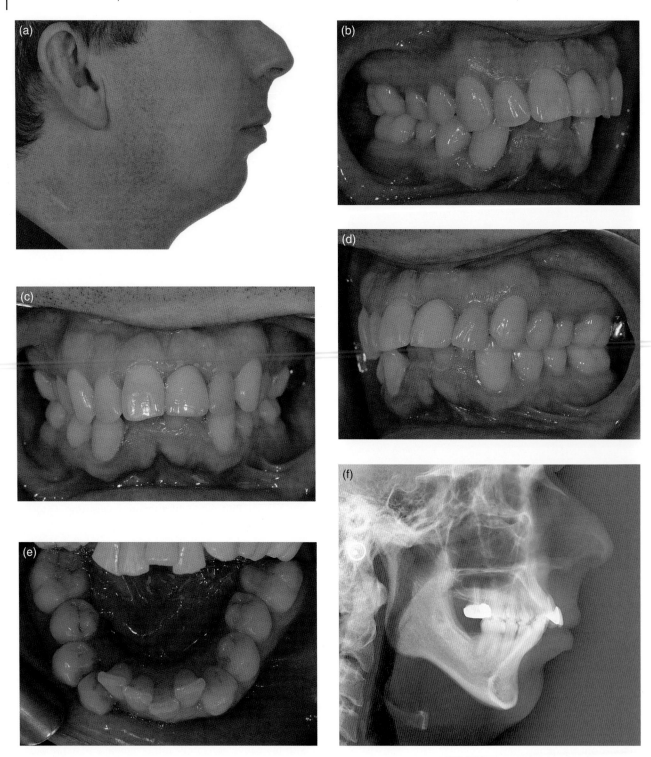

Figure 8.3 (a–f) Pretreatment photographs and lateral cephalogram showing the Class II division 1 malocclusion, Class II skeletal base, reduced lower anterior face height, proclined lower incisors, and severe anterior mandibular crowding. (g) The pretreatment OPG confirms absence of the lower second and third molar teeth. (h) OPG taken after placement of the mandibular body miniplates. (i–k) Views taken at the start of elastomeric traction from the miniplates to the lower molar attachments. (l–o) Photographs taken when space had been opened and the lower anterior teeth were bonded. (p–s) Presurgical views of the dentition and dentoskeletal pattern. These views highlight the distalised position of the lower molar teeth and lower incisor decompensation. (t) A postoperative OPG showing the fixation plates which replaced the modified miniplates. (u–z) Debond facial and intraoral photographs and the final cephalometric appearance.

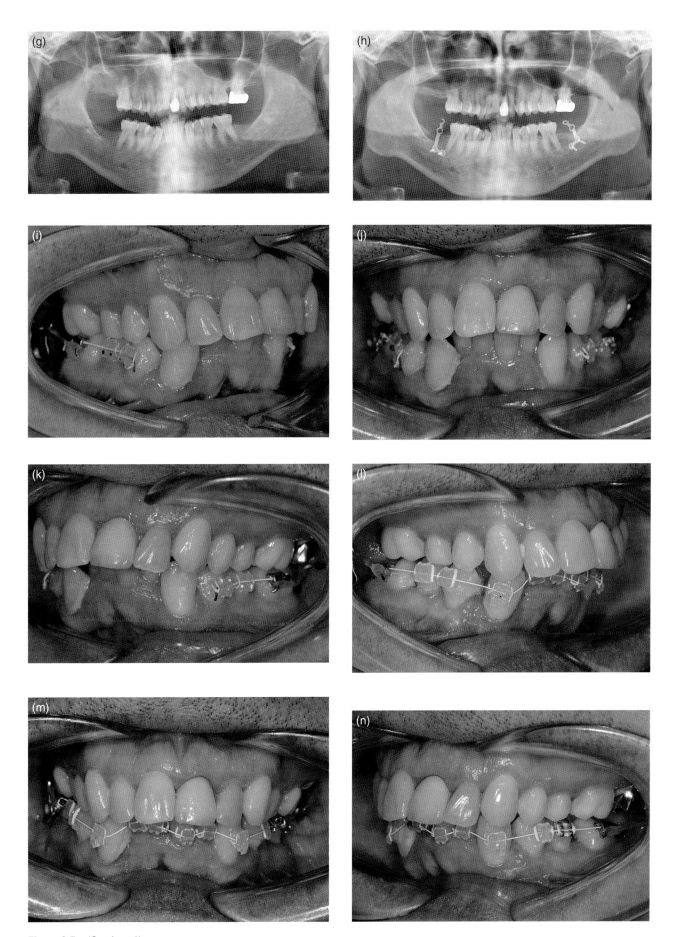

Figure 8.3 (Continued)

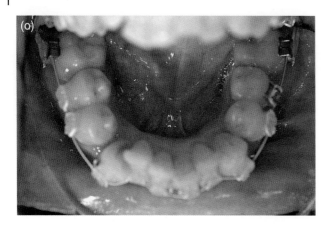

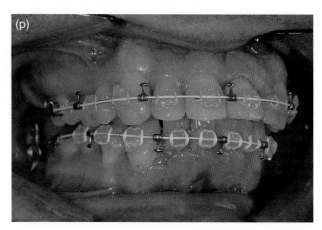

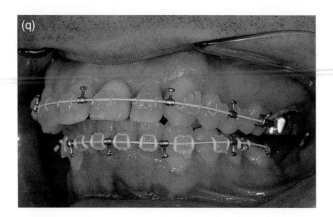

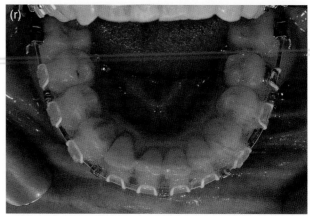

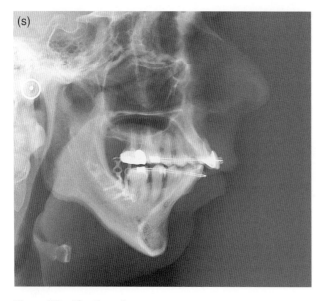

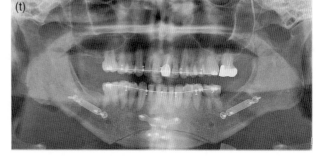

Figure 8.3 (Continued)

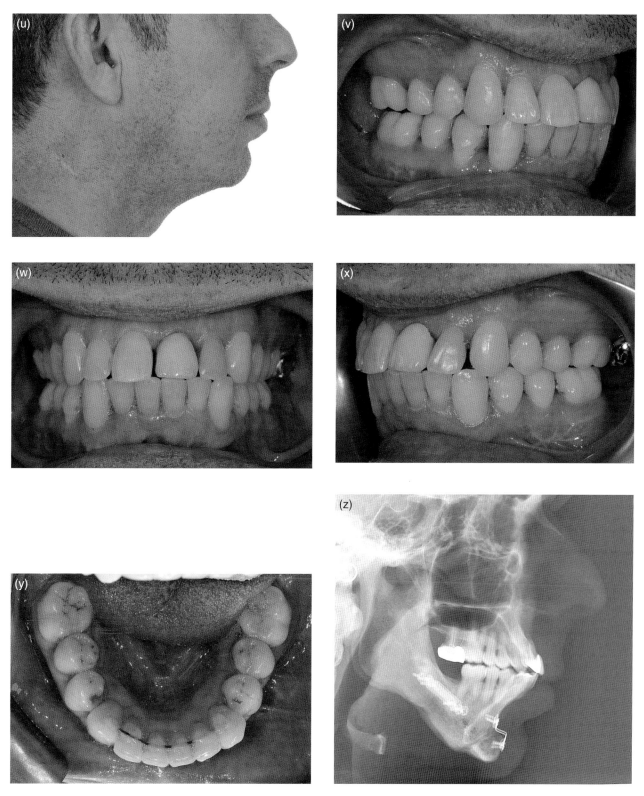

Figure 8.3 (Continued)

8.4 Key Treatment Planning Considerations

- The molar, canine and skeletal relationships, after allowing for relative changes in the buccal segment relationship during treatment.
- Eruptive status of the second molars: there is much less resistance to molar distalisation before eruption of the second molars, but also a greater tendency to molar tipping (rather than bodily movement) [12].
- Presence/absence of third molars: consider their removal (before orthodontics) if they are likely to interfere with distalisation.
- Absence of posterior teeth and possibly also the alveolar ridge (due to previous extractions or hypodontia).
- Depth and shape of the palatal vault; a high-arched palate makes access difficult for midpalate insertion of both mini-implants and a distaliser.
- Distalisation distance required and whether this differs for each side of the arch.
- Maxillary buccal alveolar insertions provide a very limited range of distalisation movements, especially in the maxillary arch, given the proximity of the buccal roots and restrictive interproximal spaces [13]. In addition, this approach often requires resiting of the mini-implants after molar distalisation and before the second-phase retraction of the premolar teeth.
- Sufficient interproximal space is available between the maxillary palatal roots for both insertion and up to half a unit distalisation of teeth (before the mini-implant is approximated by roots mesial to it).
- Midpalate anchored distalisers require more initial clinical, and especially laboratory, time due to their fabrication and fitting requirements. However, once *in situ*, they are simple to reactivate and provide the best range for distalisation. They may also provide optimum bodily molar movements, followed by simple retraction of the anterior teeth [14–17].

8.5 Biomechanical Principles

- Forces applied at the coronal level of the molars will tend to tip their crowns distally during distalisation, then risk anchorage loss as the molars upright whilst the anterior teeth are being retracted [5,18].
- Distalising forces directed at the vertical level of the molar's root furcation will produce molar bodily movement [5].
- First molars tend to distally tip when the second molars are unerupted (Figure 8.3) [12].
- There is a tendency to molar cross-bites as the molars distalise. This is exacerbated when a rigid transpalatal arch (TPA) is used, or when insufficient compensatory transverse co-ordination is incorporated in the fixed appliance archwires or a distaliser appliance's wire frame.
- Maxillary molars may be either pushed or pulled distally. On first thought, most orthodontists will think of pushcoil to deliver a distalising force. However, it is also feasible for molars to be retracted using closing coil or elastomeric traction (Figure 8.13). This has the advantage of longer ranges of activation feasible with NiTi closing coils [19].

8.6 Midtreatment Problems and Solutions

- If there are signs of distal molar tipping then elect to overcorrect their distalisation, in anticipation of molar relapse during retraction of the anterior teeth.
- It may be necessary to accept buccal cross-bites, especially if a rigid TPA is used, until after the anchorage requirements have been met. However, if alveolar mini-implants are being used for direct traction then arch co-ordination can be attempted, for example by expansion of the maxillary archwire.
- Patients should alert the orthodontist as soon as they become aware of the breakage of any components to prevent anchorage loss or unfavourable tooth movements.

8.7 Mandibular Arch Distalisation

This involves mini-implant insertion in posterior interproximal sites, the retromolar area, or the buccal shelf.

8.7.1 Clinical Steps for Mandibular Distalisation

8.7.1.1 Preinsertion

1) For buccal insertion sites, for example mesial to the first molar, increase the interproximal space by root divergence. This involves adding mesial tip to the lower second premolar bracket at bond-up.
2) Level and align the arch to be ready for the working archwire, e.g. a 0.019 × 0.025 in. rectangular stainless steel wire.
3) Determine the optimum insertion site, for example distal to the terminal molar (Figure 8.4) or in the buccal shelf area distobuccal to the first molar (Figure 8.2). This decision depends on the ease of access to the retromolar site, the available interproximal space, and the mobility and thickness of the overlying soft tissues, respectively. The retromolar site may not be suitable if the third molar is present or if it has been removed within the previous few months.

4) Consider fabrication of a stent, especially if the insertion site is difficult to access or deliberately close to a molar root, by taking either an impression or intraoral scan 1–2 weeks preinsertion. For a dental impression, remember that the fixed appliance brackets may be blocked out with soft wax except those adjacent to the insertion site, and ideally the clinical level of the mucogingival junction should be measured or photographed.

8.7.1.2   Mini-implant Selection

5) Alveolar sites: select a narrow, short neck mini-implant (e.g. Infinitas 1.5 mm diameter, 6 or 9 mm length). The length selection depends on the patient's age, the anticipated cortical bone thickness and height of attached gingiva (and hence the mini-implant's inclination and final depth of insertion). For example, a long body length is required in the retromolar area and where

there is limited height of attached gingiva in buccal sites. This is when incomplete insertion will occur. A short length is appropriate in the buccal alveolus in adult patients with reasonable height of attached tissue, enabling 'horizontal' insertion of the mini-implant at a relatively apical insertion level.

Buccal shelf: select a relatively long and wide mini-implant version, e.g. 2 mm diameter, 9 mm length (long neck) Infinitas. This allows for the relatively thick cortical bone layer and incomplete insertion of the mini-implant.

8.7.1.3   Insertion

6) Identify the insertion point in the retromolar (Figure 8.4), alveolar interproximal site or buccal shelf (Figure 8.2). Any interproximal insertion should be made just mesial to the first molar roots to allow for

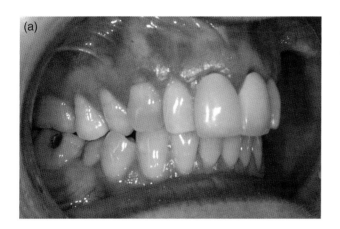

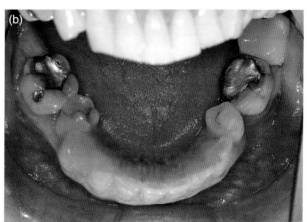

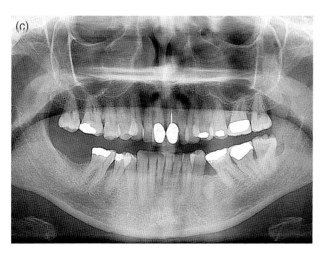

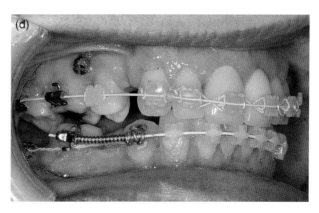

Figure 8.4   (a,b) Pretreatment view of an adult patient showing a Class II malocclusion with absent lower right second and third molars, moderate crowding and lingual displacement of the lower right second premolar. (c) Pretreatment panoramic radiograph confirming absence of the two lower right molar teeth and a heavily restored dentition. (d–f) A mini-implant inserted distobuccal to the lower right first molar provides indirect anchorage via a ligature wire to the first premolar bracket, whilst a compressed coil spring distalises the first molar. (g,h) Bonding and alignment of the lower right second premolar after molar distalisation had created sufficient space. (i) Full alignment of this premolar was achieved after 14 months of treatment, and this continued through to the debond stage (j).

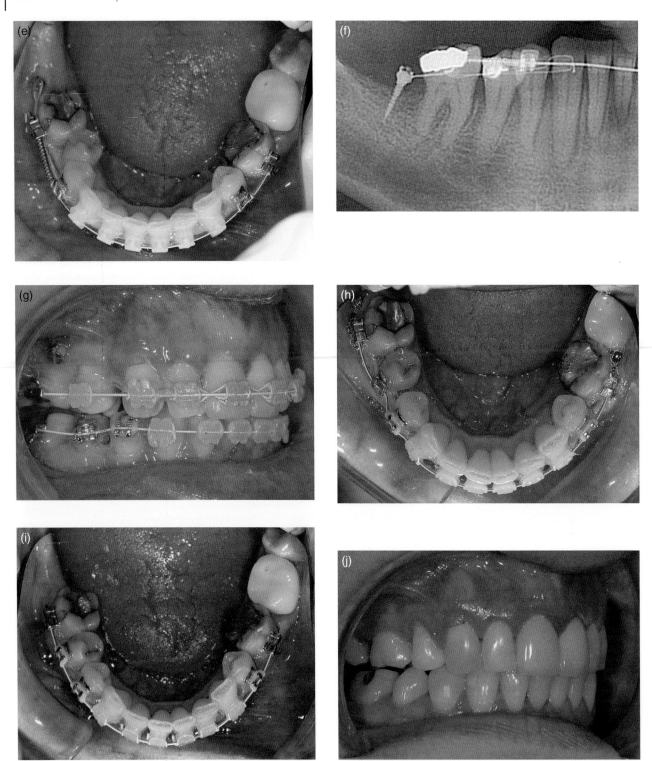

Figure 8.4 (Continued)

subsequent distal movement of the adjacent premolar towards the mini-implant (Figure 8.5). Ideally, the insertion should be through attached gingiva but if this is not feasible then use a soft tissue punch to first remove a circle of loose mucosa.

7) Superficial anaesthesia of the insertion site.

8) Determine the angle of insertion (in the vertical plane): an interproximal mini-implant is inserted relatively perpendicular to the buccal surface; a retromolar one is placed at a small oblique angle from the axial plane such that the head is slightly buccal to its body position; a buccal shelf mini-implant is relatively

'upright' or oblique to avoid penetration of the tooth-bearing alveolar area.

9) Manual insertion is feasible where there is sufficient physical access, that is, adequate stretching of the cheek and buccal sulcus. Otherwise, contra-angle handpiece insertion is recommended, especially in the retromolar area, but with resultant loss of full tactile control.

10) Limited predrilling (e.g. using a 2 mm cortical bone punch) is recommended prior to mini-implant insertion, except in adolescent patients with less dense mandibular cortex.

11) For alveolar sites, complete the insertion to the point where the mini-implant neck is partially submerged but its head is fully accessible for traction purposes. This is best performed gradually and with intermittent release of the screwdriver during the final turns, so that overinsertion is avoided. If the cortex gives rise to high insertion torque then remember to offset this by partial derotation of the mini-implant (provided that more than 1 mm of insertion range remains).

12) For the buccal shelf, complete the insertion when the head of the mini-implant is several millimetres coronal to the MGJ, in order to keep it completely accessible and relatively close to the fixed appliance level.

13) For alveolar insertions, percuss the adjacent teeth to gauge root proximity and take an intraoral radiograph if a problem is suspected.

8.7.1.4 Postinsertion

Immediately load the mini-implant with *light* traction for the first 5–6 weeks, for example with a lightly stretched power-chain. Subsequently apply *direct* traction to either an anchor tooth or the archwire using a NiTi coil spring or elastomeric attachment, or alternatively *indirect* anchorage may be performed by connecting the anchor tooth and mini-implant with a ligature wire or traction auxiliary (Figure 8.4b,c).

8.7.2 Case Examples

1) **Single mandibular molar distalisation (Figure 8.4)**

- An adult with a Class II division 2 malocclusion with absent lower right second molar and lingual displacement of the lower right second premolar tooth (Figure 8.4a).
- The lower arch, except the right second premolar, was aligned ready for insertion of a 0.019 × 0.025 in. steel archwire (Figure 8.4b).
- A 1.5 mm diameter, 9 mm body length, long neck Infinitas mini-implant was inserted on the buccal aspect of the alveolar ridge and distal to the lower right first molar. It was used to indirectly anchor the right premolar then canine teeth (Figure 8.4b–d).
- Anchorage was discontinued once molar distalisation had created space for alignment of the second premolar (Figure 8.4e,f).

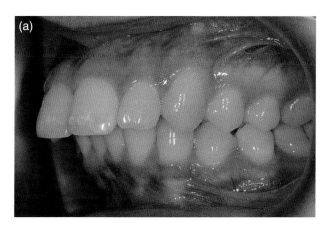
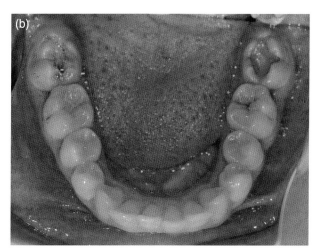

Figure 8.5 (a,b) Intraoral photographs of a 17-year-old female presenting with a Class II division 1 malocclusion and heavily restored lower left second molar tooth. (c) Panoramic radiograph showing that this molar had a periapical radiolucency and that the lower left third molar was present and viable. (d) Periapical radiograph showing a mini-implant sited mesial to the lower left third molar. (e,f) Intraoral photographs showing the lower fixed appliance *in situ* with a sigmoid powerarm crimped on the archwire distal to the lower left canine. Transparent elastomeric traction connected this powerarm to the mini-implant. (g) A panoramic radiograph taken five months into the direct traction phase shows distal movement of the lower left first molar, and also mesial tipping of the mini-implant. (h,i) Photographs at the end of the presurgical phase, showing the shortened powerarm, increased Class II left molar relationship and approximation of the lower left second molar crown and mini-implant head. (j,k) Lateral cephalograms taken at the start of traction and seven months later, showing the unilateral lower molar distalisation and lower incisor decompensation. (l–n) The posttreatment intraoral and cephalometric results, with good left molar occlusal contacts and partial eruption of the lower left third molar.

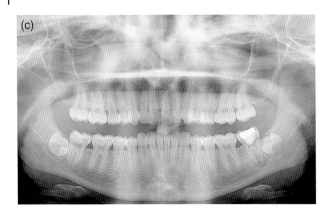

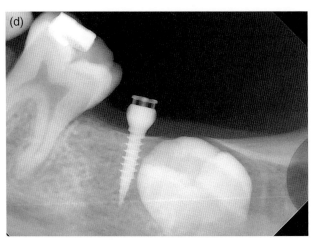

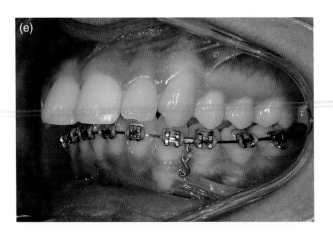

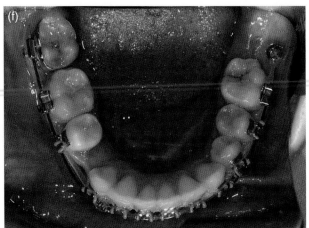

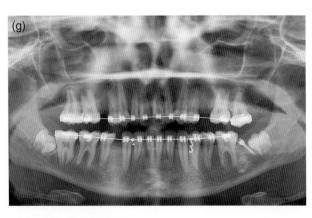

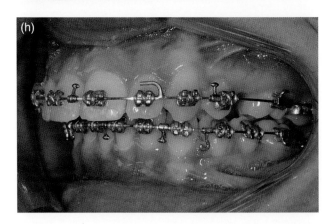

Figure 8.5 (Continued)

2) *En masse* **mandibular arch distalisation (Figure 8.5)**

- A 17-year-old female presented with a Class II division 1 malocclusion (Figure 8.5a). She required lower arch decompensation prior to a mandibular advancement osteotomy. The lower left second molar was heavily restored and had a periapical abscess (Figure 8.5b,c),

so it was decided to create space by extraction of this tooth and the lower right first premolar. The premolar space was planned for closure using conventional traction and anchorage. Posterior buccal shelf mini-implant anchorage was required on the left side for *en masse* retraction of the left buccal segment and incisor teeth.

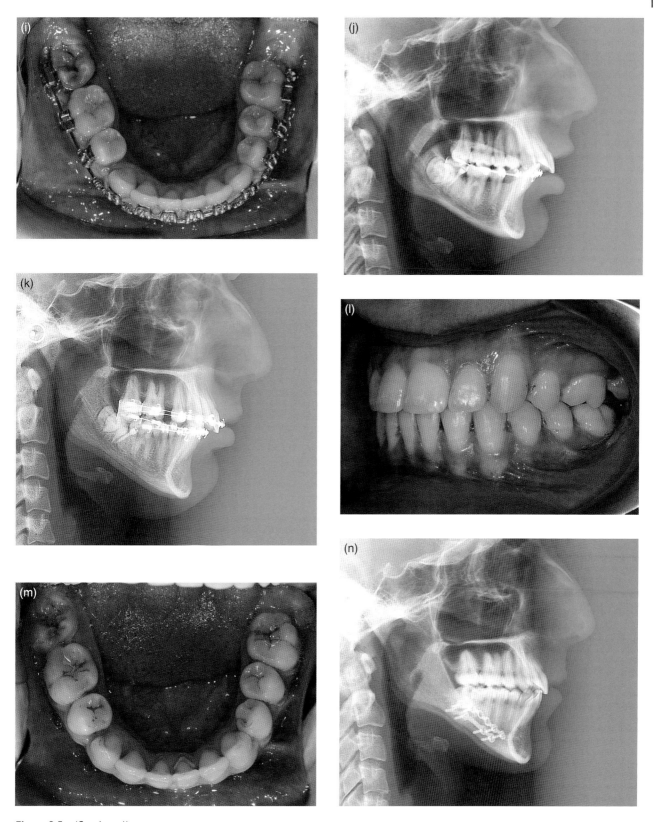

Figure 8.5 (Continued)

- Orthodontic treatment commenced, following the extractions with arch alignment to the stage that a 0.019×0.025 in. stainless steel archwire was inserted. An Infinitas mini-implant, with a 2 mm diameter, 9 mm body length and long neck, was inserted in the buccal shelf in the area distobuccal to the second molar extraction site (Figure 8.5d).
- Direct traction was applied to a crimpable powerarm on the archwire (Figure 8.5e,f).
- Traction was discontinued after seven months and the powerarm length was shortened, for subsequent use as a surgical hook. *En masse* distalisation of the lower left quadrant teeth had been achieved and the left first molar approximated the mini-implant (Figure 8.5h,i). This was partly due to mesial tipping of the mini-implant, perhaps as a result of the adjacent regional accelerated phenomenon as the molar socket healed.
- The bilateral traction had enabled full lower incisor decompensation, as evidenced by comparison of lateral cephalograms taken at the start and end of traction (Figure 8.5j,k).
- The patient then underwent a mandibular advancement osteotomy resulting in correction of her Class II features (Figure 8.5l–n).

8.8 Maxillary Arch Distalisation

The insertion site and biomechanics depend on the amount of distalisation required and the ease of accessibility of the midpalate (i.e. the palatal vault depth).

8.8.1 Clinical Steps for Palatal Alveolar Distalisation

8.8.1.1 Preinsertion

1) Band the first molars at the start of treatment if a TPA is planned for indirect molar distalisation.
2) Level and align the arch to be ready for a minimum of 0.018 in. steel archwire, but more typically a 0.019×0.025 in. rectangular wire.
3) Determine the optimum insertion site, mesial or distal to the first molar, depending on whether the second molars have erupted, the arch length, the available interproximal space, and the ease of access.
4) Consider fabrication of a stent, especially if the insertion site is difficult to access or distally offset in the interproximal space (i.e. close to the more distal palatal root), by taking an impression 1–2 weeks before insertion. Note that the fixed appliance brackets may be fully waxed out (from a gingival direction) since the insertion site and stent coverage only involve the occlusal and palate surfaces.

8.8.1.2 Mini-implant Selection

5) Use a relatively narrow mini-implant diameter, given the interproximal nature of the insertion. The neck needs to be long enough to traverse the thick mucosa; for Infinitas, use the 1.5 mm diameter, 9 mm body length, long neck version.

8.8.1.3 Insertion

6) Identify the palatal alveolar insertion point, just mesial to the first or second molar palatal root. This initially close proximity facilitates distal movement of the premolar/first molar before this root approximates the mini-implant.
7) Superficial anaesthesia of the insertion site.
8) Use a mucotome to remove a circle of mucosa from the insertion site.
9) Determine the angles of insertion. Palatal alveolar mini-implants are generally inserted perpendicular to the surface in the anteroposterior direction. In the vertical plane, they may be inserted at either 90° (perpendicular to the surface) or obliquely angled by inclining the screwdriver in an apical direction. This is appropriate to limit insertion depth if the palatal roots are relatively superficial.
10) A cortical bone punch (perforation) step is recommended in adult patients.
11) Contra-angle handpiece insertion is recommended because of the limited physical access, especially to avoid the path of insertion being angled towards the distal molar root (rather than horizontally neutral).
12) Complete the insertion to the point where the mini-implant neck is partially submerged but the head is fully accessible. This is best performed gradually and with intermittent release of the screwdriver during the final turns, so that overinsertion is avoided.
13) Percuss the adjacent teeth to gauge root proximity and take an intraoral radiograph if a problem is suspected.

8.8.1.4 Postinsertion

14) Direct traction: bond an attachment (either a hook or a modified powerarm) to the first premolar or canine tooth's palatal surface. A powerarm has the advantage of enabling a more horizontal vector of traction (Figure 8.6). Indirect traction: fit a modified TPA (fitted on the first molars).
15) Immediately load the mini-implant with *light* traction for the first 5–6 weeks, for example with a lightly stretched powerchain. Subsequently apply traction using a NiTi coil spring or elastomeric auxiliary.

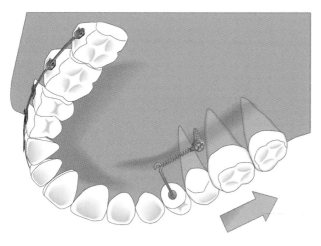

Figure 8.6 Diagram showing traction from a mini-implant, inserted in the palatal alveolus mesial to the first molar palatal root, to a powerarm bonded on the first premolar.

8.8.2 Case Examples

1) **Direct palatal alveolar traction (Figure 8.7)**
   - A 13-year-old girl with a Class II division 1 malocclusion (Figure 8.7a–c). The overjet was 7 mm and both the molar and canine were in asymmetrical Class II relationships: quarter and half unit on either side.
   - All the maxillary second premolars were hypoplastic and the second molars had been extracted. The upper incisors had short roots, contraindicating Class II intermaxillary traction.
   - An upper fixed appliance was used for initial alignment and levelling.
   - 1.5 mm diameter, 9 mm length, long neck mini-implants were inserted mesial to the first molar palatal roots (Figure 8.7d,e) and immediate traction was applied to the first premolars' palatal cleats (Figure 8.7c).

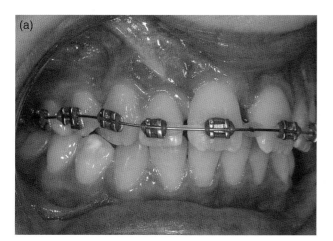

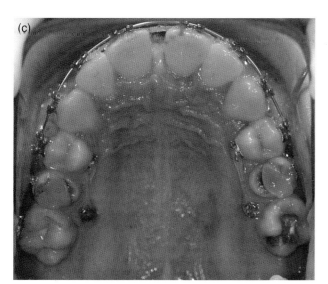

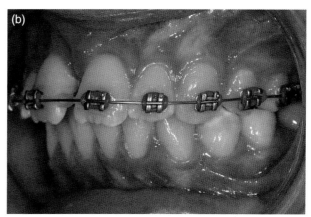

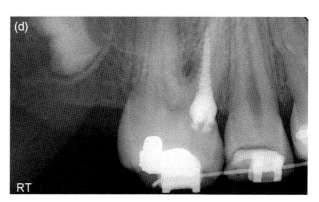

Figure 8.7 (a,b) Intraoral photographs showing the Class II malocclusion with a 7 mm overjet, asymmetrical Class II buccal segment relationships, and absent upper second molars. (c) A palatal view showing bilateral palatal alveolar mini-implants, positioned mesial to the first molar palatal roots, and with traction to first premolar palatal cleats. (d,e) Intraoral radiographs of the posterior teeth and mini-implants after insertion. (f–h) Photographs taken after five months of direct traction. The second premolar crowns appear close to the mini-implant heads following premolar and molar *en masse* distalisation. (i–k) Intraoral photographs taken two years after debond, showing the stable Class I buccal segment relationships.

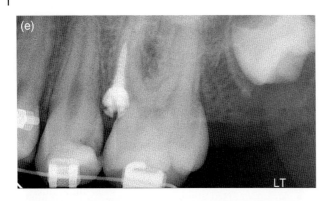

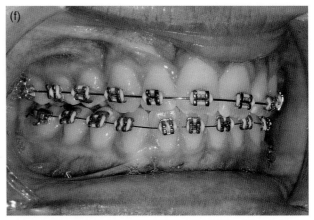

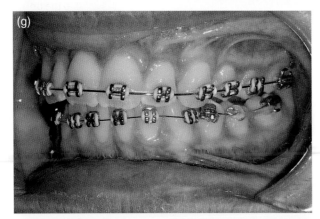

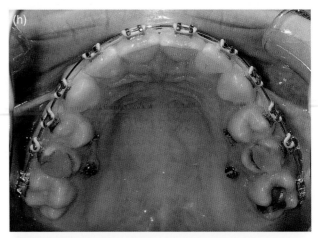

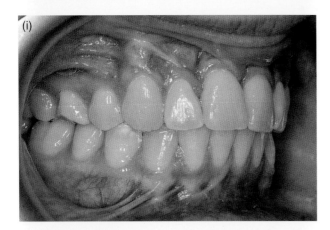

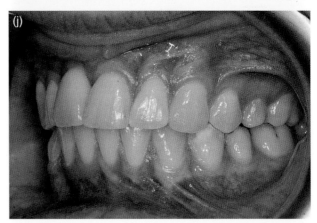

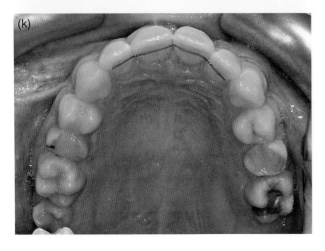

Figure 8.7 (Continued)

- Up to half a unit of asymmetrical distalisation was achieved such that the premolar crowns approximated the mini-implant heads (Figure 8.7f–h). The anterior teeth were retracted towards the premolars using indirect anchorage of the latter teeth.
- The mini-implants were explanted prior to debond (Figure 8.7i–k).

2) **Indirect palatal alveolar traction to a TPA (Figure 8.8)**
   - A 17-year-old male with a Class III malocclusion on a severe skeletal III base required presurgical orthodontics prior to bimaxillary surgery. There was severe maxillary arch crowding, impaction of the upper left canine and a substantial centreline shift to the left side, despite absence of the maxillary first premolars (Figure 8.8a,b).
   - Consequently, more than half a unit bilateral maxillary molar distalisation was required. However, the patient's palate was narrow and deeply vaulted, making it impossible to access the midpalate for mini-implant insertions.
   - The first molars were banded and a fixed appliance bonded on the more anterior maxillary teeth for arch alignment and levelling.
   - 1.5 mm diameter, 9 mm length, long neck mini-implants were inserted in the palatal alveolus mesial to the upper first molars and then a modified TPA was fitted (Figure 8.8c). Immediate traction was applied to bilateral hooks soldered on the anterior part of the TPA.

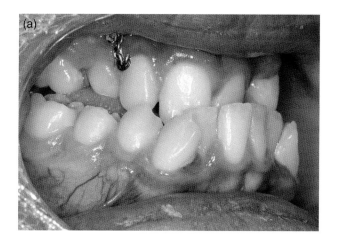
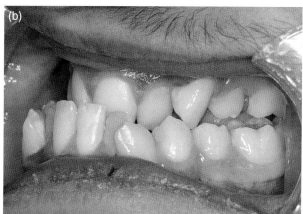
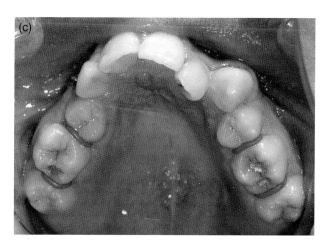
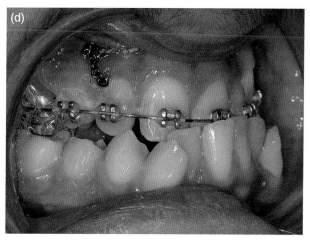

Figure 8.8 (a–c) Pretreatment views showing the severe Class III malocclusion, absent upper first premolars and impacted upper right canine. (d,e) The upper arch has been aligned with a fixed appliance. (f,g) Palatal views showing two palatal alveolar mini-implants, inserted mesial to the first molars. Elastomeric traction has been applied to two consecutive and differing designs of modified TPA. (h–j) Sufficient space created for the impacted canine following bilateral molar distalisation and centreline correction. (k) Cephalometric superimposition of the presurgical orthodontic changes (*red pretreatment, green presurgery*) showing the molar distalisation achieved, without extrusion.

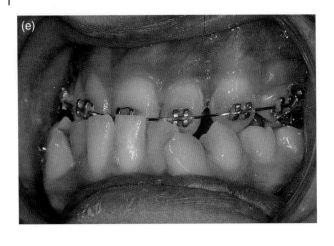

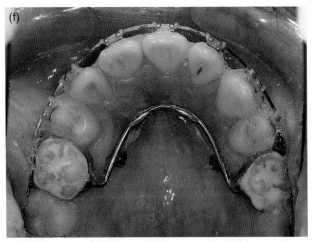

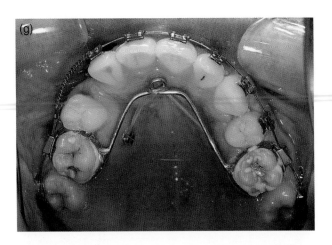

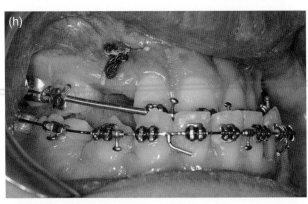

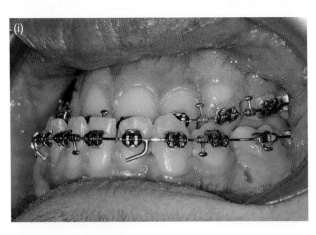

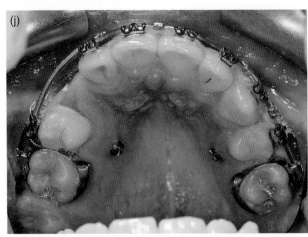

Figure 8.8 (Continued)

- The initial TPA was replaced after eight months of distalisation, when it started to overlap the mini-implant heads. A new TPA provided further clearance and traction distance, using an anterior midline hook, and was used for the final seven months of traction (Figure 8.8d).

- The second TPA was removed preoperatively once sufficient space had been created for the absent canine tooth and centreline correction (Figure 8.8e,f). Cephalometric superimposition (Figure 8.8g) shows the extent of molar distalisation over 15 months and only modest incisor proclination.

(k)

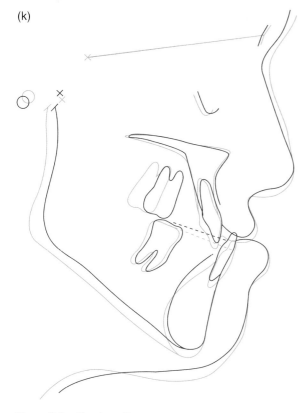

SKELETAL			SOFT TISSUES		
SNA	°	−1.5	Lip Sep	mm	−2.0
SNB	°	−0.5	Exp UI	mm	1.0
ANB	°	−1.0	LS-E	mm	0.0
SN/MxP	°	−2.0	LI-E	mm	0.0
MxP/MnP	°	3.0	NLA	°	8.5
LAFH	mm	4.5	LLA	°	−7.5
UAFH	mm	−1.0	Holdaway	°	−0.5
LAFH/TAFH	%	2.0			
LPFH	mm	2.5	NOSE PROMINENCE		
UPFH	mm	−1.0			
PFH	mm	1.5	Nose tip	mm	−2.5
Wits	mm	−3.5	Nose angle	°	−5.0

TEETH			CHIN PROMINENCE		
Overjet	mm	−0.5	Chin tip	mm	−3.5
Overbite	mm	0.5	B-NPo	mm	0.0
UI/MxP	°	−3.0	LADH	mm	0.0
LI/MnP	°	1.5			
IIangle	°	−1.5			
LI-APo	mm	0.5			
LI-NPo	mm	0.5			

Figure 8.8 (Continued)

3) **Indirect palatal alveolar traction to a quadhelix (Figure 8.9)**
   - A 36-year-old female presented with a Class II malocclusion on a skeletal I base, with absence of the first premolars and upper third molars. There was mild residual crowding, the maxillary archform was tapered and the canine relationships were three-quarter unit Class II (Figure 8.9a–g).
   - A modified removable quadhelix was fitted on the upper second molar teeth, with immediate activation (Figure 8.9j).
   - Bilateral palatal alveolar mini-implants (1.5 mm diameter, 9 mm length, long neck versions) were inserted, distal to the intermolar contact point and relatively close to the second molar palatal root (Figure 8.9h,i). Immediate traction was applied to bilateral hooks soldered on the anterior aspects of the quadhelix.
   - The traction and maxillary arch expansion continued simultaneously, although there were initial problems with distopalatal rotation of the second molars as a side-effect of the traction on the flexible quadhelix wire. This was fully controlled when the labial fixed

appliance was bonded. In hindsight, initial bonding of the first molars, and connection of the first and second molars with a rigid sectional archwire on each side would have reduced this rotational side-effect.
   - Treatment progressed onto full labial fixed appliances and the mini-implants and quadhelix were removed after 23 months of treatment. The maxillary archform had been successfully expanded and the Class II canine relationships corrected by this stage (Figure 8.9k–n).
   - The fixed appliances were debonded two months later, with scope for subsequent uprighting and occlusal settling of the overexpanded molar positions in the longer term (Figure 8.9o–t).

8.9 Midpalatal Distaliser Options

A midpalate anchored distaliser has two potential advantages: the cortical bone support offers some of the best results for mini-implant stability, especially at a young age [20], and the mini-implants are separate from the dentition and hence will not limit molar and premolar tooth

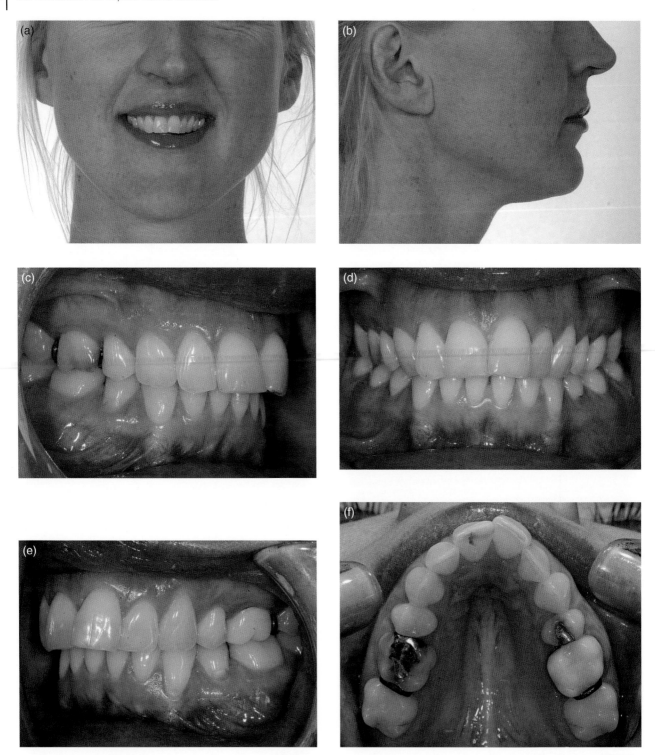

Figure 8.9 (a–f) Pretreatment photographs showing this adult patient's dentofacial features, especially her Class II malocclusion, tapered maxillary archform, absent first premolars and three-quarter unit Class II canine relationships. (g) Pretreatment panoramic radiograph confirming absence of all first premolars and the upper third molars. The upper left first molar had been endodontically treated. (h,i) Intraoral radiographs showing bilateral palatal alveolar mini-implants, inserted just mesial to the second molar palatal roots. (j) Photograph of the modified quadhelix appliance, fitted on the second molars, and with elastomeric traction connected between soldered hooks and the mini-implants. (k–n) Photographs taken once both a Class I occlusion and maxillary arch expansion had been achieved. The mini-implants had just been explanted. (o–t) Debond stage photographs, illustrating the overexpanded positions and residual buccal inclination of the second molars.

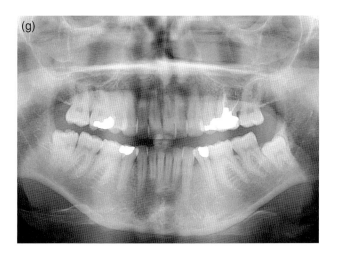

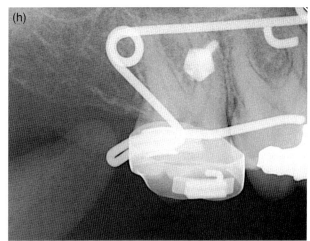

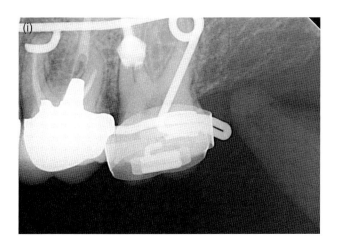

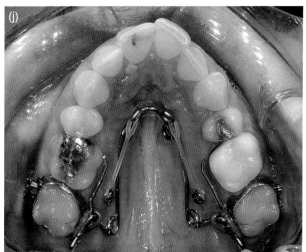

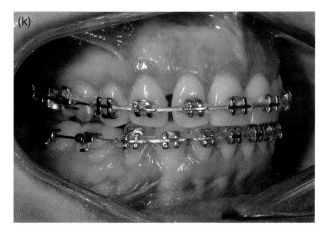

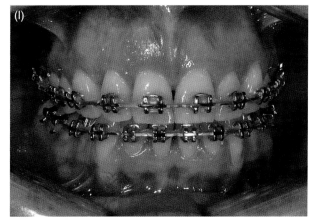

Figure 8.9 (Continued)

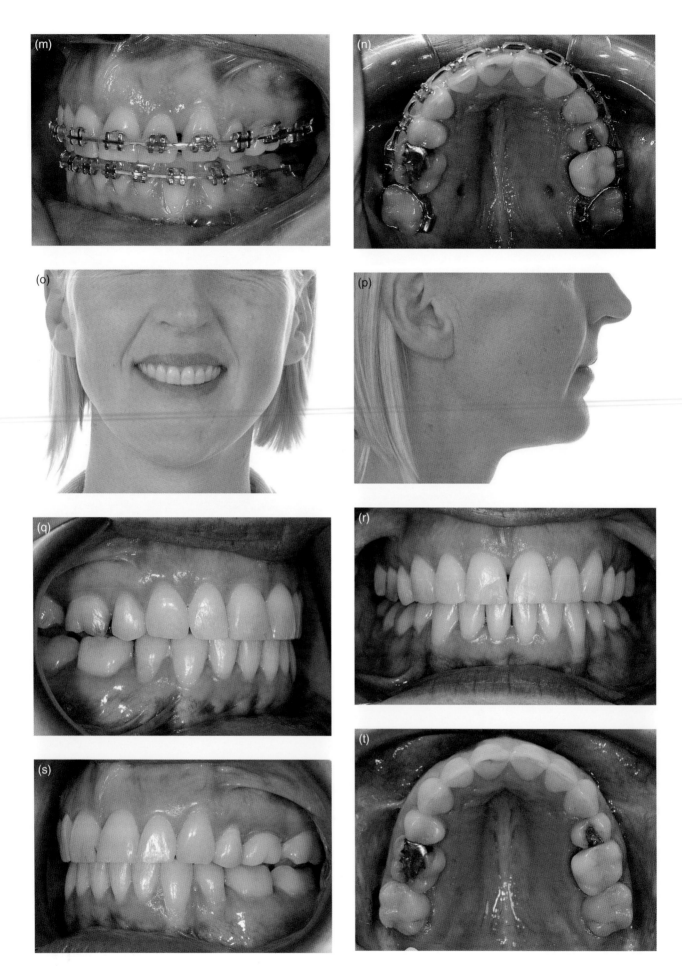

Figure 8.9 (Continued)

movements. However, midpalate distalisers are technically more demanding in terms of appliance design and insertion. There are several factors to consider.

- The method of connection between the mini-implants and the distaliser. For example, the distaliser may be attached to the mini-implant heads by the following methods.
  - Direct insertion of the distaliser wire through the mini-implant heads (Figure 8.10a). This provides a 'clean' connection, but requires alignment of the mini-implant head cross-slots for the distaliser wire to be inserted. Crucially, it also limits the size of the distalising wire frame, in this example to a 0.019 × 0.025 in. archwire size, which in turn provides incomplete control over the molar movements due to the loose fit of the wire within the molar's palatal headgear tube.
  - 'U' shaped or circular wire loops which encircle the mini-implant heads. Each wire loop's internal circumference needs to be large enough for it to seat around the respective mini-implant head. The gap between the wire and head is then sealed, after appliance seating, with composite resin (Figure 8.10b). This design provides a relatively simple, cost-effective means of attachment. In practical terms, there is no need to fully align the mini-implant heads with one another at insertion, although peri-implant hygiene is slightly restricted. It also enables a guidance stent and distaliser to be made simultaneously on the same working model (Figure 8.10c). The seal is removed with a diamond bur at the end of the distaliser usage.
  - Customised screw or abutment cap fittings. These lock the distaliser wire onto the mini-implant heads (Figure 8.10d). However, the more tightly the cap fits onto the mini-implant head, the less freedom/tolerance there is when it comes to seat several caps at once. This is illustrated in Figure 8.10d where one cap was seated but the path of insertion prevented easy fitting of the left cap, instead necessitating interposition of a wire mesh and composite resin to secure the wire and mini-implant on this side.

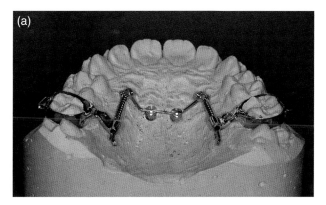

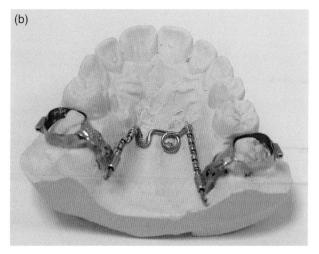

Figure 8.10 (a) A pushcoil distaliser with a 0.019 × 0.025 in. steel archwire frame inserted in the transverse cross-slots of the parallel parasagittal mini-implant heads. The distaliser frame is contoured over the palate, has Gurin locks anteriorly and pushcoil springs, and its distal ends pass through soldered 'flying' headgear tubes. (b) A 1 mm stainless steel wire distaliser frame inserted through the flying headgear tubes and carrying bilateral pushcoils. The main wire has been bent into a 'U' shape on the patient's right side and a circular loop on the left side, to fit around the mini-implant head locations. (c) A 'double-barreled' guidance stent, shown on the right side, has been made using the same working model as the distaliser on the left side of the photograph. Please note that the medial aspects of the guidance cylinders have been trimmed to enable their close approximation. The working model features Infinitas mini-implant analogues in parasagittal positions and the distaliser loops have been contoured around these analogues. (d) A steel wire frame has been attached to a free-rotating abutment cap on the patient's left side, but the right cap was removed as it was difficult to simultaneously seat it. It was replaced by interposition of a wire mesh and composite resin to secure the wire and mini-implant on this side. (e) The 1 mm diameter wire frame of a 'palatal clip' distaliser, with the addition of a soldered 0.7 mm steel wire extending around the lateral and distal aspects of the mini-implant analogues (in this working model). (f) The 0.7 mm wire 'clip' is then cinched into a closed position in the mini-implant recesses, using pliers, once the distaliser has been seated. (g) A 'traction' distaliser with a 1.0 mm steel wire frame formed into loops around the parasagittal mini-implant heads and posterior circular hooks. Traction will be applied from these posterior hooks to hooks on the free-sliding (headgear) tube on the distaliser frame, creating a distaliser force on the adjacent first molar.

(c)

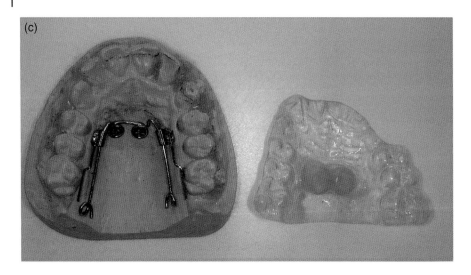

(d)

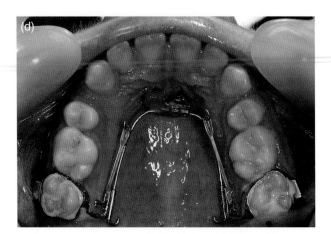

(e)

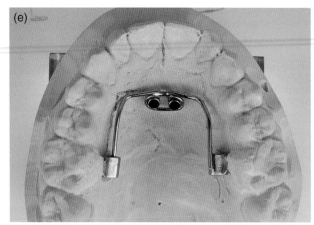

(f)

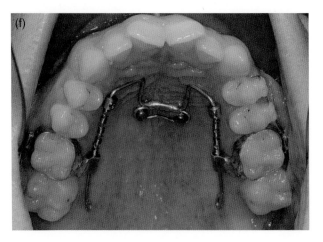

(g)

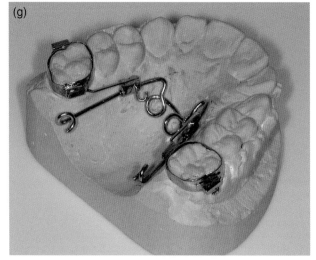

Figure 8.10 (Continued)

- A 'palatal clip' wire attachment locking into a recess in the mini-implant heads or necks (Figure 8.10e). This is a relatively simple adaptation where a thin (e.g. 0.6 or 0.7 mm) auxiliary stainless steel wire is soldered to the main distaliser wire and then crimped into the mini-implant recesses after seating of the distaliser (Figure 8.10f). It also enables a guidance stent and distaliser to be made simultaneously on the same working model.
- An acrylic Nance button with holes in it so that it seats over the mini-implants (similar to the acrylic button shown in Figure 8.10g). These holes are then in-filled in the mouth with either acrylic or composite resin.
- The means of distalising force delivery.
  - There are two strategies to choose from: the use of pushcoil springs, fitted on the distaliser frame, to push the molars distally (by shunting the flying headgear tube soldered to the molar band (Figure 8.10a,b) or the application of traction from a posterior hook to a sliding tube, to pull the molar back (Figure 8.10g). The key advantages and disadvantages of each approach are summarised in the following sections.

8.9.1 Pushcoil Distaliser

This distaliser design (shown in Figure 8.10a,b) has the advantage of using several standard components.

- A 1 mm stainless steel wire, forming the distaliser frame. If a smaller diameter wire (e.g. 0.7 mm round or 0.019×0.025 in. rectangular) is used to fabricate the frame, it will lack rigidity. This results in potential anchorage loss due to flexing of the frame. It also means that the distaliser frame fits loosely into headgear tubes, resulting in incomplete rotational control of the molars.
- Flying headgear tubes soldered to the palatal aspects of molar bands. A 1 mm wire fits neatly inside these tubes, providing bodily control of the molar movements without excessive friction.
- Nickel titanium pushcoil as the active component, but bearing in mind that standard-diameter pushcoil is designed to only fit onto 0.019×0.025 in. rectangular wire. Therefore wide-diameter pushcoil is required to fit onto the 1 mm wire frame.
- Gurin (or other) locks, or freehand additions of composite resin, which act as adjustable stops for reactivation of the pushcoil and adjustment appointments.

8.9.2 Traction Distaliser

The avoidance of pushcoil means that this design readily facilitates the use of 1 mm diameter distaliser wire, which in turn provides favourable rigidity. The active component is a NiTi closing spring, which attaches onto hooks rather than directly onto the wire frame (Figure 8.10g). This traction component also provides a longer range of activation and hence requires less frequent reactivation than pushcoil.

8.9.3 Clinical Steps for a Midpalatal Distaliser

8.9.3.1 Preinsertion

1) Place separators adjacent to the maxillary first or second molars for one week.
2) Take an alginate impression with sized molar bands *in situ* or an intraoral scan, then replace the separators.

8.9.3.2 Laboratory Distaliser Fabrication

3) Cast or 3D print a working model and add appropriately sized molar bands.
4) Mark two parasagittal insertion points: 6–9 mm distal to the incisive foramen and 3–6 mm lateral to the midline (suture). This is typically in the same transverse plane as the premolars.
5) Drill the first pilot hole in the model, angled at 20–30° inclination towards the incisors.
6) Insert the first analogue and then fit an abutment onto this analogue.
7) Drill a second hole and insert the second analogue in a mirror image position on the other side and at the same inclination as the first one (Figure 8.11a). This parallel alignment is assisted by using the first abutment as a reference plane for the second drilling direction.
8) If it is planned that the distaliser will directly engage the mini-implant cross-slots then align the analogues to make these parallel. It is also worth forming an alignment wire from a piece of 0.019×0.025 in. steel archwire to fit into the analogue and mini-implant heads (Figure 8.11b). This is very useful at the clinical stage, to help with paralleling the cross-slots during final seating of the mini-implants (rather than repeatedly taking the whole distaliser in and out).
9) Solder headgear tubes onto the palatal aspect of the molar bands for the pushcoil version (Figure 8.10a,b), or to a wire extending anteriorly from the molar bands for the traction version (Figure 8.10g).
10) Form the distaliser frame by bending a 1.0 mm round wire with anterior loops to encircle the mini-implant positions, or by soldering an auxiliary 'clip' wire to the main wire, or by using a 0.019×0.025 in. steel archwire to fit through both the analogue slots and headgear tubes. Ideally, make the latter (narrow) wire frame more rigid by adding wire struts or metal tubing to the corner sections.

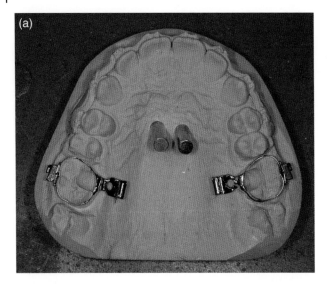
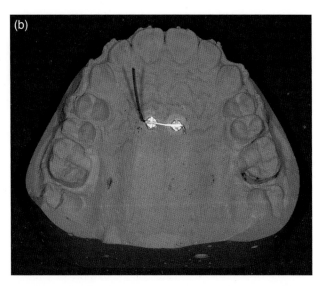

Figure 8.11 (a) Photograph of a working model showing two metal abutments placed onto midpalate implant analogues (already inserted in this model). These analogues were inserted parallel to each other, as reflected by the matching tilt of their abutments. Molar bands with 'flying' headgear tubes have been placed on the maxillary first molars. (b) A piece of 0.019 × 0.025 in. stainless steel archwire has been bent to fit into the cross-slots of two midpalate mini-implant heads. This wire may be used clinically to help line up parasagittal mini-implants so that their profiles (heights) and orientation correspond.

11) Traction version: solder a hook to the headgear tube then slide it (and the molar band assembly) onto the main distaliser wire. Pushcoil version: add a Gurin lock(s) and passive open coil spring(s) to the distaliser frame.

12) Leave an adequate length of the distaliser frame distal to the molars to provide sufficient distalisation range then coil the terminal ends (to avoid tongue irritation).

13) Make a stent (on the same dental model) according to the normal fabrication process, except that the median side of the guidance cylinders may need to be trimmed to enable both cylinders to seat on the model simultaneously (Figure 8.10c).

8.9.3.3 Mini-implant Selection

14) A short, wide-diameter mini-implant is indicated since the palate is an edentulous site with limited depth; for example, for Infinitas use the 2 mm diameter, 6 mm length, long neck version.

8.9.3.4 Insertion

15) Superficial anaesthesia of the insertion sites either directly or using nasopalatine and greater palatine blocks.

16) Fit the guidance stent.

17) Remove a punch of mucosal tissue from the insertion sites.

18) Perforate the cortical plate using a cortical punch.

19) Insert two mini-implants using a contra-angle handpiece.

20) If parallel cross-slots are required then use the alignment wire (Figure 8.11b) to check that these are level and parallel with one another on final seating (by small repeated clockwise rotations using the handpiece or a mini-screwdriver).

21) Cement the distaliser bands onto the molars and simultaneously seat the wire frame into or around the mini-implant heads. The active components should be passive at this point. The wire frame is secured by adding composite resin, by cinching the 'palatal clip' closed, or by adding ligature wires to the mini-implant heads.

22) Activate the distaliser by compressing the coil spring(s), through advancement of the Gurin lock(s) or adding crimpable stops onto the distaliser frame or by adding traction in the form of elastomeric chain.

8.9.3.5 Postinsertion

23) Check and if necessary reactivate the active components every 6–8 weeks; switch to NiTi closing springs for prolonged traction activity, or recompress the NiTi coil spring(s).

24) After the distalisation phase, use the distaliser to anchor the molar positions, as the premolar and anterior teeth are retracted.

25) Once anchorage is no longer required, trim the composite resin to separate the mini-implants and the distaliser frame, then remove the latter.

26) Explant the mini-implants using a contra-angle handpiece with counter-clockwise rotations.

8.9.4 Case Examples

1) **Midpalatal pushcoil distaliser – 'palatal clip' design (Figure 8.12)**

   - This case was treated by Dr Lars Christensen, an orthodontist in Oxford, UK.
   - A 24-year-old man presented with a Class II division 2 malocclusion on a mild skeletal II base with mild lower facial asymmetry (Figure 8.12a–h). The chin and the lower centreline were to the left side and he had asymmetrical buccal segment relationships: one-quarter II on the right and three-quarters II on the left sides. The third molars had erupted.
   - The aims of treatment were to achieve full alignment, Class II corrections and centreline correction.
   - Treatment options discussed included space provision by extraction of the upper premolars or upper third molars. The latter would require a bone-anchored distaliser with asymmetrical activation, followed by left Class II traction (to correct the lower dental centreline). The patient elected to have the distaliser treatment option.
   - 6 mm length IMT (long neck) Infinitas mini-implants were inserted parasagittally, in line with the first premolars. These were selected so that a 0.6 mm auxiliary section of steel wire could be added to the main 1 mm distaliser wire, creating a 'clip' to engage the external undercuts of the IMT heads (Figure 8.12i). This ovoid clip design also allowed for minor differences in the positions of the mini-implants and incomplete duplication of their heads in the working model.
   - The relatively distal insertion position was chosen for the mini-implants because the palatal mucosa was relatively thick more anteriorly. Consequently, the shape of the distaliser frame was modified to provide sufficient length for the pushcoil springs (Figure 8.12i).
   - The distaliser was seated passively and the auxiliary wire clip crimped to engage the mini-implant undercuts. The pushcoils were activated using Gurin locks on the 1 mm distaliser frame (Figure 8.12j).
   - The upper left premolars were bonded at the same time as distalisation began, to initiate their early alignment.
   - The rest of the upper fixed appliance, excluding the second molars, was bonded as distalisation progressed. The distalisation phase lasted nine months, by which time there had been asymmetrical distalisation to Class I on the left and one-quarter II on the right (Figure 8.12k–m). Most of the left side wire

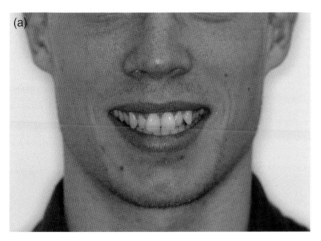
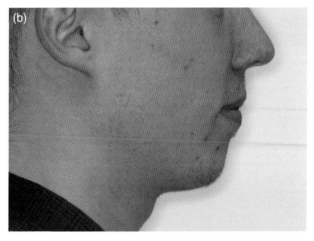

Figure 8.12 (a–f) Photographs showing a Class II division 2 malocclusion on a mild skeletal II base with mild lower facial asymmetry. The chin and lower centreline were displaced to the left side and the patient had asymmetric buccal segment relationships: one-quarter II on the right and three-quarters II on the left sides. There was mild dental crowding and the third molars had erupted. (g,h) Pretreatment radiographs, confirming the presence of all permanent teeth and the Class II features. (i) Working model made after the (IMT head) mini-implants had been inserted, and featuring the 'palatal clip' distaliser design. This has a 1 mm diameter wire frame and a 0.6 mm auxiliary section of steel wire soldered on its anterior aspect. Flying extraoral traction (EOT) tubes have been soldered on first molar bands, and bilateral pushcoil springs and Gurin locks added. Reservoir lengths of wire project distal to the EOT tubes, with their ends formed into a circular loop. (j) Distaliser fitted with the auxiliary wire 'clip' compressed between the mini-implants to engage their external undercuts. The pushcoils were activated using Gurin locks on the 1 mm distaliser frame. (k–n) Photographs taken at the end of the active distalisation phase and after the rest of the upper fixed appliance had been bonded. The buccal segment relationships were Class I on the left and one quarter II on the right sides. The left side of the distaliser had almost exhausted the wire reservoir on this side. Mild mucosal overgrowth was evident around the anterior 'elbows' of the distaliser frame. (o–r) Photographs taken several months after removal of the distaliser, and with full fixed appliances in place. Source: Case illustrations kindly provided by Dr Lars Christensen, Oxford, UK.

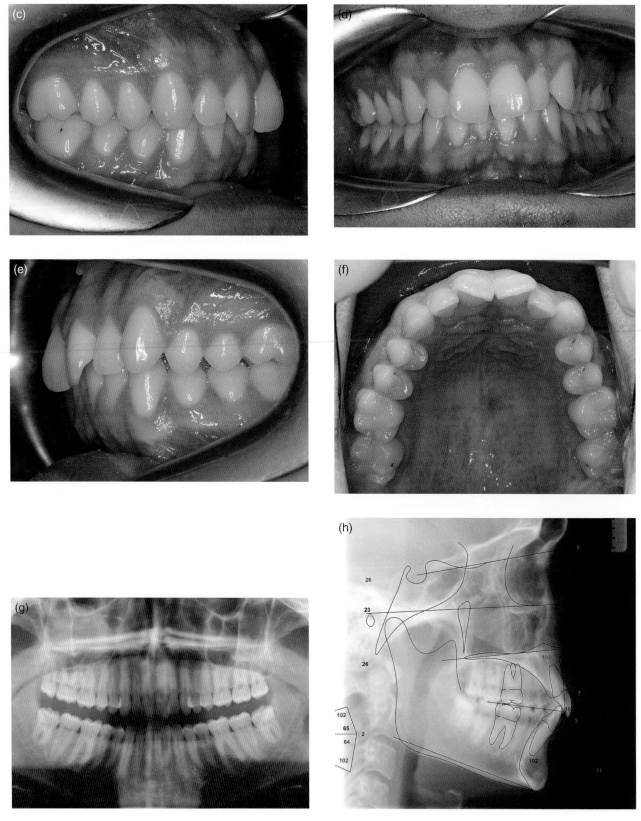

Figure 8.12 (Continued)

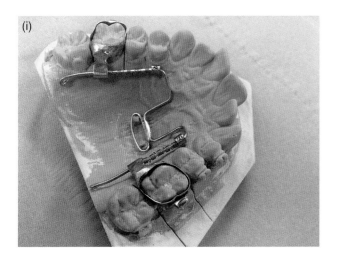

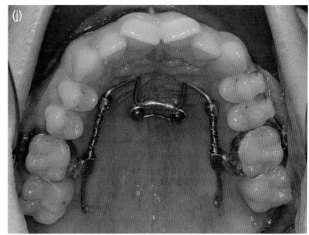

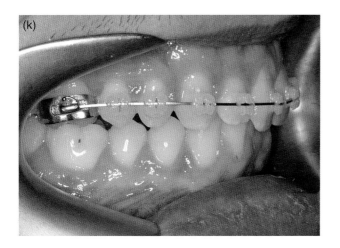

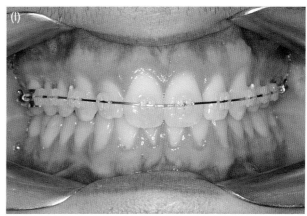

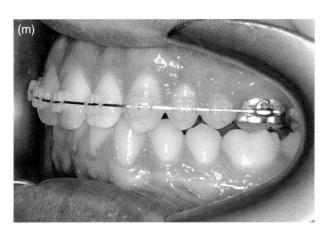

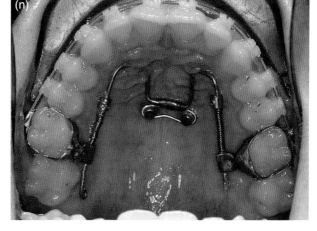

Figure 8.12 (Continued)

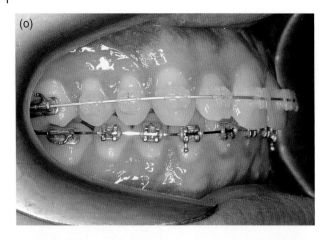

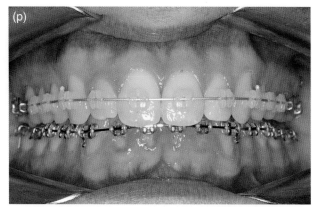

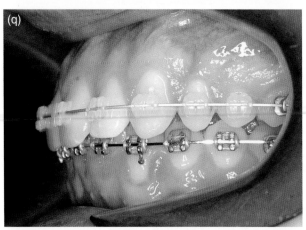

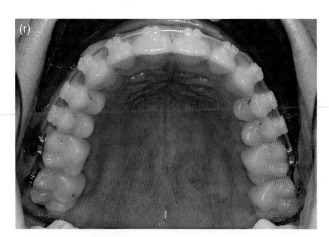

Figure 8.12 (Continued)

reservoir had been used during this distalisation (Figure 8.12n). There was mild mucosal overgrowth around the anterior 'elbows' of the distaliser frame.

- The distaliser and mini-implants were removed four months later, and conventional treatment continued with full fixed appliances, progressing to the stage of left Class II intermaxillary traction for final centreline and Class II corrections (Figure 8.12o–r).

2) **Midpalatal traction distaliser (Figure 8.13)**
   - A 16-year-old male presented with a Class III malocclusion on a moderate skeletal III base, and impacted upper second molars. His treatment plan involved fixed appliance alignment, with partial decompensation, and a maxillary advancement osteotomy. The impacted molars were removed during surgery, in order to avoid a second surgical procedure, and the immediate postoperative occlusion was planned to be Class II (Figure 8.13a–c). This would then be corrected by maxillary molar distalisation.
   - Two palatal mini-implants (Infinitas 2.0 mm diameter, 6 mm length, long neck versions) and a 'traction' distaliser were inserted two months after surgery (Figure 8.13d). This was fabricated to correct

a one-quarter and one-half unit Class II canine relationship on the right and left sides respectively, using NiTi coil spring traction. The first molars were banded and the distaliser loops were secured around the mini-implant heads with composite resin.

- Class I canine relationships were achieved after four months (Figure 8.13e,f). The molar relationships had been overcorrected and intrusion of the upper first molars was noted. The right limb of the distaliser was sectioned to allow settling, whilst the left side was retained for active anchorage during conventional retraction of the upper labial segment (Figure 8.13g).
- The distaliser was removed and the mini-implants explanted (after six months *in situ*) when it was obvious that some anchorage loss could be afforded during final space closure and finishing stages (Figure 8.13h–j). The fixed appliances were debonded, accepting the need for gradual settling of the intruded and distally tipped upper first molar positions (Figure 8.13k–m). This occurred during the retention period, as observed in final photographs taken two years later (Figure 8.13o,p).

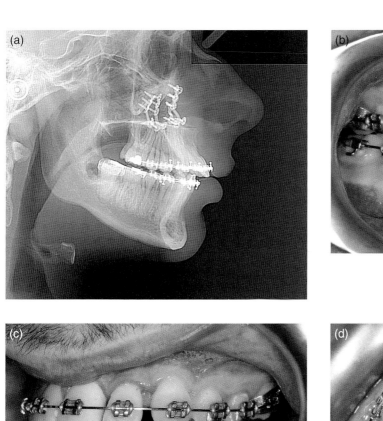
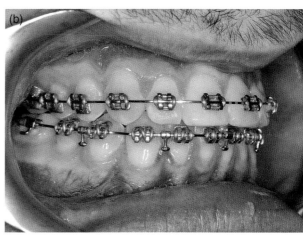
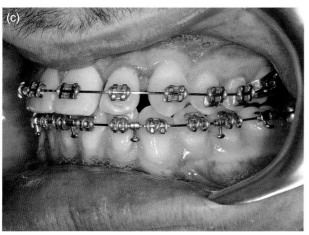
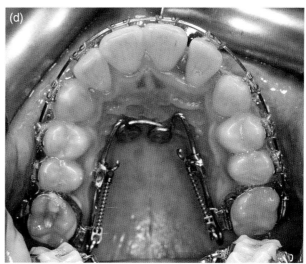
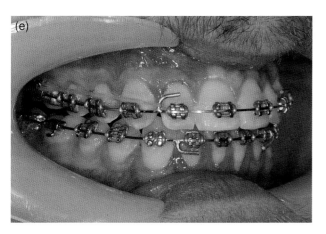
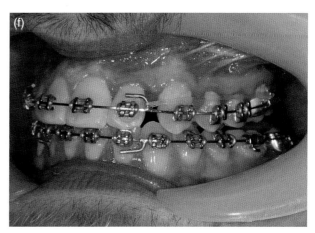

Figure 8.13 (a–d) Molar distalisation beginning after a maxillary advancement osteotomy (to an overcorrected Class II incisor relationship) and surgical removal of impacted upper second molars. (e,f) Molar intrusion occurred during distalisation with the 'traction' distaliser. At the same time, intra-arch elastomerics were used to retract the incisor teeth and move the centreline to the left. (g) The right side of the distaliser frame was cut off and unilateral traction continued on the left side. (h–k) End of the distaliser phase, with Class I canines and incisors, and a corrected maxillary centreline. The distaliser components and mini-implants were removed, and upper molars bonded to facilitate vertical settling. (k–m) Debond views showing a Class I occlusion, with incomplete occlusal contacts of the terminal molars. (n) Final cephalogram, showing the Class I parameters and distalised maxillary molar positions. (o,p) Photographs taken two years after debond, showing how the upper first molars have settled into a stable occlusion.

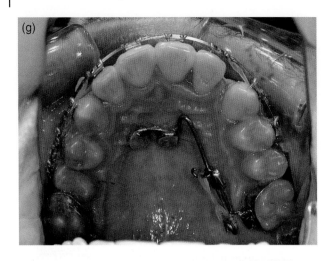

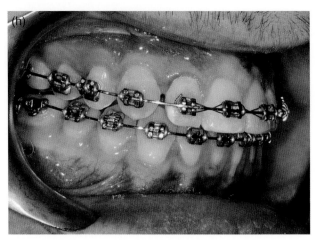

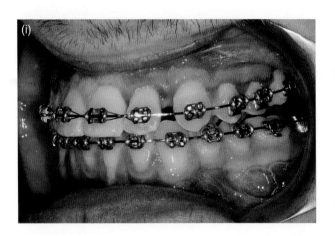

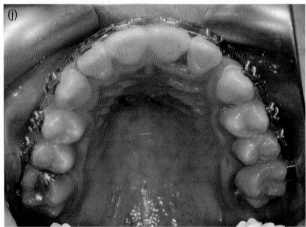

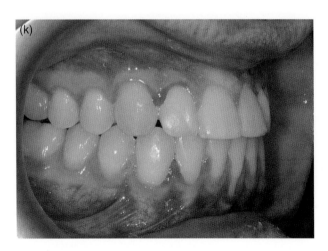

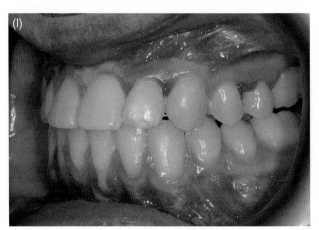

Figure 8.13 (Continued)

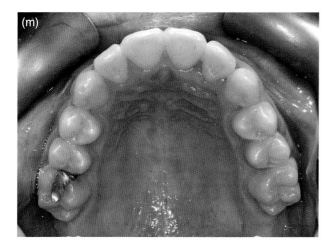
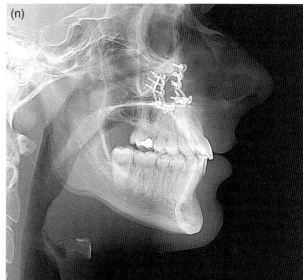
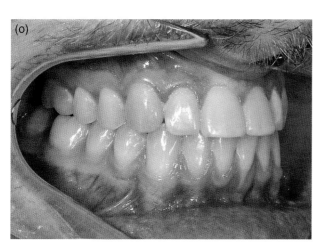
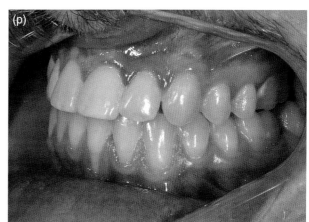

Figure 8.13 (Continued)

References

1 Da Costa Grec, R.H., Janson, G., and Branco, N.C. (2013). Intraoral distalizer effects with conventional and skeletal anchorage: a meta-analysis. *Am. J. Orthod. Dentofac. Orthop.* 143: 602–615.

2 Manni, A., Mutinelli, S., Pasini, M. et al. (2016). Herbst appliance anchored to miniscrews with 2 types of ligation: effectiveness in skeletal class II treatment. *Am. J. Orthod. Dentofac. Orthop.* 149: 871–880.

3 Von Bremen, J., Ludwig, B., and Ruf, S. (2015). Anchorage loss due to Herbst mechanics – preventable through miniscrews? *Eur. J. Orthod.* 37: 462–466.

4 Elkordy, S.A., Abouelezz, A.M., Salah Fayed, M.M. et al. (2016). Three-dimensional effects of the mini-implant–anchored Forsus Fatigue Resistant Device: a randomized controlled trial. *Angle Orthod.* 86: 292–305.

5 Gelgor, I.E., Karaman, A.I., and Buyukyilmaz, T. (2007). Comparison of 2 distalization systems supported by intraosseous screws. *Am. J. Orthod. Dentofac. Orthop.* 131: 161.e1–161e8.

6 Escobar, S.A., Tellez, P.A., Moncada, C.A. et al. (2007). Distalization of maxillary molars with the bone-supported pendulum: a clinical study. *Am. J. Orthod. Dentofac. Orthop.* 131: 545–549.

7 Sar, C., Kaya, B., Ozsoy, O., and Ozcirpici, A.A. (2013). Comparison of two implant-supported molar distalization systems. *Angle Orthod.* 83: 460–467.

8 Nienkemper, M., Wilmes, B., and Pauls, A. (2014). Treatment efficiency of mini-implant-borne distalization depending on age and second-molar eruption. *J. Orofac. Orthop.* 74: 1–14.

9 Chang, C., Sean, S.Y., Liu, W., and Roberts, W.E. (2015). Primary failure rate for 1680 extra-alveolar mandibular buccal shelf mini-screws placed in movable mucosa or attached gingiva. *Angle Orthod.* 85: 905–910.

10 Nucera, R., Lo Giudice, A., Bellocchio, A.M. et al. (2017). Bone and cortical bone thickness of mandibular buccal shelf for mini-screw insertion in adults. *Angle Orthod.* 87: 745–751.

11 Elshebiny, T., Palomo, J.M., and Baumgaertel, S. (2018). Anatomic assessment of the mandibular buccal shelf for miniscrew insertion in white patients. *Am. J. Orthod. Dentofac. Orthop.* 53: 505–511.

12 Kinzinger, G.S.M., Fritz, U.B., Sander, F., and Diedrich, P.R. (2004). Efficiency of a pendulum appliance for molar distalization related to second and third molar eruption stage. *Am. J. Orthod. Dentofac. Orthop.* 125: 8–23.

13 Oh, Y., Park, H., and Kwon, T. (2011). Treatment effects of microimplant-aided sliding mechanics on distal retraction of posterior teeth. *Am. J. Orthod. Dentofac. Orthop.* 139: 470–481.

14 Kinzinger, G., Gulden, N., Yildizhan, I. et al. (2008). Anchorage efficacy of palatally-inserted miniscrews in molar distalization with a periodontally/miniscrew-anchored distal jet. *J. Orofac. Orthop.* 69: 110–120.

15 Kinzinger, G.S.M., Gulden, N., Yildizhan, I., and Diedrich, P.R. (2009). Efficiency of a skeletonized distal jet appliance supported by miniscrew anchorage for noncompliance maxillary molar distalization. *Am. J. Orthod. Dentofac. Orthop.* 136: 578–586.

16 Oberti, G., Villegas, C., Ealo, M. et al. (2009). Maxillary molar distalisation with the dual-force distalizer supported by mini-implants: a clinical study. *Am. J. Orthod. Dentofac. Orthop.* 135: 282e1–282e5.

17 Polat-Ozsoy, O., Kırcelli, B.H., Arman-Özçırpıcı, A. et al. (2008). Pendulum appliances with 2 anchorage designs: conventional anchorage vs bone anchorage. *Am. J. Orthod. Dentofac. Orthop.* 133: 339.e9–339.e17.

18 Kook, Y., Bayome, M., Trang, V.T.T. et al. (2014). Treatment effects of a modified palatal anchorage plate for distalization evaluated with cone-beam computed tomography. *Am. J. Orthod. Dentofac. Orthop.* 146: 47–54.

19 Longerich, U.J.J., Matthias Thurau, M., and Kolk, A. (2014). Development of a new device for maxillary molar distalisation with high pseudoelastic forces to overcome slider friction: the Longslider – a modification of the Beneslider. *Oral Surg. Oral Med. Oral Pathol. Oral Radiol.* 118: 22–34.

20 Di Leonardo, B., Ludwig, B., Lisson, J.A. et al. (2018). Insertion torque values and success rates for paramedian insertion of orthodontic miniimplants. *J. Orofac. Orthop.* 79: 109–115.

9

Molar Protraction

Space closure in patients with either hypodontia or premature loss of buccal teeth is often difficult to manage with conventional orthodontics if the labial segment position needs to be preserved. This is particularly the case in uncrowded Class II cases with missing lower posterior teeth where conventional treatment results in worsening of the Class II features and facial profile. Instead, in these situations, the ideal space closure movement involves mesialisation (protraction) of the buccal teeth. However, conventional anchorage provides very limited options for anterior anchorage reinforcement during molar protraction, especially in the mandibular arch. This is because the anterior teeth form an inadequate anchorage unit, since the incisor teeth have a small total root surface area. Consequently, many orthodontists are historically reluctant to attempt closure of large posterior spaces, especially if retained deciduous molars are infraocclusal (indicating a vertical alveolar deficiency) or alveolar necking is present. Notably, these bone deficiencies also cause problems for dental implant treatment, so 'passing the buck' to the restorative dentist is not necessarily in the patient's interest either.

Fortunately, mini-implant anchorage now means that many more such patients can be treated orthodontically, and during adolescence (rather than delaying treatment for a restorative plan). However, one still needs to be realistic in terms of the difficulties posed by alveolar deficiencies. Therefore, it is crucial that each patient is assessed regarding their feasibility for space closure in terms of both the anchorage requirements and the edentulous site anatomy. In lieu of surgical alveolar ridge augmentation, substantial reductions in alveolar height and width may severely limit mesial movement of the posterior teeth, especially in hypodontia cases (where the alveolus is hypoplastic) or long-standing edentulous sites (where it has atrophied). Furthermore, remember that the molar which is immediately distal to such an alveolar deficiency is very prone to mesial tipping problems, although there are now biomechanical solutions for this problem whereby bodily movement can be promoted.

Having said that, remember that biomechanical side-effects may sometimes be beneficial, such as for reduction of a deep overbite. Therefore, this chapter aims to provide an understanding of how best to make mini-implant biomechanics work in individual cases, depending on their overbite.

> Assess the feasibility of space closure in terms of both the anchorage requirements and the edentulous site anatomy.

Mini-implant sites for molar protraction in the mandibular arch are limited to the buccal aspect of the alveolus. However, there are options for maxillary protraction. This can utilise options of either buccal or palatal alveolar sites for direct traction or the midpalate for both direct and indirect anchorage set-ups. Therefore, anchorage reinforcement for molar protraction may be subdivided into the following categories.

- *Direct buccal anchorage.* This involves the application of traction from the mini-implant head to a molar hook (Figure 9.1) or a powerarm (Figure 9.2a). It is relatively simple to apply at any stage of treatment and may be adjusted independent of other fixed appliance changes. Oblique traction to a standard molar hook may cause minimal vertical side-effects when the second premolar is present (Figure 9.1), but typically causes such problems when the edentulous space is immediately mesial to the target molar tooth. This will be discussed in detail in the following biomechanics section. In addition, if the anchorage site needs to be mesial to the canine (e.g. when space closure is required on the distal aspect of the canine) then the traction may impinge on the soft tissues adjacent to the canine as it traverses over the canine eminence (Figure 9.2a).
- *Indirect buccal anchorage.* The simplest version of this is to anchor the nearest canine or a premolar tooth to the mini-implant using either a ligature wire or a bonded

The Orthodontic Mini-Implant Clinical Handbook, Second Edition. Richard Cousley.
© 2020 John Wiley & Sons Ltd. Published 2020 by John Wiley & Sons Ltd.

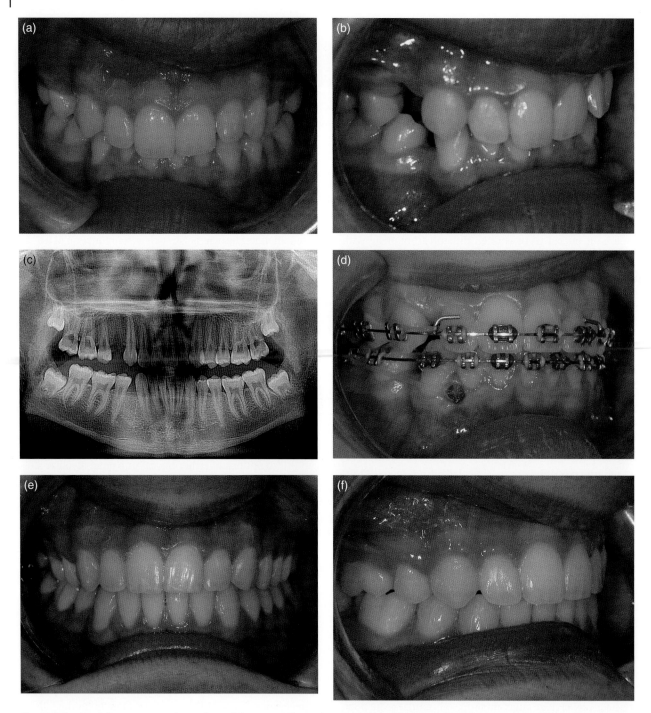

Figure 9.1 (a–c) Pretreatment views of an adolescent patient who presented with absent upper and lower right first premolar teeth. He had a deep overbite and lower centreline shift to the right side, so lower right molar protraction was indicated. (d) Oblique traction was applied from a mini-implant, inserted mesial to the canine, to the first molar hook. (e,f) Space closure was achieved without molar tipping side-effects, probably because the lower right second premolar buttressed the first molar tooth.

wire strut (Figure 9.2b). Alternatively, a cross-tube (two 0.028 × 0.025 in. rectangular tubes welded perpendicular to one another) provides a means of connecting a wire strut from the mini-implant to the archwire (Figure 9.2c). Traction is then applied from this vertical wire strut to

a molar hook, in a similar biomechanical fashion to conventional traction. This approach has the advantage of forming a vertical rigid link to a mini-implant where it has been inserted at a relatively apical level, as may be necessary when there is vertical alveolar hypoplasia

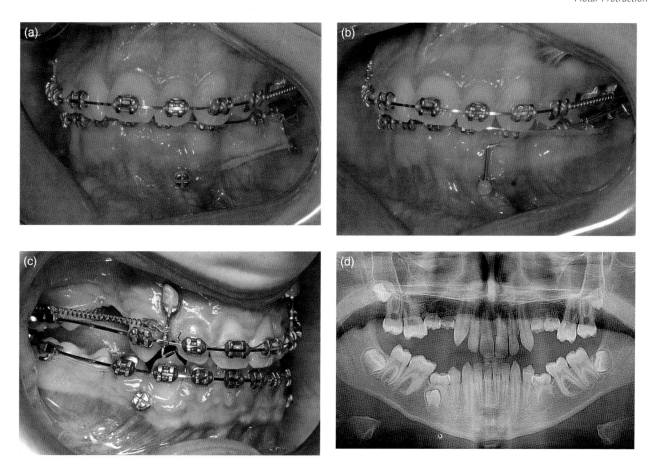

Figure 9.2 (a) The mini-implant was inserted mesial to the lower left canine in this adult patient, but the elastomeric traction caused mucosal trauma adjacent to the canine eminence. (b) The anchorage method was changed from direct to indirect, using a 0.019 × 0.025 in. steel wire to anchor the canine. Traction was then applied between the canine bracket and the molar hook. (c) Indirect anchorage using a vertical section of 0.019 × 0.025 in. wire connected to the main archwire via a cross-tube. A NiTi closing coil was attached between this vertical wire strut and the molar hook. (d) The pretreatment panoramic radiograph of the patient shown in (c), illustrating the vertical alveolar hypoplasia in this hypodontia patient, necessitating insertion of the mini-implants at relatively apical levels.

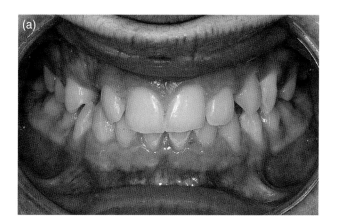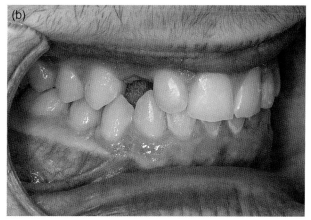

Figure 9.3 (a,b) Pretreatment views of a 14-year-old boy with a Class I malocclusion, an absent right maxillary canine, a small upper centreline shift to the right side and a Class I right molar relationship. (c,d) A lateral cephalogram and clinical view showing a 6 mm length midpalatal mini-implant and a 0.019 × 0.025 in. steel wire connection between the mini-implant and the palatal surfaces of the maxillary incisors. (e,f) Fixed appliances *in situ* with a wire ligature undertied from the upper lateral incisor to the left first molar. Elastomeric traction has been applied between the right lateral incisor and right molar teeth. (g,h) Photographs taken at debond showing the right maxillary space closed, full unit right Class II molar relationship and maintenance of the original small centreline discrepancy.

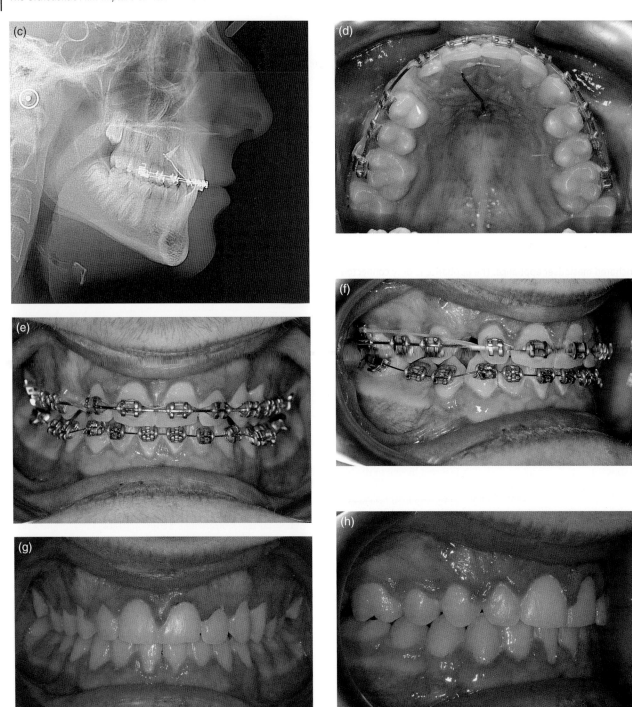

Figure 9.3 (Continued)

(Figure 9.2d). However, this cross-tube arrangement makes it very difficult to adjust other aspects of the fixed appliance (such as changing the archwire) during the traction phase.

- *Indirect palatal anchorage.* The simplest approach in utilising midpalate anchorage involves using one or two midpalatal mini-implants to anchor the anterior teeth. This requires a connecting wire bonded to the palatal surfaces of incisor teeth and a mini-implant head (Figure 9.3). However, it is possible that a rotational moment will affect a single mini-implant and that anchorage loss may occur due to distortion/bending of the connecting wire.

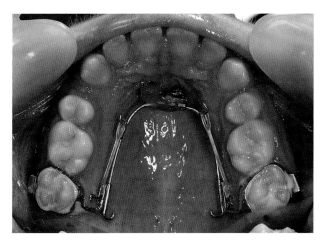

Figure 9.4 Direct palatal anchorage in the form of a bone-anchored mesialiser appliance. The appliance is only connected to the midpalatal mini-implants and the target molar teeth. Elastomeric traction provides the active component.

- *Direct palatal anchorage*. This typically involves a prefabricated midpalate appliance capable of molar protraction without involvement of any teeth in the dental arch (except the target teeth) (Figure 9.4). However, it is also feasible to add a 'T' bar component which acts as an anterior extension to contact and stabilise the palatal surfaces of the upper incisors [1]. A directly anchored mesialiser appliance requires one or two midpalate mini-implants to anchor the mesialiser appliance and traction components. It has the benefit of avoiding a fixed appliance during this phase, but does require more preparatory steps.

9.1   Clinical Objective

- To prevent distal movement of the anterior teeth during molar protraction for closure of a posterior space (e.g. a second deciduous molar or permanent molar site).

9.2   Treatment Options

- Buccal alveolar mini-implant anchorage (direct or indirect) in either arch.
- Palatal alveolar mini-implant (direct) anchorage.
- Indirect anchorage of upper incisors using midpalate mini-implants.
- Midpalate mini-implant protraction appliance (mesialiser).
- Indirect anchorage using buccal mini-implants for intermaxillary traction.
- Conventional anchorage, for example protraction headgear or intermaxillary elastics.

- Alteration of the skeletal base by orthognathic surgical or orthopaedic appliance treatments, in order to offset anterior anchorage loss (incisor retraction).

9.3   Key Treatment Planning Considerations

- The molar, incisor and centreline relationships.
- The quantity (volume) and quality of the alveolar ridge in the edentulous space. If a deciduous tooth is still present, is it ankylosed, or did infection or other pathology cause bone loss?
- The depth and shape of the palatal vault, since a high-arched palate makes it difficult to insert mini-implants in the midpalate region.
- The interproximal bone volume at the proposed mini-implant (alveolar) site, in terms of both the mesiodistal space (root divergence) and buccolingual alveolar depth. Limitations in both dimensions mean that an oblique angle of mini-implant insertion and possibly a shorter body length are preferable. Alternatively, as suggested by expert German orthodontist Dr Björn Ludwig, a long mini-implant may be inserted perpendicular to the surface with the aim of bicortical engagement. This option requires additional lingual anaesthesia and then composite resin coverage of the mini-implant tip, if it projects beyond the lingual tissues, risking tongue irritation. In addition to the benefit of bicortical anchorage support [2], this lingual projection may also be used to provide supplementary traction to the lingual side of the molar, hence reducing the risk of molar rotation during mesialisation. However, in practical terms, it is difficult to manage bicortical engagement, meaning that it is not a routine option.
- The amount of mesialisation required and whether this differs on each side of the arch.

9.4   Biomechanical Principles

- Hypodontia cases may have limited alveolar bone width and/or height at the mini-implant insertion site. The alveolus may be vertically underdeveloped (Figure 9.2d) or narrow and lacking a canine eminence (if the canine erupted in an ectopic position).
- Prepare the fixed appliance ready for mini-implant insertion (by divergence of adjacent roots) and the simultaneous initiation of space closure by progressing to a rigid working archwire, for example a 0.019 × 0.025 in. stainless steel one.
- If a lengthy period of initial alignment is required, then consider delaying any extractions, especially of ankylosed

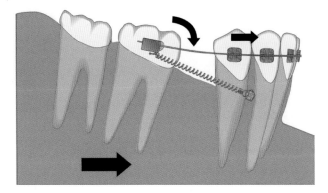

Figure 9.5 Diagram of the side-effects of oblique traction from an anterior mini-implant to the first molar hook and a reduction in the adjacent alveolar height. Molar tipping causes archwire binding and advancement, resulting in incisor protraction and intrusion.

deciduous molars, until the arch is ready for the immediate start of space closure. Otherwise, alveolar resorption will occur at an already compromised site and quickly limit space closure.

- Indirect anchorage of an anterior tooth means that the traction is limited in terms of bodily control of the molar since it is applied at the coronal level (in a similar manner to conventional traction) (Figure 9.2b).

- Forces applied at the coronal level will tip molars mesially during protraction, especially if there is a vertical alveolar deficiency on the mesial aspect of the molar (Figure 9.5). This also tends to be worse if a second molar is unavailable or not attached to the fixed appliance to help control the first molar alignment.

- Mesial tipping of molar teeth causes archwire binding within the molar tube. This manifests clinically as protraction (mesial shunting) of the entire dental arch, and incisor proclination and intrusion. This is detected as a reduction in overjet and overbite (Figure 9.6). It may be counteracted by supplementary (conventional) traction which provides a retractive force on the incisors (Figure 9.6c,d).

- The use of a posterior powerarm, to apply traction at the molar furcation level, assists bodily movement of the molar and protraction-type space closure (Figure 9.7) [3]. Powerarms provide the best form of bodily control when either connected to the molar tube or bonded directly onto a molar crown (Figure 9.8). The former approach involves placement of a double tube attachment on at least one molar per dental quadrant, and then fabrication of a steel powerarm from a piece of rigid archwire, for example 0.021 × 0.025 in. size.

- Traction on the buccal side of the target tooth causes a molar rotation side-effect, and hence archwire binding, although this is less of an issue than mesial tipping problems. Therefore, it is ideal if supplementary traction is applied simultaneously on the lingual aspect of the

molar crown, by the addition of a lingual cleat (Figure 9.9). A finite element analysis study has shown that the lingual force should be approximately one-third of the buccal force level [3]. I find it easiest to use 'powerchain' for this purpose, which delivers a lower force level than the buccal elastomeric traction.

> Consider delaying any extractions, especially of ankylosed deciduous molars, until the arch is ready for the immediate start of space closure.

9.5 Midtreatment Problems and Solutions

- Bond or band the second molar, in each relevant quadrant, prior to space closure, since this helps to control mesial tipping of the first molar and enables direct closure of any intermolar spaces.

- Ideally, apply traction to a buccal powerarm, balanced with lingual traction, in order to optimise bodily molar movement.

- A shallow posterior buccal sulcus depth may prevent initial placement of a powerarm, especially on the terminal molar, but this can be added once sufficient mesial movement of the molar moves it into an area with more sulcus depth.

- If there are signs of unfavourable incisor intrusion then add a bite-closing curve to the archwire.

- If incisor advancement and proclination occur, as a result of archwire binding, then add supplementary traction from a molar hook to either an anterior archwire hook or the linked block of anterior teeth (Figure 9.2b,c).

> The use of a posterior powerarm, to apply traction at the molar furcation level, assists bodily molar movement and unidirectional space closure.

9.6 Clinical Steps for Molar Protraction Using Alveolar Site Anchorage

9.6.1 Preinsertion

1) Determine the optimum mini-implant insertion site(s), for example mesial or distal to the first premolar, depending on whether the second premolar is present. It is preferable to avoid insertions mesial to the canines because of limited interproximal space here and the risk

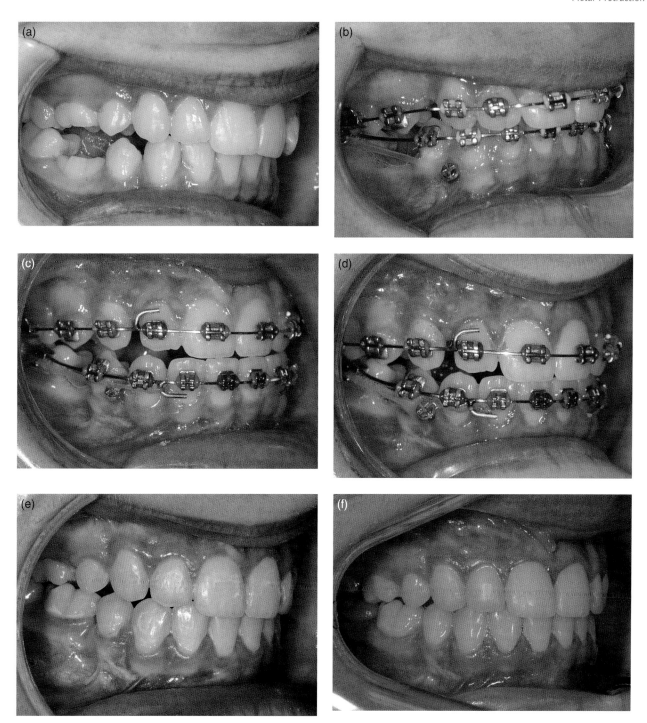

Figure 9.6 Right buccal photographs of (a) an adolescent girl who presented with a Class II division 2 malocclusion and absent second premolars. (b) An oblique vector of elastomeric traction applied from the mandibular mini-implant, inserted mesial to the first premolar, directly to the first molar hook. This resulted in (c) a reduction in the overjet and overbite as the lower incisors proclined and intruded. Elastomeric traction was then added between the molar and archwire hooks, to prevent mesial movement of the archwire. (d) Control of the incisor relationship had been achieved after eight weeks of combined traction and this continued during the complete phase of molar protraction. (e) The occlusion at debond and (f) a view of the stable, settled occlusion 18 months later.

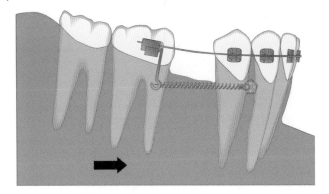

Figure 9.7 Diagram of bodily molar protraction utilising a powerarm connected to the molar tube to achieve a horizontal vector of traction.

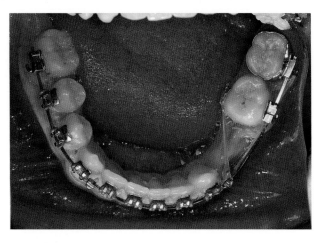

Figure 9.9 Supplementary elastomeric traction applied from the (buccal) archwire hook to a lingual cleat on the left mandibular first molar.

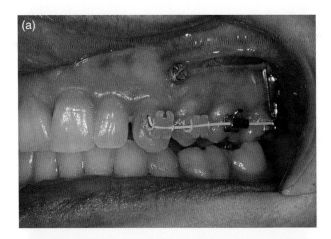

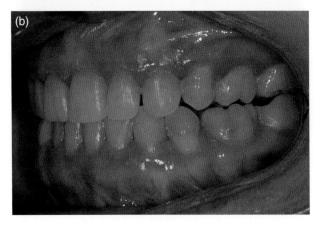

Figure 9.8 (a) An adult patient with a double molar tube bonded on the upper left second molar. A 0.019 × 0.025 in. steel wire has been used to fabricate a powerarm which engages the auxiliary molar tube and matches the vertical level of the mini-implant. (b) Debond view showing mesialisation of the left maxillary dentition without vertical side-effects (e.g. a lateral openbite).

of the traction auxiliary traumatising the soft tissue over the canine eminence/'corner' of the arch (Figure 9.2a).

2) Increase the available interproximal space by bonding the adjacent teeth at altered attachment tips; for example, for an insertion distal to the canine add mesial tip to the canine bracket, causing the root to move mesially (away from the insertion site) during initial alignment.

3) Bond a double tube on either the first or second molar(s).

4) Align and level the arch ready for insertion of a 0.019 × 0.025 in. stainless steel archwire.

5) Arrange the extraction of retained posterior teeth, for example ankylosed deciduous molars, with a view to commencing space closure immediately (before alveolar resorption occurs). It is helpful to request that the buccal and lingual sides of the extraction socket should not be compressed (as is customary following extractions), so that the alveolar width is not actively restricted.

> Request that the buccal and lingual sides of the extraction socket should not be compressed (as is customary following extractions), so that the alveolar width is not actively restricted.

9.6.2 Mini-implant Selection

6) Maxilla: use a long mini-implant especially if the alveolus appears to be diminutive at the insertion site, for example a 1.5 mm diameter, 9 mm length, short neck Infinitas™ version.

7) Mandible: the length selection depends on the anticipated cortical depth and density; select a long (9 mm) body length in an adolescent patient or if angulated insertion is indicated (because of limited attached

gingival height). A short (e.g. 6 mm Infinitas version) is usually sufficient in adults if there is sufficient attached gingival depth and cortical density to enable the insertion to be vertically perpendicular to the bone surface.

9.6.3 Insertion

8) Superficial anaesthesia of the insertion site.
9) Identify the ideal buccal alveolar insertion point, through attached gingiva (which precludes the need for a soft tissue punch step), and either mesial or distal to the first premolar.
10) Determine the angles of insertion. All mini-implants are inserted into the interproximal space and perpendicular to the surface in the horizontal plane. In vertical terms, maxillary mini-implants may be inserted either perpendicular to the surface or at an oblique angle (up to 30° in an apical direction). Mandibular insertions are generally perpendicular to the vertical plane unless a lack of attached gingival height necessitates an oblique (apically directed) angle of insertion.
11) Manual screwdriver insertion is normally feasible where physical access (e.g. stretching of the cheek) is sufficient for correct screwdriver orientation. A cortical bone punch is recommended as the first step for mandibular buccal sites in adult patients.
12) Take an intraoral radiograph if close root proximity is suspected.
13) Complete insertion to the point where the mini-implant neck is partially submerged but the head is fully accessible.

9.6.4 Postinsertion

14) Ideally, add a powerarm, formed from a 0.019 or 0.021×0.025 in. rectangular steel wire, through the molar auxiliary tube, with an appropriate length to create a horizontal line of traction (parallel to the occlusal plane). The exception to this occurs if the buccal sulcus depth is too shallow for a powerarm to be comfortable.
15) Immediately load the mini-implant with a low force level (approximately 50 g) for the first 5–6 weeks, using a lightly stretched powerchain. Subsequently apply traction using a NiTi coil spring or elastomeric auxiliary.
16) Bond a lingual cleat (Figure 9.9) on the lingual surface of the target molar crown. Apply light (e.g. powerchain) traction from this to either the buccal aspect of the fixed appliance or a lingual cleat on the ipsilateral canine tooth. This supplementary traction will reduce archwire winding effects and promote bodily molar movement.
17) Add supplementary (conventional) buccal traction and/or a bite closing archwire curve if the incisor

relationship changes unfavourably in terms of incisor proclination and intrusion. The simplest form of additional traction is from a posted archwire hook to the molar (Figure 9.6b–d).
18) Discontinue the traction and consider explanting the mini-implant once sufficient space closure has occurred and the protracted teeth are upright.

9.7 Case Examples

1) **Direct molar protraction: example 1 (Figure 9.10)**
   - A 17-year-old female with a Class II division 2 malocclusion, an absent upper left second premolar and retained second deciduous molar, Class I molar relationships, and left Class II canine relationship. The dental centrelines were coincident but both displaced to the left side by 2 mm (Figure 9.10a–f). The upper third molars were present and unerupted (Figure 9.10g). The treatment plan involved extraction of the retained maxillary deciduous molar and closure of its space by molar protraction (to finish to a full unit left Class II molar relationship and coincident dental centrelines).
   - The arches were aligned with fixed appliances, and the upper left space reduced to a single unit space by conventional retraction of the upper left canine into a Class I position (Figure 9.10h–k). A buccal mini-implant (Infinitas 1.5×9 mm version) was then inserted distal to the upper left canine and oblique elastomeric traction applied to a conventional molar hook (Figure 9.10j).
   - The mini-implant was explanted once the upper left molar had been mesialised into a three-quarter unit Class II relationship and there was scope for anchorage loss. This was due to mesial movement of all the upper left buccal teeth as a side-effect of the oblique traction. There was an associated movement of the upper centreline to the right and opening of a partial left lateral openbite (Figure 9.10k–o). This allowed scope for final conventional space closure, accompanied by right Class III traction to correct the lower centreline.
   - The fixed appliances were debonded once final space closure and Class I features and coincident centrelines had been achieved (Figure 9.10p–t).
   - Superimposition of the pretreatment (brown) and debond (green) digital models of the maxillary arch showed one unit mesial movement of both upper left molar teeth (Figure 9.10u,v).
2) **Direct protraction: example 2 (Figure 9.11)**
   - A 15-year-old hypodontia patient with a Class II division 2 malocclusion on a mild skeletal II base with a reduced mandibular plane angle. She had absence of six teeth: right maxillary canine, left mandibular first

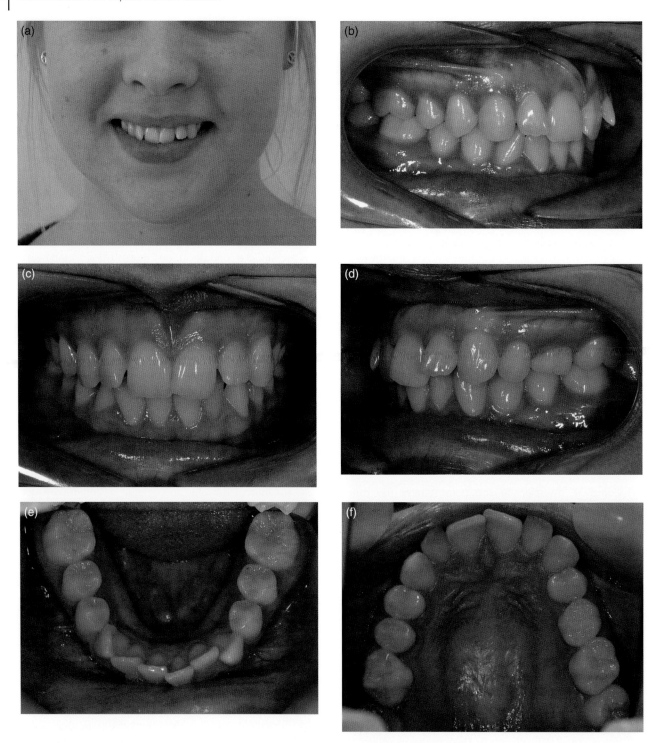

Figure 9.10 (a–f) Pretreatment views showing the Class II division 2 malocclusion with mild anterior crowding and a retained upper left second deciduous molar. The left canine and molar relationships were Class II and Class I respectively. The dental centrelines were coincident but both displaced to the left side by 2 mm. (g) A panoramic radiograph shows that the upper left second premolar was absent but the upper third molars were present. (h–k) The arches were aligned with fixed appliances, and the upper left space reduced to a single unit space by conventional retraction of the upper left canine into a Class I position. (j) A buccal mini-implant (Infinitas 1.5 × 9 mm version) was inserted distal to the upper left canine and oblique elastomeric traction applied to a conventional molar hook. (k–o) The mini-implant was explanted once the upper left molar had been mesialised into a three-quarter unit Class II relationship. The oblique vector of traction and archwire binding had resulted in mesial movement of all the upper left buccal teeth, opening of a partial left lateral openbite, and an associated movement of the upper centreline towards the right side. (p–t) The debond views showing full space closure, with Class I features and coincident centrelines. (u) The pretreatment (*brown*) and debond (*green*) digital models of the maxillary arch. Their superimposition (v) showed one unit mesial movement of both upper left molar teeth.

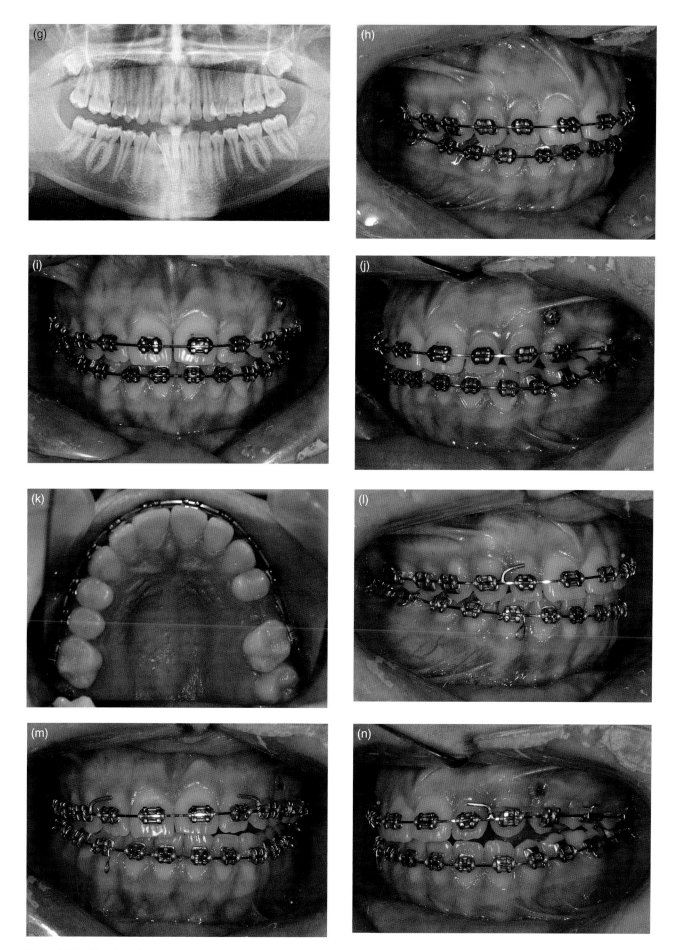

Figure 9.10 (Continued)

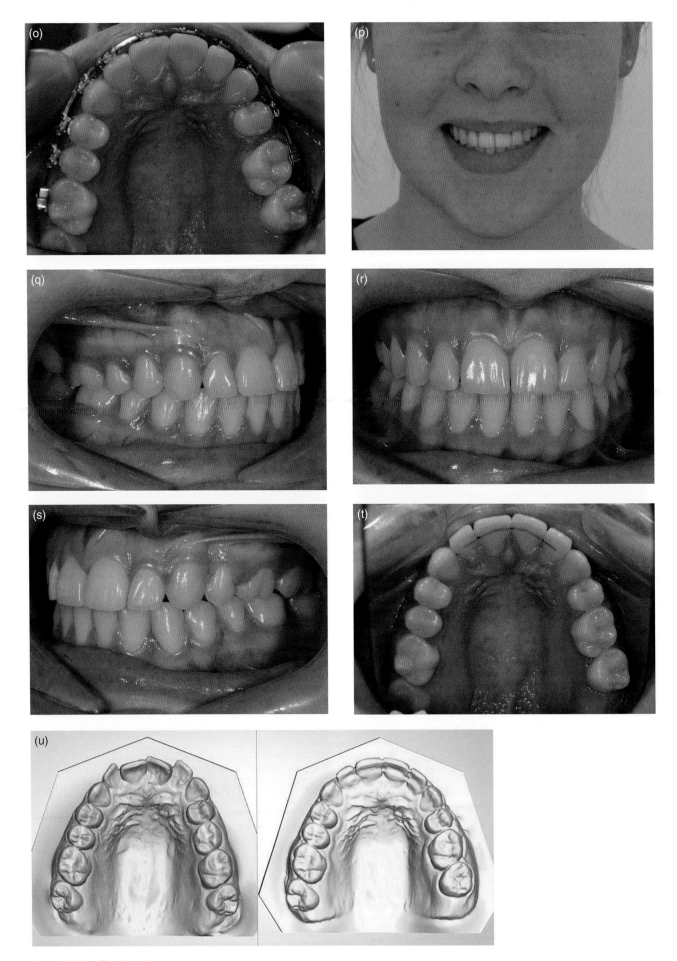

Figure 9.10 (Continued)

(v)

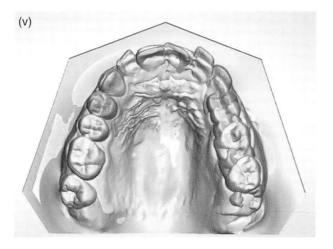

Figure 9.10 (Continued)

premolar and all second premolars. The retained lower second deciduous molars were ankylosed (Figure 9.11a–h). The treatment goals included achieving a Class I occlusion and closure of four quadrant premolar spaces. Ideally, this required lower molar protraction rather than lower incisor retraction (and a worsening of the Class II features and deep overbite).

- Both arches were aligned and levelled with fixed appliances (Figure 9.11i–l). Indeed, overcorrection of the deep overbite had been achieved although partly by premature contact on extruded premolar teeth.
- The two ankylosed lower deciduous molars were extracted once the appliances had 0.019×0.025 in. steel archwires *in situ*, ready for space closure (Figure 9.11k).
- Bilateral buccal mini-implants (Infinitas 1.5×9 mm version) were inserted distal to the mandibular canine and immediate light elastomeric traction applied (Figure 9.11i–k).
- Supplementary buccal traction was applied, from the archwire hooks to lower molar hooks, in order to prevent expression of excessive proclination and intrusion side-effects on the mandibular incisors.
- Supplementary traction was later applied to lingual cleats on the lower first molars (rather than the buccal molar hooks). This was balanced with the buccal traction to achieve substantial molar protraction, without lingual movement of the lower incisors, as seen after one year of traction (Figure 9.11n–p).
- An increase in the forces applied to the lower molar lingual cleats resulted in a deepening of the overbite, through deliberate uprighting of the lower incisor positions (Figure 9.11q,r).
- Treatment was completed after approximately two years of molar traction and a settling phase, achieving a Class I finish in terms of both the occlusion and

facial profile. Potential spaces were retained in the upper right canine and lower left first premolar sites. The mandibular molars had been protracted by more than a unit and the overbite greatly reduced (Figure 9.11t–x). Space was also now available for normal eruption of the lower third molar teeth and these teeth had spontaneously migrated into favourable mesial positions (Figure 9.11s and x).

3) **Direct protraction: example 3 (Figure 9.12)**

- This case illustrates when the side-effect of oblique traction for molar protraction is favourable. This 47-year-old hypodontia patient had previously had orthodontic treatment to close her lower second deciduous molar spaces, but this had resulted in retraction of the lower labial segment and an increased overjet, which the patient now wished to have corrected. She presented with a Class II division 2 malocclusion on a mild skeletal II base with a reduced mandibular plane angle. She had absence of the right maxillary first premolar and first molar teeth and the second premolars in the other three quadrants. The overjet was 7 mm and the overbite was deep, although the patient habitually postured her mandible to camouflage this overjet (Figure 9.12a–f).
- Treatment was complicated by a dental implant restoration in the right maxillary premolar region. It was therefore agreed to avoid maxillary arch treatment, and ideally correct the increased overjet and overbite features by whole lower arch protraction.
- The lower arch was aligned and levelled with a fixed appliance, then the premolar spaces were reopened with pushcoil springs until the incisors and canines were essentially in Class I positions. The mandibular canine brackets were then repositioned to diverge the canine and first premolar roots (Figure 9.12g–i).

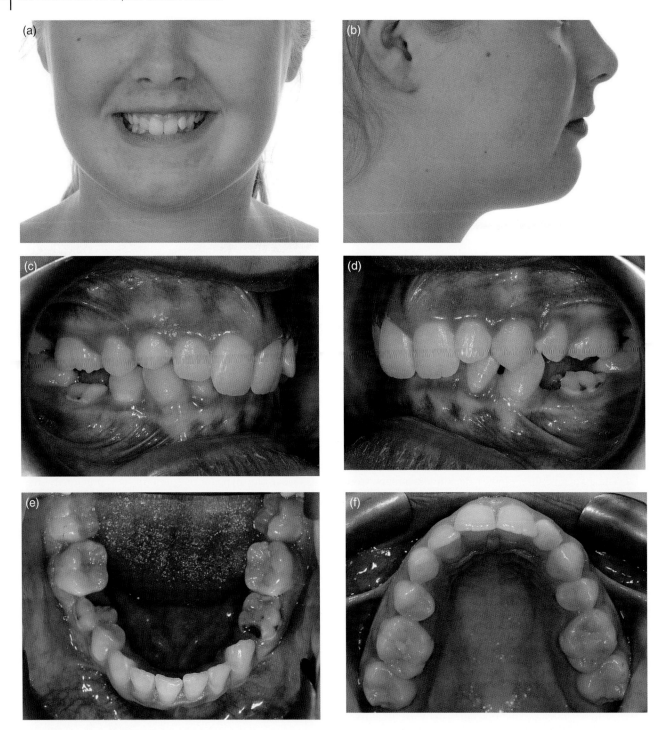

Figure 9.11 (a–f) Pretreatment views showing this Class II division 2 malocclusion on a mild skeletal II base with a reduced mandibular plane angle. The upper right deciduous canine and lower second deciduous molars were present, with ankylosis of the latter. (g,h) Pretreatment radiographs confirmed these clinical features and absence of the upper right canine, lower left first premolar and all second premolars. However, all third molars were present. (i–m) Photographs of the dentition and a lateral cephalogram taken after extraction of the ankylosed lower second deciduous molars and at the time of mini-implant insertions distal to the lower canine teeth. Light elastomeric traction connected the mini-implants and first molar hooks. (n–p) Photographs showing lingual cleats on the lower first molars and two forms of supplementary traction: from anterior archwire hooks to buccal molar hooks and to the lingual cleats. (q,r) An increase in the overjet and overbite was seen two months later. (s) A panoramic radiograph taken at the end of space closure, showing mild mesial tipping of the lower first molars and substantial improvements in the positions of the developing third molars. (t–x) Debond photographs showing a Class I finish in terms of both the occlusion and facial profile. Potential spaces were retained in the upper right canine and lower left first premolar sites.

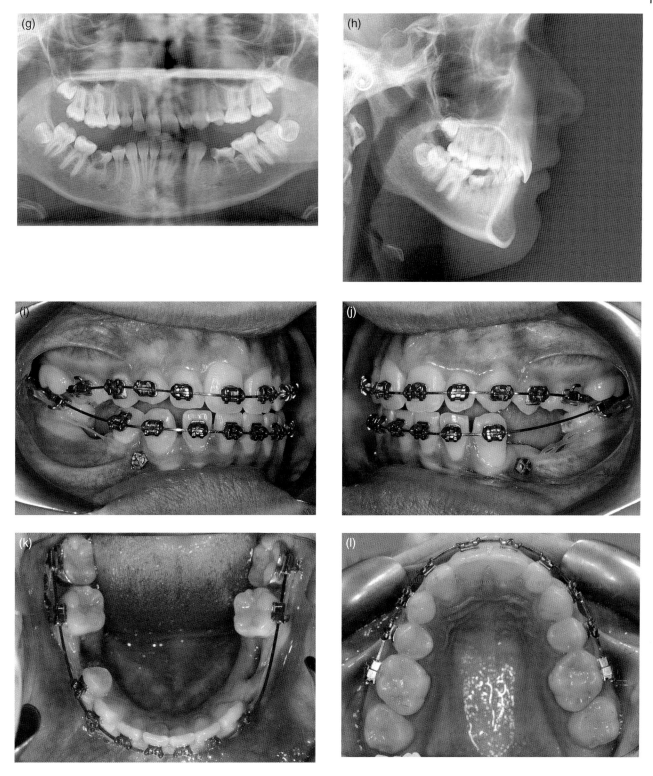

Figure 9.11 (Continued)

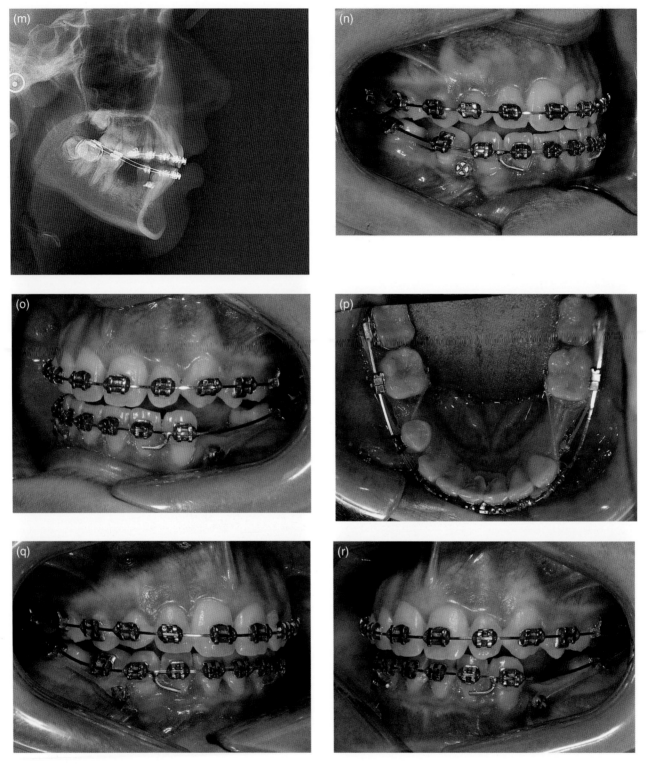

Figure 9.11 (Continued)

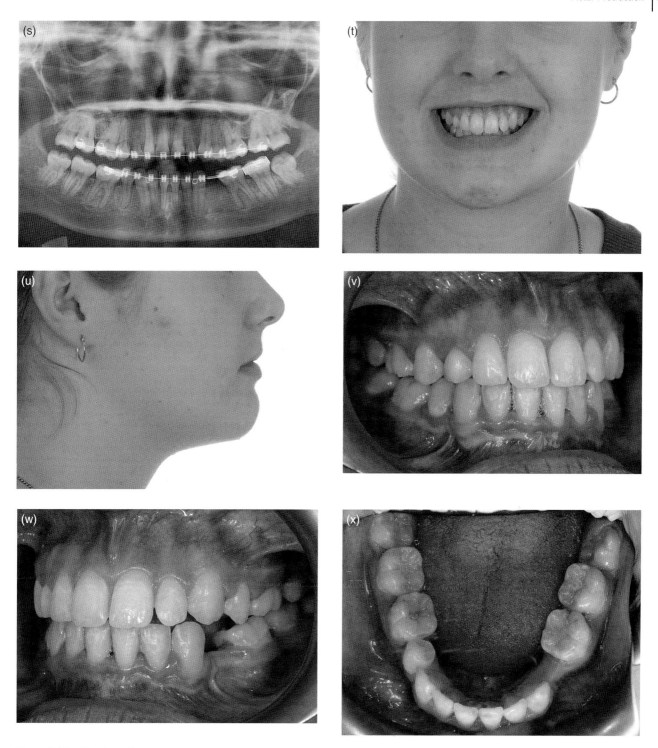

Figure 9.11 (Continued)

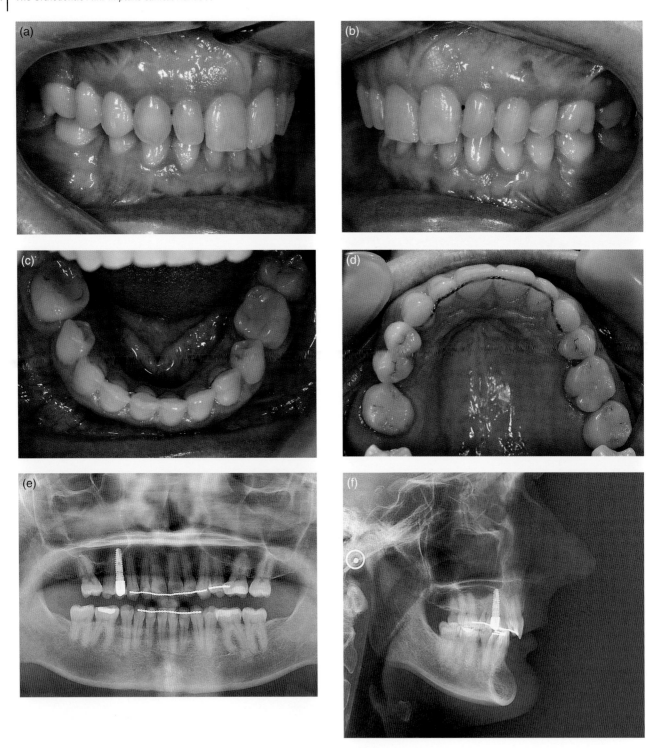

Figure 9.12 (a–f) Pretreatment views showing this Class II division 2 malocclusion on a mild skeletal II base with a reduced mandibular plane angle. The overjet was 7 mm in the retruded contact position and the overbite was deep. (e) The pretreatment panoramic radiograph confirms absence of the right maxillary first premolar and first molar teeth and the second premolars in the other three quadrants. It also shows a restored dental implant restoration in the right maxillary premolar region. (g–i) The lower arch had been initially aligned and levelled with a fixed appliance, then the premolar spaces had been reopened. These photographs show that the canines were essentially in Class I positions and the mandibular canine brackets had additional mesial tip. (j–l) Views taken after insertion of the bilateral buccal mini-implants, distal to the mandibular canine and the oblique elastomeric traction applied to the first molars. (m–o) Photographs taken when the mandibular spaces had been closed and the canine brackets replaced to reflect the distally tipped canine angulation. (p–r) Debond views showing Class I incisor and canine relationships.

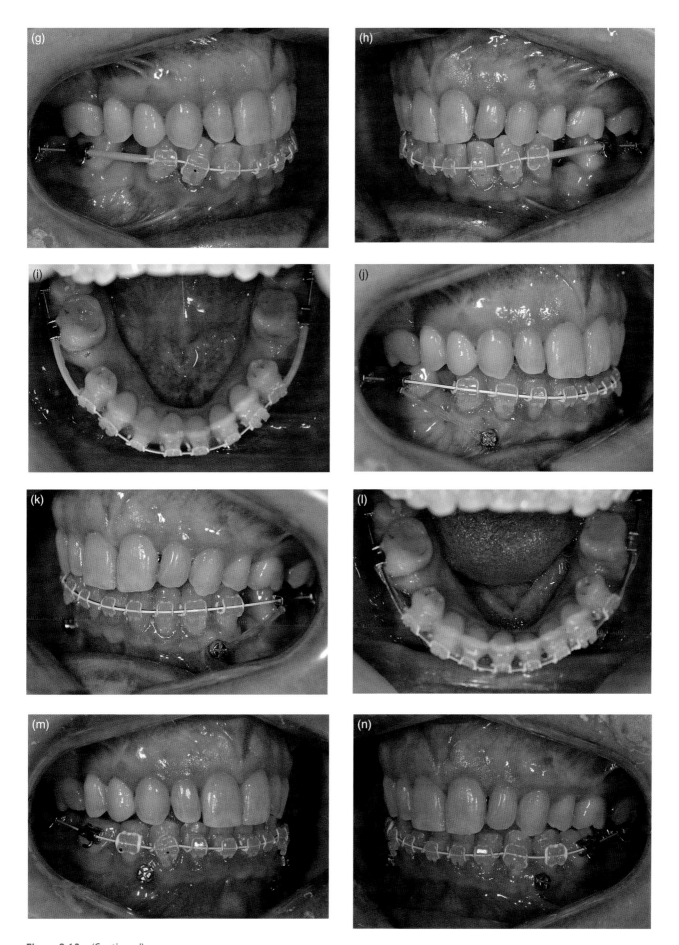

Figure 9.12 (Continued)

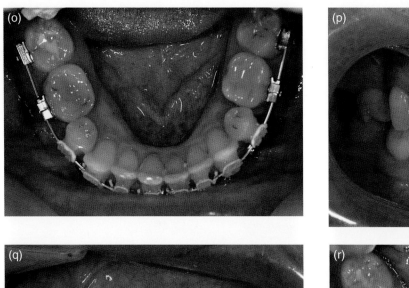

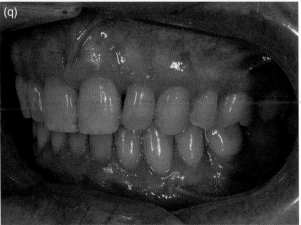

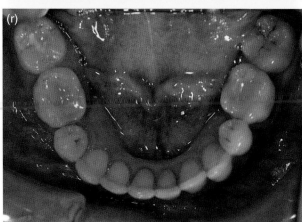

Figure 9.12 (Continued)

- Bilateral buccal mini-implants (Infinitas 1.5×9 mm version) were inserted distal to the mandibular canine and immediate oblique elastomeric traction applied to the first molars (Figure 9.12j–l). This was then switched to the second molar hooks, but no supplementary traction was applied to the lingual aspects or the labial segment.
- The canine brackets were replaced, to reflect the distally tipped canine angulation, once space closure had been achieved and the molars were in Class III positions (Figure 9.12m–o). Uprighting of the tipped canines would then move their crowns into Class I positions, ready for debond three months later (Figure 9.12p–r).

4) **Direct protraction: example 4 (Figure 9.13)**
   - This case illustrates the difficulties which occur when the only suitable mini-implant insertion site is in a space due for closure. This 14-year-old boy presented with a Class I malocclusion with bimaxillary proclination. The mandibular canine teeth were severely ectopic (Figure 9.13a) and required surgical removal. The lower second molar teeth were impacted and required space for alignment. Loss of the lower canines was to be balanced by extraction of the upper second premolar teeth for alignment and incisor retraction purposes (Figure 9.13b–f).

- Both arches were aligned and levelled with fixed appliances and maxillary arch anchorage was assisted with a Nance palatal arch (Figure 9.13g–j).
- Bilateral buccal mini-implants (Infinitas 1.5×9 mm version) were inserted distal to the mandibular lateral incisor and immediate light elastomeric traction applied to the first molar hooks (Figure 9.13k–o). The mode of traction was then changed to molar power-arms, after replacement of the standard molar tubes with double tubes (Figure 9.13l–p).
- Powerarm traction allowed a thinner NiTi archwire to be used, which in turn enabled extension of the fixed appliance to the impacted second molars (Figure 9.13l–p).
- Despite the use of powerarm traction, the lower incisors were proclined during the molar protraction phase. However, this meant that the final mandibular arch space closure could be achieved after removal of the mini-implants, clearing the way for space closure (Figure 9.13q–u).
- Treatment was completed once the spaces had been closed and Class I incisors, canines and molar positions achieved (Figure 9.13v–z). The mandibular second molars had been fully aligned, although ironically, the third molars were now impacted.

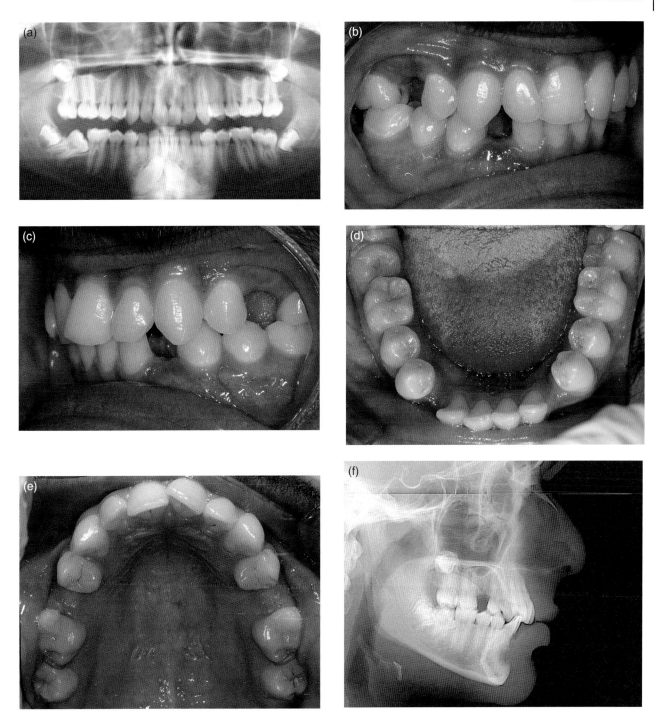

Figure 9.13 (a) Panoramic radiograph of this 14-year-old boy showing the severely ectopic mandibular canine teeth and impacted lower second molar teeth. (b–f) Clinical views and a lateral cephalogram taken after surgical removal of the lower canines, and extraction of the lower deciduous canines and upper second premolar teeth. These show the Class I malocclusion with bimaxillary proclination. (g–j) Photographs taken during alignment of both arches with fixed appliances and a Nance palatal arch *in situ*. Bilateral buccal mini-implants had just been inserted distal to the mandibular lateral incisor and elastomeric traction applied to the first molar hooks. (k) A lateral cephalogram showing Class I incisors with normal inclinations at the time of mini-implant insertions. (l–p) The biomechanics were changed after nine months, when the lower second molars were bonded and a 0.018 NiTi archwire inserted. A double tube was bonded on each first molar and a powerarm was formed from 0.019×0.025 in. steel archwire. (q–u) These views show a Class III incisor relationship and were taken immediately after removal of the mini-implants, after 12 months of use. Small residual spaces remain in the upper and lower anterior areas. (v–y) Debond photographs, showing closure of all spaces, a Class I occlusion and fully erupted/aligned mandibular second molars. (z) A posttreatment panoramic radiograph showing reasonable angulation of all teeth except the impacted lower third molars.

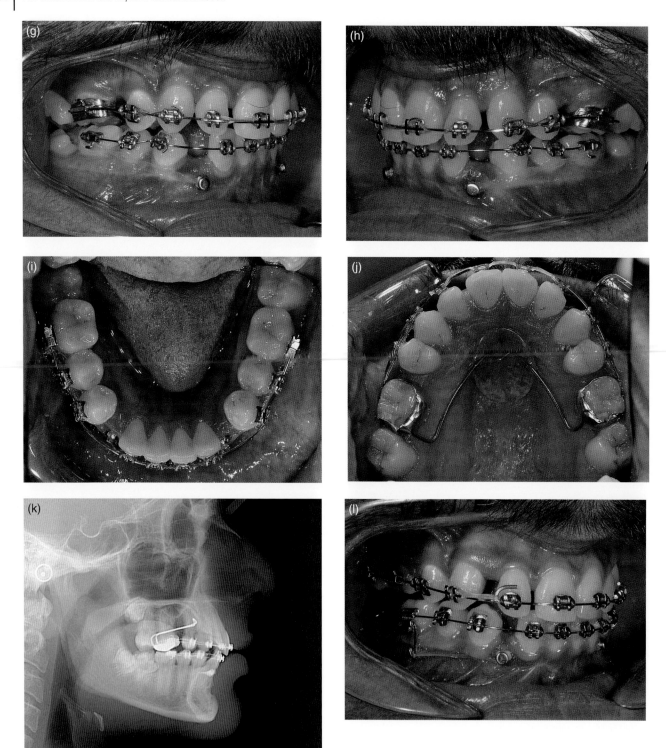

Figure 9.13 (Continued)

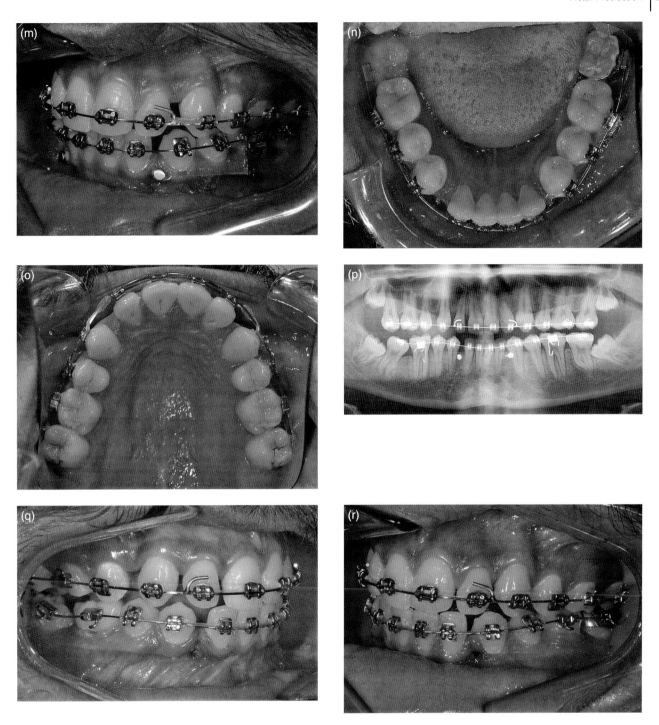

Figure 9.13 (Continued)

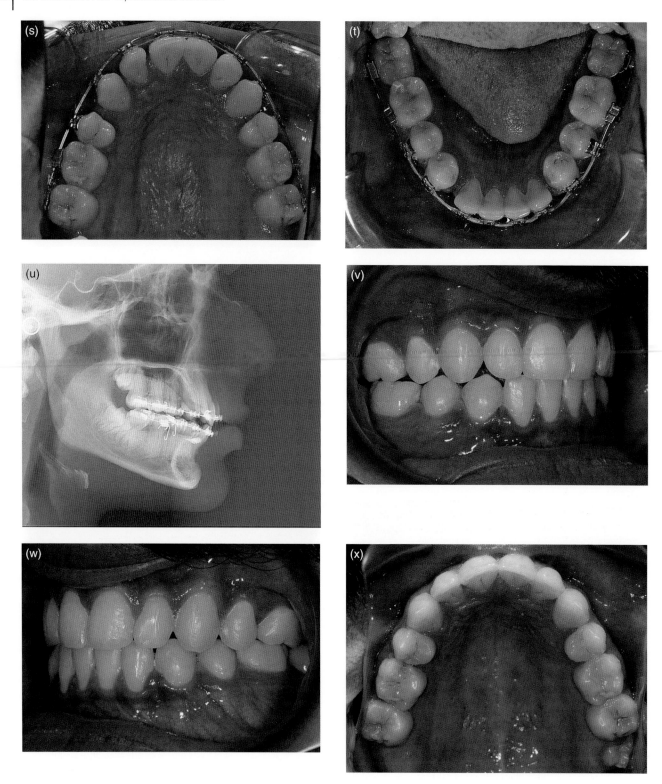

Figure 9.13 (Continued)

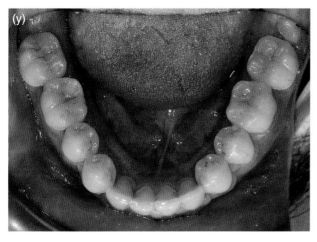

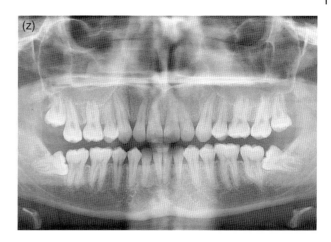

Figure 9.13 (Continued)

9.8 Clinical Steps for Midpalate (Indirect) Anchorage (Figure 9.3)

9.8.1 Preinsertion

1) Align and level the maxillary arch ready for insertion of a passive 0.019×0.025 in. steel archwire. It may be ideal to undertake finishing adjustments, in terms of repositioning the central incisor brackets, at this stage since this then enables the indirect anchorage to be applied to these teeth until the completion of treatment (or even into retention).

2) Evaluate the anterior palatal depth on a lateral cephalogram or cone beam computed tomography (CBCT).

9.8.2 Mini-implant Selection

3) If bilateral traction is required then a single mini-implant may provide sufficient anchorage to prevent palatal movement of the incisor bloc. However, if the space closure and hence traction is unilateral, then a single mini-implant may be affected by counter-clockwise rotational moments, resulting in anchorage loss and a centreline shift (Figure 9.14a). The auxiliary palatal wire may also be deflected in the direction of traction. The addition of a second mini-implant, either in the same transverse plane or in series, will mitigate this rotational side-effect (Figure 9.14b).

4) Choose a short length mini-implant, given the limited palatal bone depth; for example, for Infinitas use a 2.0 mm diameter, 6 mm body length, long neck version (Figure 9.3c).

9.8.3 Insertion

5) Superficial anaesthesia of the insertion site.

6) The insertion site should be at the anteroposterior level of the premolars, to provide adequate bone depth while avoiding close proximity to the nasopalatine canal.

7) The insertion angle should be 20–30° to the vertical plane, angled towards the anterior nasal spine, since this both directs the implant through the optimum bone depth and avoids the contra-angle handpiece contacting the incisal edges at the final insertion stage [2]. A guidance stent may be useful in this respect.

8) Us a slow speed (e.g. 128:1 speed reduction ratio) contra-angle handpiece insertion to overcome the restricted physical access.

9) Use the soft tissue if the attached mucosa appears thick. Use the cortical bone punch in adult patients.

10) Complete insertion to the point where the mini-implant neck is partially submerged but the head is fully accessible. Note that if the patient has a limited depth of palatal bone then they may experience sensitivity on the nasal side and this may prevent full-depth insertion.

9.8.4 Postinsertion

11) Bond a passive auxiliary wire (e.g. 0.019×0.025 in. steel) through the mini-implant head and onto the palatal surfaces of the central incisor crowns. This wire requires a preformed step or addition of a crimpable stop to prevent slippage through the mini-implant head, and hence anchorage loss. It should also be contoured over the palate surface and form a rest on the incisors'

(a)

(b)

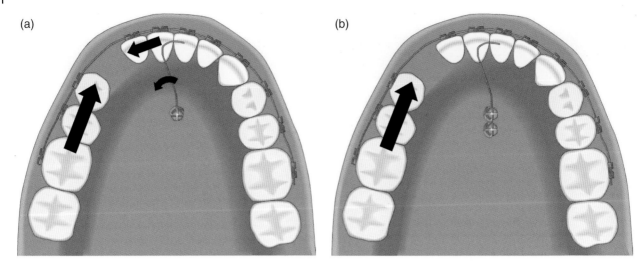

Figure 9.14 (a) Diagram of counter-clockwise (CCW) rotational side-effects occurring when right-sided unilateral traction is applied to a midpalatal (clockwise threaded) mini-implant. The CCW moment partially loosens the mini-implant, resulting in unilateral movement of the incisor teeth. This anchorage loss may be exacerbated if the auxiliary wire flexes under traction. (b) The addition of a second palatal mini-implant stabilises the first against CCW rotational moments, reducing anchorage loss.

palatal surfaces. These features are best achieved if this wire is preshaped using a recent plaster model (with the mini-implant position evident).

12) Immediately apply traction from the anterior (anchor) teeth to the molar(s). Use *light* (approximately 50 g) traction for the first 5–6 weeks, for example using a lightly stretched powerchain, then apply full traction using a NiTi coil spring or elastomeric.

13) Remove the auxiliary wire +/− explant the mini-implant once the anchorage requirements have been met. This may entail air rotor trimming of the mini-implant head to free the wire, but this is not problematic for Infinitas mini-implant removal since the screwdriver engages its (intact) neck section.

9.9 Direct Palatal Anchorage Example (Figure 9.15)

- A 13-year-old boy presented with a Class I malocclusion with hypodontia. Both maxillary lateral incisors were absent and the central incisors had a history of repeated trauma (Figure 9.15a–d). It was therefore desirable to space close by molar protraction (rather than allocate spaces for later incisor implants) and with as limited bracket and force application on the central incisors as possible.
- Parasagittal midpalatal mini-implants (Infinitas 2.0×6 mm version) were inserted with the assistance of a premade

guidance stent. A mesialiser appliance was also premade on the same working model. This appliance involved a 1 mm 'U'-shaped steel wire frame which had circular loops around the mini-implants. It was inserted through palatal extraoral traction (EOT) tubes on the first molars.

- The mesialiser was first seated (with glass ionomer cement) on the first molars and passively over the mini-implant heads. The gap between the wire loops and mini-implant heads was filled with composite resin and immediate light elastomeric traction applied from anterior (soldered) hooks to the first molar hooks (Figure 9.15e–g).
- Substantial space closure was achieved by molar protraction and indirect spontaneous mesialisation of the premolars, to the extent that the retained left deciduous canine exfoliated (Figure 9.15h–j).
- Full fixed appliances were then bonded. Final, conventional space closure then took place once the mesialiser was removed, the upper molar bands replaced with bondable tubes and 0.019×0.025 in. archwires were inserted (Figure 9.15k–m).
- Treatment was completed once the spaces had been closed, the incisor relationship was Class I and the canines Class II (Figure 9.15n–p). Standard vacuum-formed retainers were provided.
- The maxillary central incisors were provisionally restored soon after debond (Figure 9.15q,r), and then re-restored two years later without any reopening of the lateral incisor spaces (Figure 9.15s,t).

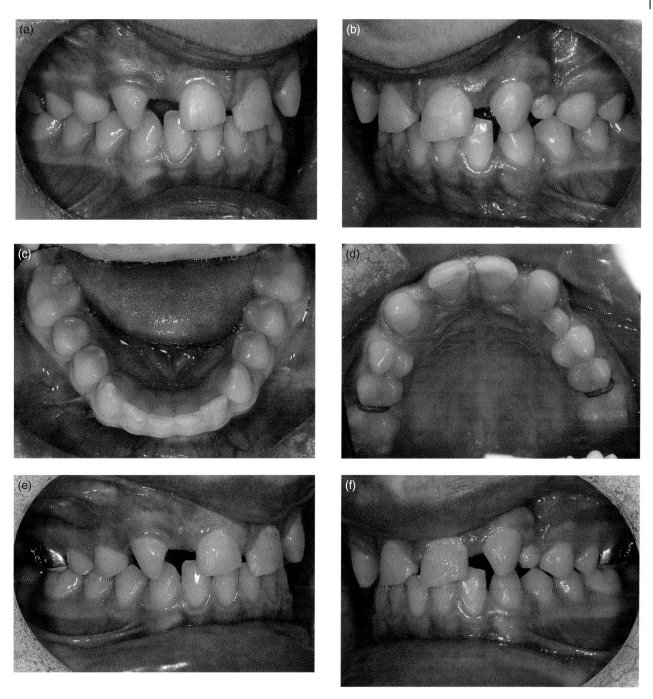

Figure 9.15 (a–d) Pretreatment view showing this Class I malocclusion and absent upper lateral incisors. The upper left deciduous canine is retained, distal to the permanent canine, and there is generalised upper anterior spacing. The upper central incisors are seen in a provisionally restored state. (e–g) Photographs taken after insertion of the two palatal mini-implants and the mesialiser appliance. Notably, composite resin covers the mini-implant heads and elastomeric traction has been applied between anterior hooks and the palatal molar hooks. (h–j) Substantial mesial movement of the upper first molars can be seen to have occurred, with spare appliance wire projecting distal to the palatal molar tubes. The upper left deciduous canine has exfoliated as the buccal teeth have been shunted mesially. (k–m) Views taken after removal when full archwires were in place, the mesialiser appliance having been removed previously, and the upper first molars instead bonded. Conventional elastomeric traction was being used for closure of small residual spaces. (q,r) Photographs taken at the debond stage and then (s,t) two years later once the upper central incisors had been re-restored. Notably, there had been no reopening of the lateral incisor spaces.

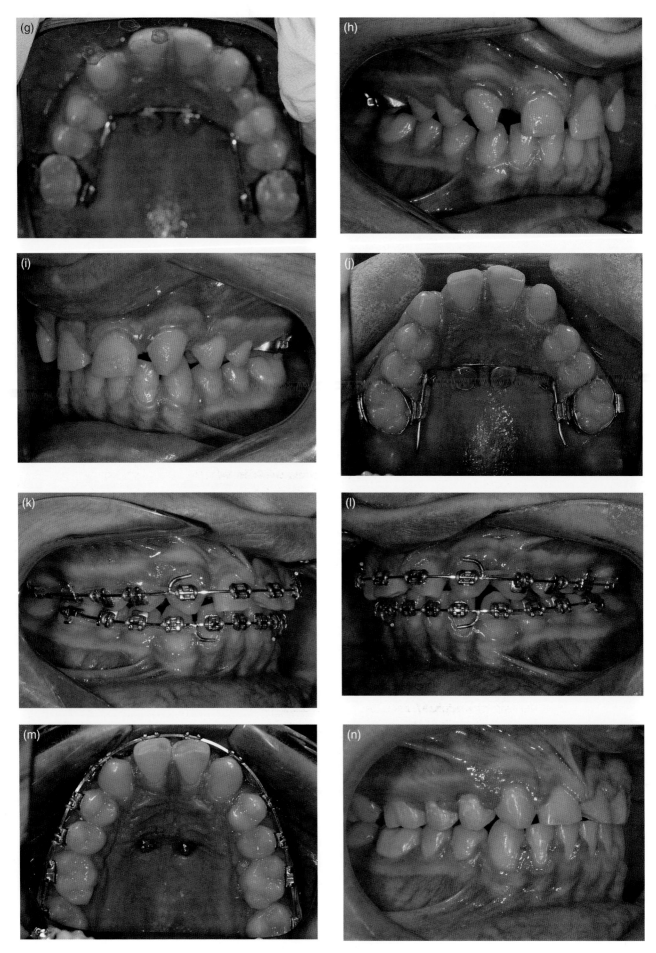

Figure 9.15 (Continued)

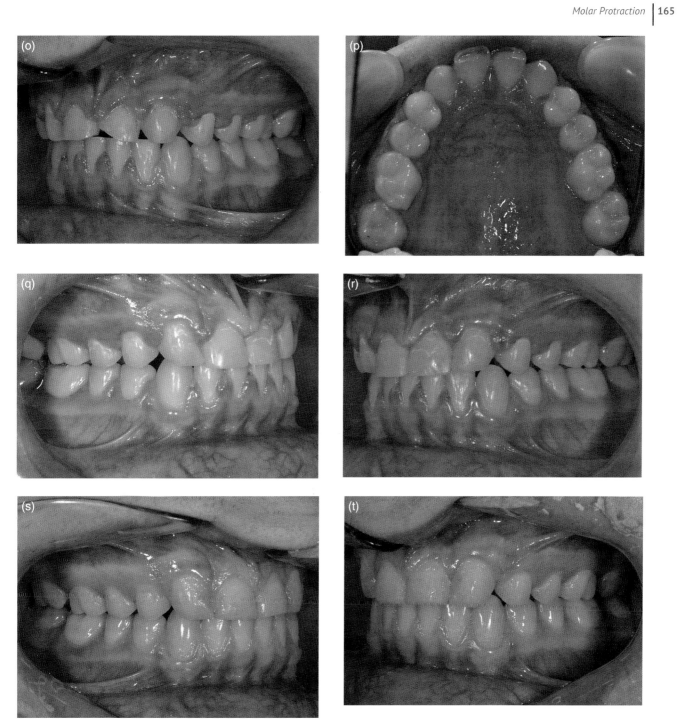

Figure 9.15 (Continued)

References

1 Kanavakis, G., Ludwig, B., Rosa, M. et al. (2014). Clinical outcomes of cases with missing lateral incisors treated with the 'T'-Mesialslider. *J. Orthod.* 41: S33–S38.

2 Brettin, B.T., Grosland, N.M., Qian, F. et al. (2008). Bicortical vs monocortical orthodontic skeletal anchorage. *Am. J. Orthod. Dentofac. Orthop.* 134: 625–635.

3 Nihara, J., Gielo-Perczak, K., Cardinal, L. et al. (2015). Finite element analysis of mandibular molar protraction mechanics using miniscrews. *Eur. J. Orthod.* 37: 95–100.

10

Intrusion and Anterior Openbite Treatments

Vertical control of the dentition has always been one of the most difficult problems in orthodontics. It's relatively easy to extrude teeth (even when we don't want to), but this comes at the cost of unpredictable stability. However, it's much more difficult to intrude teeth such that, before the advent of bone anchorage, the accepted wisdom in orthodontics was that excess vertical growth problems could only be effectively corrected with orthognathic surgery.

Therefore, the ability to effectively intrude teeth (and also avoid extrusion of anchor unit teeth) is one of the most revolutionary applications of mini-implant anchorage. For the first time in orthodontics, it is realistic to intrude single or multiple anterior and posterior teeth, albeit with the caveat that the periodontium needs to be healthy in order to avoid an exacerbation of pocket depth. Consequently, many orthodontists now consider (non-surgical) molar intrusion approaches as the first line of treatment for anterior openbite (AOB) in Class I and Class II cases. As will be demonstrated in this chapter, the expectation is that we can not only correct the malocclusion, but also provide a significant improvement in the facial profile, lip closure and soft tissue contour. The latter is what I affectionately call an 'orthodontic chin-lift' (Figure 10.1). The exception is Class III cases where counter-clockwise rotation of the mandible worsens the incisor relationship. However, these cases may still benefit from molar intrusion by altering their management from a bimaxillary surgical plan to a more conservative one of molar intrusion (to first reduce the vertical excess) and either a mandibular setback or maxillary advancement osteotomy. Such combinations of intrusion and surgery will be discussed in more detail in Chapter 14.

Molar intrusion has many benefits over a maxillary impaction osteotomy and I've never seen an AOB patient elect for maxillary surgery rather than molar intrusion when purely vertical changes are being considered. Patients readily grasp the concept that molar intrusion is a gradual biological process which is equivalent to the surgeon removing a segment of maxillary bone, but without the morbidity and costs (both to the patient and the health system) involved with surgery. Furthermore, improvements in the lower facial profile (Figure 10.1) can be achieved without the unfavourable nasal changes (alar widening and upturn of the nasal tip) which result from maxillary impaction movements, reducing the scope for long-term patient complaints. Finally, remember that both orthognathic correction and orthodontic camouflage treatment of skeletal AOB still have relatively high relapse rates [1–4].

So how does skeletal anchorage create tooth intrusion and is it safe? The biological mechanism for molar intrusion was established at an early stage by Sugawara and colleagues using zygomatic miniplates in a dog model [5,6]. First, they showed that the alveolar complex crest remodelled at both the crest and nasal floor levels (the dog nasal floor is equivalent to the maxillary sinus in humans). Second, when the supracrestal periodontal fibres were sectioned the molars submerged into the alveolus, but when the fibres remained intact there was a physical reduction in the alveolar height. Strictly speaking, this represents true dentoalveolar remodelling rather than simple tooth intrusion, and I have consistently observed only a limited and temporary reduction in clinical crown height and finishing with normal probing depth in over 50 clinical cases I've treated with molar intrusion therapy. Hence, we probably ought to refer to this treatment effect as *alveolar remodelling* (and dentoalveolar height reduction), but the term 'molar intrusion' has stuck in common usage to describe this form of AOB treatment and hence will be used here.

The other important finding of these and subsequent animal studies is that molar intrusion causes neither loss of pulp vitality nor a clinically significant reduction in root length [7–11]. A micro-computed tomography (CT) study of human molar teeth has corroborated this with the observation that root resorption only occurs to a clinically insignificant depth, despite the observation of resorption lacunae over large surface areas of the intruding roots [10].

The Orthodontic Mini-Implant Clinical Handbook, Second Edition. Richard Cousley.
© 2020 John Wiley & Sons Ltd. Published 2020 by John Wiley & Sons Ltd.

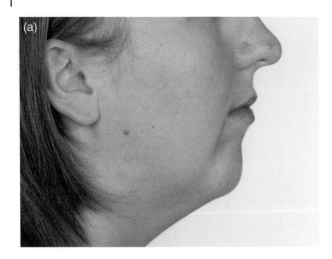
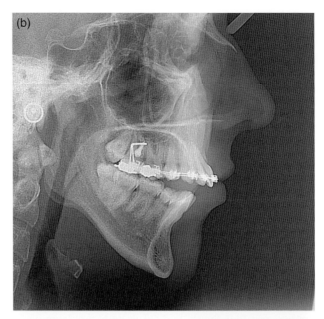
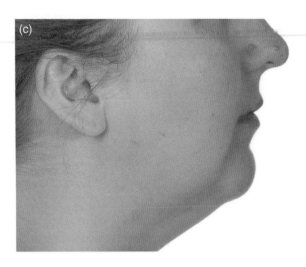
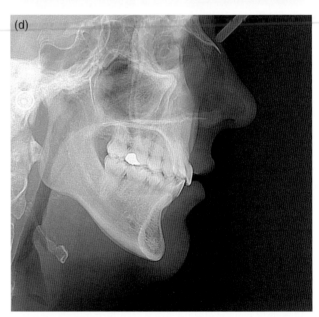

Figure 10.1 (a) Pretreatment profile view of a adult patient with a Class II malocclusion with an AOB. The lower anterior face height is increased and the soft tissue pogonion is 'flat'. (b) A lateral cephalogram taken at the start of maxillary molar intrusion. (c) A photograph and (d) lateral cephalogram of the patient's facial and dentoskeletal profile features two years after the end of treatment. These show stable, favourable improvements in the lower face height and chin-neck soft tissue contour as a result of the 'orthodontic chin-lift' effect.

This was even the situation when relatively heavy forces were applied [8,10]. Therefore, it's reassuring to conclude that mini-implant assisted tooth intrusion is both biologically sound and safe. Finally, it has been demonstrated in human subjects that molar intrusion treatment has no effects on temporomandibular joint or masticatory muscle function [12].

In the presence of normal periodontal tissues, the intrusion mechanism involves alveolar remodelling (a reduction in alveolar height) rather than actual tooth 'intrusion'.

10.1 Single-Tooth and Anterior Segment Intrusion Treatments

10.1.1 Clinical Objectives

- Intrusion of a single overerupted tooth
- or intrusion of an entire group of upper or lower incisors to correct a deep overbite and reduce excess vertical incisal display/gummy smile.

10.1.2 Treatment Options

- Conventional approaches such as the use of either bite-opening archwire curves or segmental arch mechanics.
- Maxillary impaction orthognathic surgery, especially in the presence of excessive gingival display and lip incompetence.
- Direct intrusive traction from labial or buccal mini-implants to either adjacent orthodontic brackets or the archwire (Figure 10.2). In the case of lower incisor intrusion, for true intrusion (without labial flaring) the authors of a finite element analysis (FEA) study have recommended that the mini-implants are inserted distal to the canine roots, and that traction is applied in a 'V' configuration from the mini-implants to the archwire both mesial and distal to the lateral incisors [13].
- Cantilever traction from buccal mini-implants (inserted mesial to the first molars) to anterior powerarms. This has been illustrated in Chapter 7 (Figure 7.12) and is particularly useful if space closure is also required.
- Cantilever traction from palatal mini-implants (inserted mesial in the midpalate), via a flexible wire [14].
- Indirect anchorage of a molar tooth whilst a utility intrusion arch or a cantilever wire is utilised from an auxiliary tube on the molar.
- Orthodontic aligner therapy, although the amount of actual molar intrusion achievable is small and AOB closure is largely due to incisor retroclination and extrusion changes.

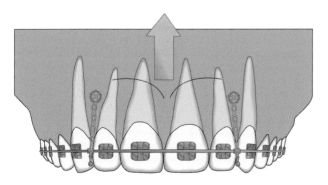

Figure 10.2 Diagram of incisor intrusion mechanics where vertical traction is applied from bilateral mini-implants, sited mesial to the canines, to the archwire or nearby brackets.

10.1.3 Relevant Clinical Details

- The incisor relationship and inclinations.
- Upper incisor vertical display (both passive and smiling) in the context of the patient's age; that is, is incisor intrusion beneficial in terms of reducing the incisal show or would this risk prematurely ageing the patient?
- Presence of vertical facial asymmetry, manifesting as an occlusal cant.
- The periodontal status since teeth must not be intruded in the presence of active periodontal disease (bleeding or pocketing).
- The height of attached gingiva adjacent to the tooth/teeth to be intruded. If this is reduced then it will limit the intrusion range for direct traction (from an adjacent mini-implant), given that the intruding teeth will move towards the mini-implant. In this situation, indirect anchorage of a posterior tooth and the use of an intrusive lever arm may be preferable.
- The root proximity of teeth adjacent to the planned insertion sites.

10.1.4 Biomechanical Principles

- Labial/buccal mini-implants may cause undesirable inclination/torque changes in the target tooth since traction applied to the labial crown surface will tip the crown labially. In some cases, this is acceptable, when the target tooth rolled in a palatal direction as it overerupted, but it is still crucial that the orthodontist is aware of this side-effect. The potential problem is reduced by the use of a low-profile mini-implant (where the traction is applied close to the gingival surface), insertion of the mini-implants distal to the canines (for incisor intrusion), and/or the addition of archwire torque. Interestingly, the same inclination effect occurs with conventional treatment options, such as an intrusion arch. However, mini-implant incisor intrusion does not result in additional molar side-effects observed with conventional treatment [15].
- If the incisors procline during intrusion then anterior spacing will develop. This is avoided by cinching back the ends of the archwire or applying traction for space closure.

10.1.5 Clinical Tips and Technicalities

- If there is a prominent labial frenum then either avoid midline mini-implant insertion or undertake a frenectomy to deter soft tissue interference or overgrowth (over the mini-implant head).
- Labial crown tipping of an intruding single tooth may also be controlled by the use of a vacuum-formed baseplate to contact the coronal aspect of the crown and with a window cut to allow for apical movement of the attachment on the tooth.

10.1.6 Clinical Steps

10.1.6.1 Preinsertion

1) Diverge the roots of teeth adjacent to the insertion site by bonding their brackets at altered tips; for example, for insertion mesial to the canine root, add mesial tip to the lateral incisor bracket and distal tip to the canine one.

2) Level and align either the whole arch with a full fixed appliance or only those teeth requiring intrusion with a sectional fixed appliance. This depends on the extent of the vertical discrepancy between the intruding and adjacent teeth, such that a large step favours segmental mechanics prior to full arch engagement.

10.1.6.2 Mini-implant Selection

3) A narrow-diameter mini-implant, e.g. Infinitas 1.5 mm version, is appropriate for interproximal sites.

4) Select a mini-implant with a short neck to reduce the risk of the traction being more buccal (distant from the surface) than the crown surface and hence increasing the tooth's inclination.

5) If there is sufficient height of attached gingiva then the insertion should be perpendicular to the surface, in which case a relatively short body length (e.g. 6 mm length Infinitas version) is appropriate and avoids the risk of lingual perforation. However, if a limited height of attached gingiva dictates that oblique insertion is required, then it may be more appropriate to select a longer body length (e.g. 9 mm) mini-implant.

10.1.6.3 Insertion

6) Aim to insert the mini-implants close to or at the mucogingival junction (MGJ) in order to both gain access to the relatively larger interproximal space and provide sufficient vertical range for continued tooth movements.

7) Insert the mini-implant 'horizontally', that is, perpendicular to the bone surface so that the traction is easily and securely applied to its head.

8) Superficial anaesthesia of the insertion sites.

9) Ideally, insert at least two mini-implants on the buccal side of the alveolus such that intrusive forces can be applied from both sides of the target tooth or group of teeth.

10) Take an intraoral radiograph if close root proximity is clinically suspected.

11) Complete insertion to the point that the mini-implant neck is partially submerged and the head has a low emergence profile yet is fully accessible.

10.1.6.4 Postinsertion

12) Apply traction from the mini-implants to adjacent brackets or an archwire hook. Use approximately 50 g (elastomeric chain) traction for the first 4–6 weeks, then increase the force to around 150 g provided that a group of teeth are being loaded.

13) Monitor treatment progress by recording key features at the start of intrusion and at subsequent appointments, such as overjet, AOB/overbite, incisor–lip relationship and buccal segment relationship.

14) Monitor oral hygiene and the periodontal condition (probing depth) of the intruding teeth during treatment.

15) Consider overcorrection of the intrusion effects to allow for possible relapse.

16) Keep the mini-implants *in situ* until it is clear that further anchorage is not required.

17) Consider an intensive initial retention regimen, such as three months full-time wear of full-coverage plastic retainers. This should prevent early vertical relapse of intruded teeth (but not of any extruded teeth).

10.1.7 Case Examples

1) **Single-tooth intrusion (Figure 10.3)**
   - A 45-year-old female with a Class II division 1 malocclusion (Figure 10.3a) complicated by mandibular retrognathia, a very low maxillomandibular planes angle (MMPA) and a compromised dentition (unsuitable for comprehensive orthodontics). A mandibular advancement osteotomy was performed (utilising mini-implant intermaxillary fixation) to correct the extremely traumatic overbite, followed by limited alignment and levelling of the lower buccal segments. This required intrusion of the overerupted upper left canine.
   - 1.5 mm diameter, 6 mm length, short neck Infinitas mini-implants were fully inserted on the buccal aspect mesial and distal to the upper left canine. Elastomeric traction was applied to a cleat on the canine's labial surface (Figure 10.3b,c). By 16 weeks, the canine had been vertically overcorrected, without labial crown tipping. The canine was allowed to settle into occlusion as the lower buccal teeth were extruded using a box elastic from the mini-implants (Figure 10.3d,e) and remained stable six years after debond (Figure 10.3f).

2) **Incisor teeth intrusion (Figure 10.4)**
   - A 24-year-old female with a Class II division 2 malocclusion with absent upper right first premolar and left canine teeth, and a history of aggressive juvenile periodontitis (Figure 10.4a). She required periodontal

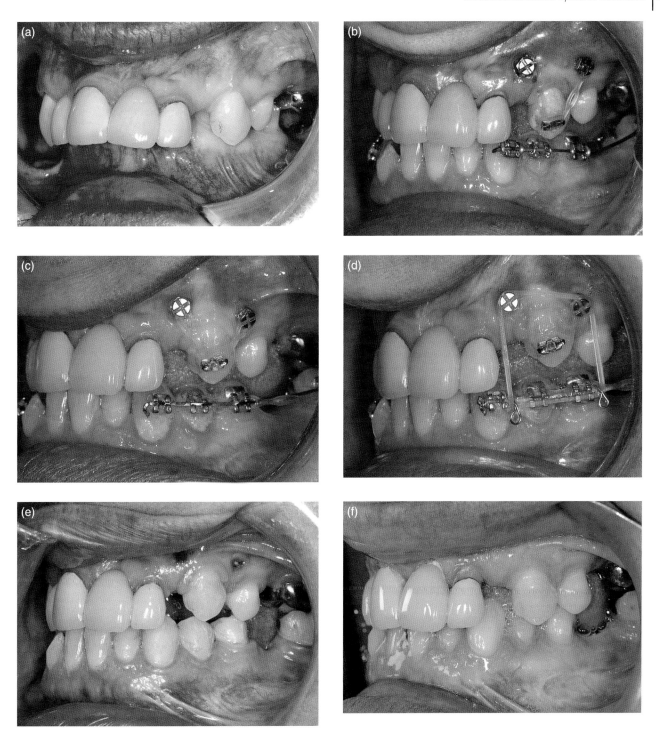

Figure 10.3 (a) Pretreatment views showing this severe Class II division 1 malocclusion complicated by overeruption of the maxillary left canine and inadequate dental support for formal fixed appliance treatment. (b) The upper left canine at the start of its intrusion, following a mandibular advancement osteotomy to correct the Class II discrepancies. Elastomeric traction is applied from mesially and distally sited 6 mm length mini-implants to a low-profile cleat. This intrusion will enable the lower buccal teeth to be levelled. (c) The canine intrusion is progressing by eight weeks and (d) by 16 weeks its level has been overcorrected, without buccal tipping. A vertical box elastic is then added to extrude the lower teeth. (e) Debond view, accepting incomplete occlusal interdigitation. (f) Photograph taken six years after debond (prior to replacement of the incisor crowns).

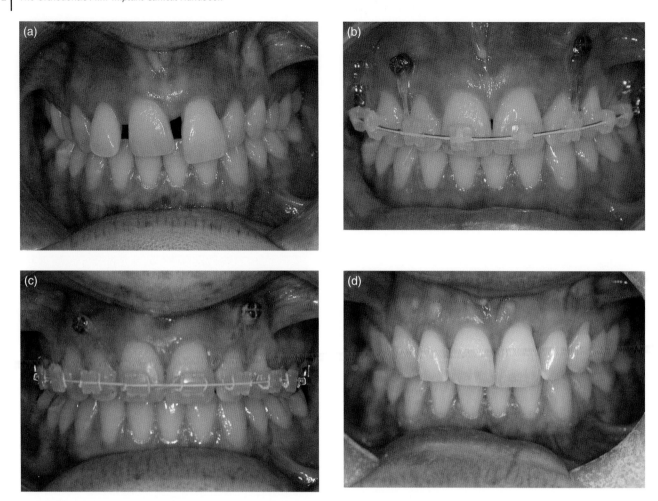

Figure 10.4 (a) Pretreatment view of this adult patient showing the overerupted upper left central incisor, absence of the upper right first premolar and left canine teeth, and anterior spacing. (b) Photograph showing a 0.019 × 0.025 in. steel archwire *in situ*. Vertical elastomeric traction has been applied from the lateral incisor brackets to bilateral mini-implants. These were inserted at the mucogingival junction and distal to the upper lateral incisors. (c) View of aligned teeth and the improved gingival contour during treatment, when the traction had been reapplied on the central incisor brackets. (d) Photograph taken four years after debond and occlusal settling.

stabilisation, then alignment and intrusion of the overerupted upper incisor teeth and the creation of interincisal clearance for a bonded retainer.

- The maxillary arch was levelled to accommodate a 0.019 × 0.025 in. NiTi archwire and then 1.5 mm diameter, 9 mm length, short neck Infinitas mini-implants were inserted on the buccal aspect of the arch, distal to the upper lateral incisors and close to the MGJ. Light elastomeric traction was applied for six months, initially to the lateral and then to the central incisor brackets (Figure 10.4b,c). The later traction vector was more oblique to limit labial crown tipping. The periodontal status and overbite remained stable over four years after debond (Figure 10.4d).

10.2 Anterior Openbite Treatment

Anterior openbite is one of the most difficult malocclusion features to treat non-surgically. Traditional orthodontic camouflage tends to extrude the incisors, but this has several key disadvantages: the risk of excessive upper incisor exposure (crown length and gingival display); unfavourable incisor retroclination; an unaesthetic effect on the nasolabial profile and smile; and a particularly high relapse risk (partly due to practical difficulties in retention) [3,4,16]. There is also a greater tendency to prescribe premolar extractions in AOB cases with the aim of limiting incisor proclination and consequently vertical incisor separation. Furthermore, it is claimed that premolar extractions enable mesial movement of the molars and consequently reduce the MMPA, but this is not supported by research evidence [4]. Therefore, extraction decisions should be based on dental factors such as crowding and centreline discrepancies, rather than the AOB *per se*. The alternative of surgical impaction of the posterior maxilla is effective, but it involves invasive and expensive treatment, it must be delayed until after completion of facial growth, it entails surgical morbidity and risks (including occlusal imprecision), and may result in unfavourable nasal changes. How much better would it be to both correct the AOB and improve dentofacial aesthetics by a more effective and patient-friendly approach?

Mini-implant molar intrusion now represents a real alternative to orthognathic surgery in Class I and II skeletal AOB cases (but not in skeletal Class III patients where mandibular autorotation would worsen the anteroposterior relationship). In effect, a reduction in dentoalveolar height causes clockwise rotation of the maxillary occlusal plane and consequently a reduction in both the MMPA and AOB [17–24]. This treatment approach is also logical since AOB patients have 'overdeveloped' posterior alveolar height as part of their trait [25]. Crucially, intrusion treatment is feasible in both adults and adolescents, and avoids the surgical morbidity and inpatient costs associated with a maxillary osteotomy. Over the last few years, I have given those AOB patients whom I think may benefit from orthognathic surgery the opportunity to discuss the options fully on a combined orthognathic clinic: none have opted for surgery on the basis of their AOB problems, and some have been desperate to avoid surgery, even accepting residual Class II facial features. I find this to be truly informed consent and would advise that such patients are given details of all options open to them. In my experience, none have regretted taking a non-surgical approach.

The biological mechanism of mini-implant anchored molar intrusion has already been outlined earlier in this chapter. However, we still need to consider issues such as the optimum techniques, clinical outcomes and long-term stability. Given that molar intrusion is a relatively new treatment modality, there are few published studies on long-term outcomes to date. In the short term, two retrospective cephalometric studies have provided almost identical short-term findings, although the North Carolina study sample (30 patients) was much more heterogenous (by including mini-implant and miniplate cases) than the study by Hart et al. [23] in which the 31 cases were treated solely with mini-implants [22,23]. Twenty-six of these consecutive cases were treated by me solely with palatal alveolar mini-implant anchorage [23]. The mean amount of upper first molar intrusion was 2.3 mm in both studies (ranging up to 5 mm in my case series), with associated reductions in the MMPA and lower anterior face height,

and increases in sella-nasion-B point (SNB). Surprisingly, the adolescent patients showed the greatest mandibular autorotation effects, whilst adults had more tilting of the occlusal plane angle. In terms of technique, both studies reported unfavourable eruption of the lower molars in adolescent patients, giving us the 'take-home' message that the vertical position of these molars needs to be controlled from the start of molar intrusion. The appropriate practical options will be discussed in this chapter and some of the key clinical 'tips' are highlighted in Table 10.1.

One of the seminal posttreatment studies involved the two year follow-up of 30 adult females who presented with a mean 4.5 mm AOB. They were subdivided into two groups: one treated with premolar extractions, headgear anchorage and intermaxillary elastics and the other with bimaxillary buccal mini-implants (producing an average of 2.3 and 0.8 mm upper and lower first molar intrusion changes). In effect, the two groups had similar occlusal

Table 10.1 Ten tips for clinical success in molar intrusion

Clinical tip	Benefit
Bond upper second molars	Optimises hygiene given that these crowns may initially submerge during intrusion
Overexpand maxillary arch	To allow for the constrictive effects of palatal traction and the transverse effects of Class II improvements
Use palatal sites, ideally distal to first molars	Applies intrusive forces to the posterior end of the arch, and enables direct traction on the second molars
Palpate posterior alveolar mucosal thickness/mobility	Avoids risk of mucosal mobility, at sites distal to the first molars, from destabilising or overgrowing the mini-implant
Fit intrusion TPA or modified quadhelix	To control or expand the intermolar width and torque, respectively
Add bite-opening curve	To control the vertical level and torque of the upper incisors (due to the rotational effect on the arch from posterior intrusive forces)
Stabilise lower molars from the start of intrusion	Either bond all lower molars early or fit a full coverage lower retainer, to prevent lower molar overeruption
Add mandibular mini-implants	If there is a marked reverse curve of Spee in the lower arch or the AOB is severe
Overcorrect AOB	To allow for some vertical relapse risks, especially if there has been any incisor extrusion
Initial three months full-time retainer wear	To provide an intrusive effect on the molar teeth

AOB, anterior openbite; TPA, transpalatal arch.

results, with positive overbites two years after debond. However, they had significantly different facial outcomes: the mini-implant group demonstrated 3.6° of anticlockwise mandibular rotation, a 3.6 mm reduction in lower face height, a 1.4° increase in SNB, better lip competence and minimal incisor extrusion. The conventional group did not [26]. Other authors have focused specifically on long-term stability. For example, Baek et al. [20] have reported a three year follow-up of nine adult mini-implant intrusion patients. and found that most of the 1 mm overbite relapse occurred within the first year and that by three years the stability of upper first molar and AOB changes was 77% and 83% respectively [20]. Similar results were reported after a four year study of 26 miniplate anchorage patients who had a mean of 3 mm upper first molar intrusion [27]. Their relapse rates were 10% and 13% relapse of the upper first molar vertical position by one and four years. Again, most (76%) of the relapse occurred within the first year, which is reassuring in terms of retention strategies. Arguably, these relapse figures include some settling of molar (openbite) overcorrections, so it may be unfair to view this all as relapse.

Finally, a prospective study of 14 adolescent AOB cases showed mean reductions (relative to controls) in the vertical positions of the upper and lower first molars, the mandibular plane angle, and the lower face height of 5.6, 2.8° and 4.3 mm, respectively. This was principally due to passive restraint of vertical dentoalveolar growth plus modest effects of active traction on the upper molars [24]. These changes remained stable by the age of 20 years and at least one year after debond. Only the upper incisors demonstrated a small amount of relapse. Notably, their retention regimen featured six months of full-time, then nightly, wear of full coverage plastic retainers.

> Intrusion treatment is feasible in both adults and adolescents, and avoids the surgical morbidity and patient costs associated with a maxillary osteotomy.

After initially utilising buccal mini-implant sites in my first cases (Figure 10.5), over the last 10 years I have found palatal insertion sites to be much more effective for maxillary molar intrusion in terms of the greater availability of interproximal space, sufficient cortical bone support and range for vertical traction [23,28]. Indeed, it is important to remember that the cortical thickness is less in 'long' face (dolichofacial) types than other patients, which favours palatal insertion sites over buccal ones [29–31]. However, the use of an appropriate speed reduction handpiece and guidance stent for palatal sites has been the 'game changer' for me in this respect. Consequently, the clinical steps out-

lined here describe the culmination of this experience with palatal mini-implants combined with an intrusion type of transpalatal arch (TPA) or a modified quadhelix.

10.2.1 Clinical Objectives

- Intrusion of the maxillary, and possibly the mandibular, molars to correct an AOB (and Class II discrepancies where present).
- Counter-clockwise mandibular autorotation.

10.2.2 Treatment Options

- Molar intrusion using mini-implant anchorage.
- Headgear to limit vertical maxillary dentoalveolar growth.
- Functional (orthopaedic) appliances or posterior bite blocks.
- Premolar or molar extractions to facilitate incisor retraction.
- Bite closing curves in archwires and intermaxillary elastics.
- Maxillary impaction osteotomy
- Aligner treatment for minor molar intrusive effects.

10.2.3 Relevant Clinical Details

- The incisor (overjet, openbite) and buccal segment relationships.
- Upper incisor vertical display relative to the passive and smiling lip level.
- Whether vertical facial asymmetry and an occlusal cant are present.
- Whether there is a vertical step in the occlusion between the anterior and posterior teeth and/or potential occlusal interferences from palatally displaced teeth.
- Eruptive status of the second and third molars.
- Maturity of the palatal alveolar mucosa, especially distal to the second molars.
- Transverse molar relationships; that is, would mandibular clockwise rotation cause posterior crossbites?

10.2.4 Biomechanical Principles

- Buccal mini-implants provide only a limited range of intrusion in many patients because of a limited height of attached gingiva both before treatment and especially when allowing for subsequent apical movement of the molar teeth.
- Posterior palatal alveolar insertion sites offer three advantages over buccal ones: greater height of attached mucosa, cortical bone thickness, and interproximal bone volume.

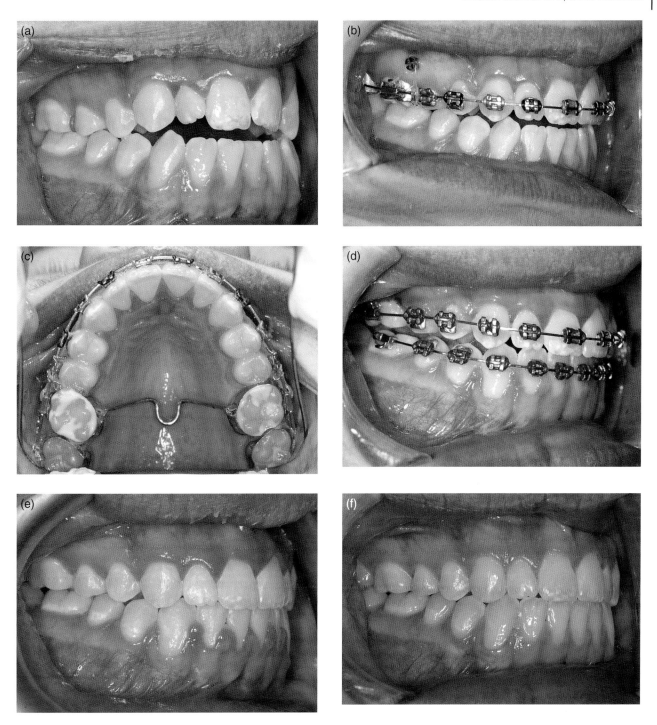

Figure 10.5 (a) Pretreatment intraoral buccal view of a 15-year-old boy showing his Class II malocclusion and AOB. (b,c) Views of an upper fixed appliance with an intrusion TPA. An inverted 'V' configuration of elastomeric traction has been applied from bilateral buccal mini-implants (mesial to the first molars) to the adjacent tooth attachments. (d) The mini-implants and TPA have just been removed after nine months of traction, when posterior openbites were present and the molars approximated the mini-implants. (e) Debond and (f) 15 months post-debond views showing the Class I finish and slight long-term relapse of the overbite correction.

- Buccal or palatal intrusion forces cause undesirable transverse side-effects, that is, buccal crown rolling or arch constriction, respectively. Therefore, the transverse arch width and molar torque should be controlled either by a modified, rigid TPA (Figure 10.6), a modified quad-helix expander or simultaneous buccal and palatal mini-implant traction.
- Molar intrusive movements, especially with traction applied to the second molars, may cause the entire dental arch to tip around its centre of rotation (in a clockwise direction in the maxilla), causing inadvertent incisor extrusion (Figure 10.7). This is countered by the use of segmental mechanics (separate buccal and labial segments) or the addition of a bite-opening curve to any steel archwires used during continuous arch mechanics.

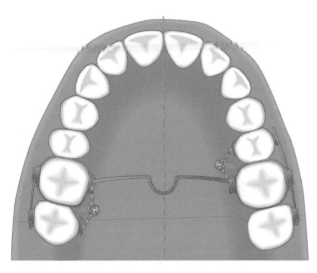

Figure 10.6 Diagram of palatal mini-implants inserted mesial and distal to the first molar palatal root, and traction to a TPA and palatal attachments.

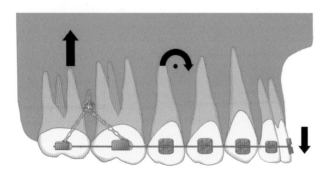

Figure 10.7 Diagram showing the biomechanical side-effects of posterior intrusion where rotation of the entire maxillary arch also results in extrusion of the incisors.

10.2.5 Clinical Tips and Technicalities

- Consider removal of erupted third molars (prior to orthodontics) since they may cause occlusal interference after intrusion of adjacent molars.
- Increase the maxillary intermolar and canine widths at the start of treatment, to allow for the combined effects of mandibular autorotation and to counteract the constrictive effects of palatal traction. If in any doubt, err towards overexpansion since it is easy to allow this to settle later in treatment, whereas it is difficult to simultaneously intrude and expand molars at the finishing stages of treatment (when relatively light wires may be more ideal). I have frequently used a removable quadhelix appliance, with some simple modifications so that the posterior loops are sufficiently mesial to the mini-implants (when sited distal to the first molars) and elevated off the palate (Figure 10.8a). The same quadhelix can then remain *in situ* during the intrusion phase. Alternatively, at that stage an intrusion TPA can be inserted, especially if the mini-implants are being inserted mesial to the first molars (Figure 10.8b). However, the means of expansion should be determined according to the amount needed, the patient's age and the orthodontist's preferences. Therefore, if needed or preferred then either rapid maxillary expansion (RME) or bone-anchored RME (see Chapter 13) appliances can be used to attain substantial expansion (Figure 10.9).
- Bond the upper second molars, rather than banding them. This is much more favourable for oral hygiene, especially if these molars become temporarily subgingival [32].
- A mini-implant insertion site mesial to the first molars is reasonably accessible, and is appropriate in adolescents with partial or non-eruption of the second molars. Traction from here tends to produce little clockwise rotation of the maxillary arch (Figure 10.8b). Alternatively, insertion distal to the first molars is feasible in adults and in some adolescents, and gives more ability to directly intrude and control the inclination (torque) of the second molars (Figure 10.10a). However, it does create a clockwise rotational moment, resulting in incisor extrusion with whole arch engagement (Figure 10.7). This may be partly negated, during the transition from a molar sectional to continuous whole archwire, by having the anterior/premolar archwire separate from the pre-existing molar archwire (Figure 10.10b).
- Always palpate the mucosa at the potential insertion sites to check that it is firmly attached, rather than feeling mobile or excessively viscoelastic. This occurs in adolescent patients if the soft tissue on the posterior aspect of the palatal alveolus is not tightly attached to the

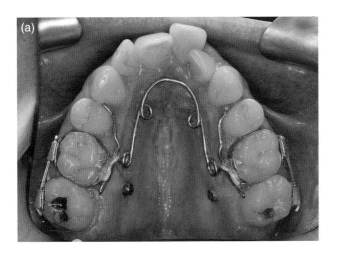
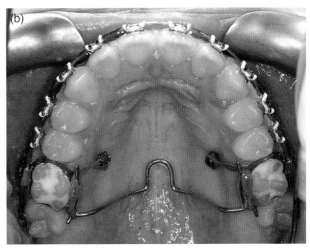

Figure 10.8 (a) A palatal photograph showing an 'intrusion' quadhelix, fitted on the first molars, for maxillary arch expansion. The distal loops of the quadhelix have been positioned more anteriorly than usual and elevated away from the palatal mucosa. There is a buccal sectional fixed appliance, using molar tubes on the second molar teeth. (b) An 'intrusion' TPA, with the bar positioned distal to the anchorage sites (mesial to the first molars) and elevated off the palate (by 5 mm in the midline). There are bilateral mini-implants, mesial to the first molars.

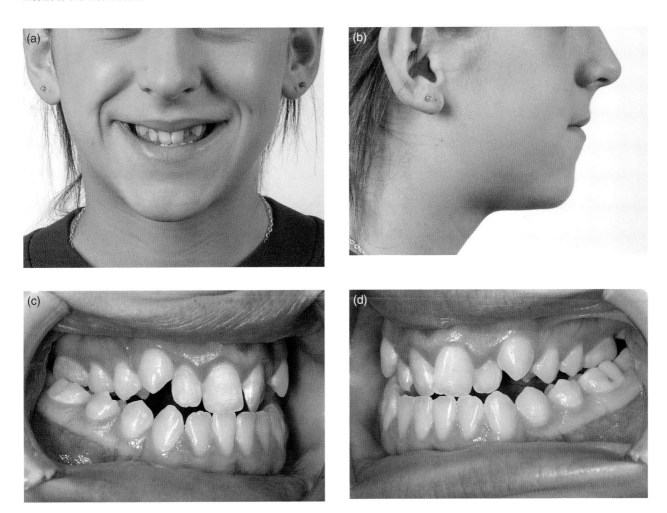

Figure 10.9 (a–e) Pretreatment photographs of a 15-year-old girl who presented with a Class III malocclusion on a skeletal Class I base with increased lower facial vertical proportions. There is a partial anterolateral openbite and bilateral buccal cross-bites. (f) Pretreatment lateral cephalogram showing the Class I skeletal base, high mandibular plane angle and bimaxillary retroclination. (g,h) Photographs taken at the end of the RME activation. (i–k) Views at the start of the intrusion phase, with the full upper fixed appliance and intrusion TPA in place. The mini-implants are mesial to the first molars and elastomeric traction connects them to the TPA. (l) A lateral cephalogram taken at the start of the intrusion phase. (m–o) Intraoral views taken after 15 months of the intrusion and lower arch alignment phase. (p) Cephalometric superimposition of the start and end of the intrusion phase. This shows the upper molar intrusion, mandibular rotation and bimaxillary proclination changes. (q–u) Photographs taken at debond. (v) A lateral cephalogram taken at the end of treatment.

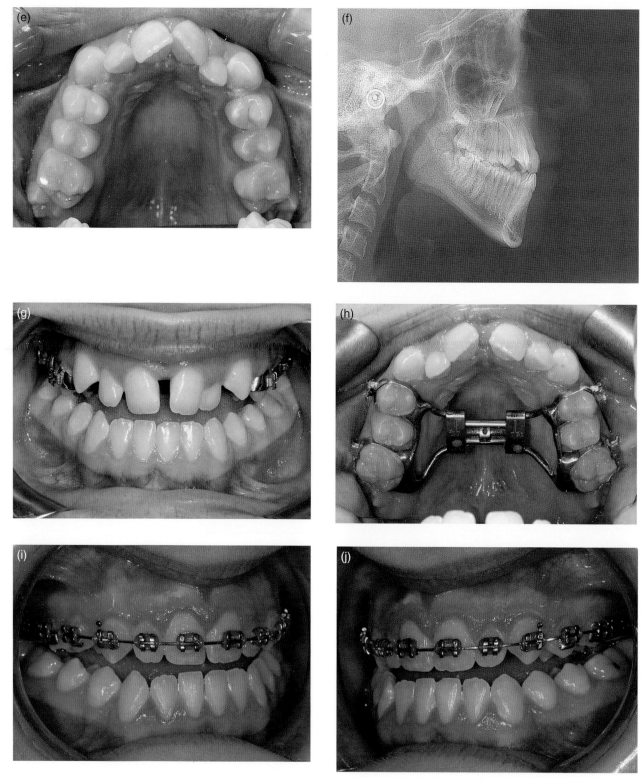

Figure 10.9 (Continued)

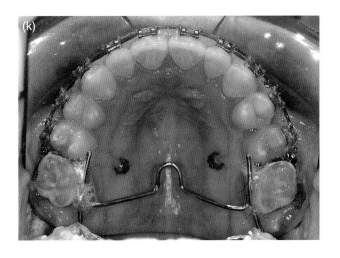
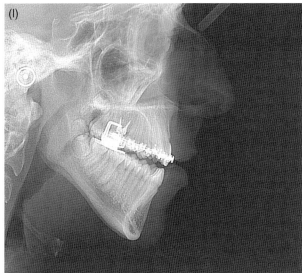
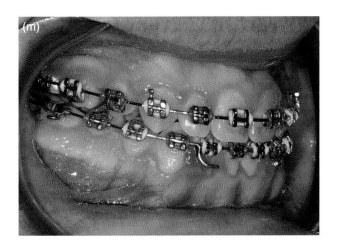
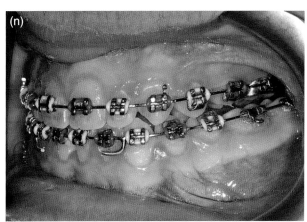
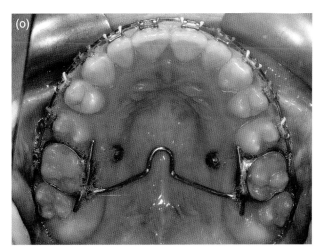

Figure 10.9 (Continued)

(p)

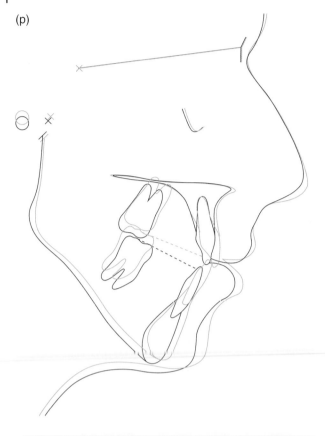

SKELETAL			SOFT TISSUES		
SNA	°	0.0	Lip Sep	mm	0.5
SNB	°	1.5	Exp UI	mm	1.5
ANB	°	−1.0	LS-E	mm	−2.0
SN/MxP	°	1.5	LI-E	mm	−1.5
MxP/MnP	°	−3.0	NLA	°	−17.5
LAFH	mm	−2.5	LLA	°	6.5
UAFH	mm	1.0	Holdaway	°	−1.0
LAFH/TAFH	%	−1.5			
LPFH	mm	−2.0	**NOSE PROMINENCE**		
UPFH	mm	0.5			
PFH	mm	0.5	Nose tip	mm	1.0
Wits	mm	1.0	Nose angle	°	−1.0

TEETH			CHIN PROMINENCE		
Overjet	mm	2.0	Chin tip	mm	3.0
Overbite	mm	3.5	B-NPo	mm	0.0
UI/MxP	°	9.0	LADH	mm	1.5
LI/MnP	°	1.5			
IIangle	°	−7.5			
LI-APo	mm	0.5			
LI-NPo	mm	0.5			

(q)
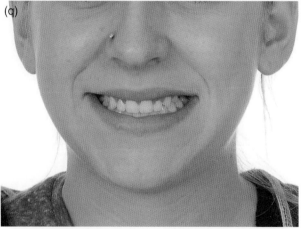

(r)
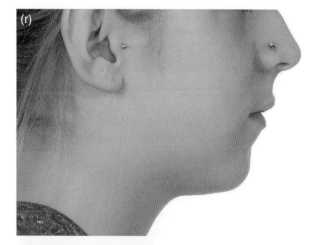

(s)
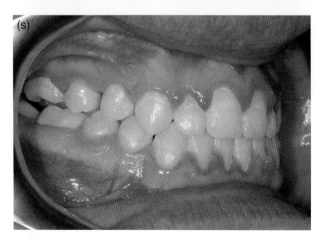

(t)
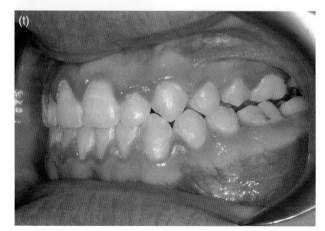

Figure 10.9 (Continued)

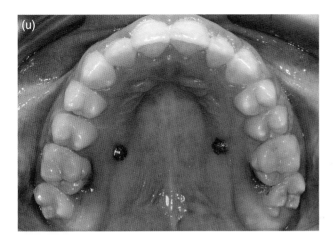
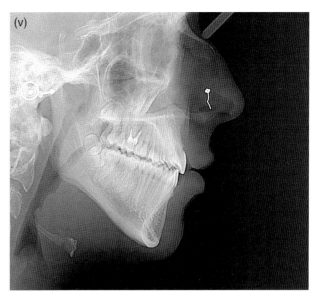

Figure 10.9 (Continued)

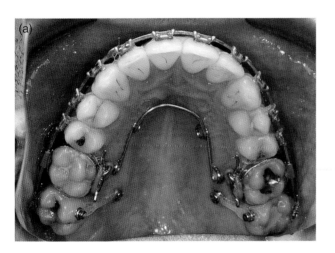
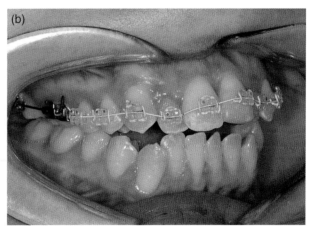

Figure 10.10 (a) Upper occlusal photograph showing an intrusion quadhelix *in situ*. Direct (elastomeric) traction has been applied between button attachments on the palatal surfaces of the second molars and the mini-implants (sited distal to the first molars). (b) The upper anterior and premolar teeth have just been bonded prior to this photograph. The coated NiTi archwire connects these ceramic brackets but the pre-existing rectangular archwire has been left in the molar areas so that the molar intrusion is separate from alignment of the rest of the maxillary arch.

periosteum or if it moves with soft palate movement. In this case, plan for the mini-implants to be inserted mesial to the first molars (Figure 10.8b).

- Preplan whether sectional (molar only) (Figure 10.8a) or full arch fixed appliance engagement is optimal at the start of treatment. I prefer to restrict the initial expansion and intrusion phases to molar engagement only and then bond the rest of the arch once an overbite has been achieved or anterior interferences arise (Figure 10.10b). This makes it easy to monitor the overjet and overbite changes, knowing that these are not due to incisor movements *per se*. Patients also prefer this for aesthetics and hygiene purposes. However, if there are palatally dis-

placed or overerupted teeth, such as canines or lateral incisors, then the whole arch should be bonded and initially aligned prior to intrusion, in order to avoid occlusal interference during AOB closure.

- I highly recommend the combined use of a speed reduction contra-angle handpiece and a guidance stent for palatal alveolar insertions since direct access is limited in the molar areas.
- If there is no rush to bond the mandibular arch during the initial intrusion phase then fit a lower full coverage plastic retainer at the start of intrusion. This prevents overeruption of the lower molars (as the upper ones intrude). Alternatively, if the lower arch is bonded then

include the second molars as early as possible in order to stabilise their vertical position. It is also helpful to create a favourable differential vertical step between the lower molars by placing the second molar tube more occlusally than the first molar one.

- If the TPA needs to be removed, to facilitate final alignment and levelling (using a molar tube on the first molars), then some vertical relapse of the first molar may occur if there is an extrusive step between it and the adjacent teeth. This may be counteracted by bonding an attachment onto the palatal surface of the first molar and applying *light* elastomeric traction or a ligature wire from the mini-implant for vertical retention. However, standard forces are not recommended if there is a risk of crossbite (from maxillary molar constriction).

> Always expand the upper arch at the start of treatment, to allow for the transverse effects of mandibular autorotation and to counteract the constrictive effects of palatal traction.

10.2.6 Simultaneous Mandibular Molar Intrusion

The maxilla is the predominant source of excessive vertical alveolar height in most AOB cases [25,31,33], so it makes anatomical sense to focus intrusion efforts in this jaw. Results from adult intrusion studies also show that lower molar intrusion is much less achievable (e.g. one-third of upper molar changes) than simultaneous maxillary changes [26]. However, mandibular molar intrusion may still be beneficial in adults requiring large AOB corrections and if there is a pre-existing reverse curve of Spee in the lower arch (Figure 10.11). In terms of adolescent AOB patients, Professor Peter Buschang's research group at Baylor College (USA) have recently demonstrated long-term benefits from supplementary mandibular anchorage in terms of limiting vertical molar growth effects [24].

Whilst passive anchorage (with a ligature or bonded connecting wire) has few transverse side-effects, active mandibular intrusion requires transverse control to avoid buccal rolling of the molars. This may be achieved using a lingual arch, which is preplanned using the following steps.

- Preparation: for interproximal insertions, first diverge the adjacent roots, by adding mesial tip to the second premolar bracket.
- Take an impression or scan, lower molar periapical radiographs or cone beam computed tomography (CBCT), and place intermolar separators.

- Fabricate a lingual arch for the first molars (to control molar arch width/torque).
- Insert bilateral lower molar mini-implants either mesial or distal to the first molars (using a 1.5 mm diameter, 6 or 9 mm length, short neck mini-implant) and as close as possible to the mucogingival junction. Alternatively, site the mini-implants in the buccal shelf (if accessible) using a 2 mm diameter, 9 mm length version (and cortical perforation step in adult patients).
- Apply 'V'-shaped elastomeric traction to the adjacent hooks/brackets, using the same principles as for maxillary intrusion.

10.2.7 Clinical Steps for Maxillary Molar Intrusion

10.2.7.1 Preinsertion

1) Palpate the mucosa distal to the first molars, to check for mobility/excess thickness and hence determine if the insertion site needs to be mesial to the first molar position.
2) Expand the maxillary arch to facilitate future arch coordination. It is highly recommended to overexpand since it is relatively easy to allow the arch to constrict towards the end of treatment, but very difficult to gain expansion in the finishing stages.
3) Band the upper first molars (and record the band sizes if it is planned to switch from an expander to an intrusion TPA later) at the start of treatment. Select a band size which enables relatively gingival seating of the band and allows for any band constriction during TPA fabrication. This makes it easier to create a favourable vertical step with the second molar tube.
4) Bond molar tubes on fully erupted upper second molars. Crucially, the avoidance of molar bands facilitates effective gingival hygiene at the posterior limit of the dental arch where a temporary reduction in crown height may occur and toothbrush access is most limited.
5) If the second molars are not fully erupted (in an adolescent) then do not bond them during initial alignment. Instead, plan to insert the mini-implants mesial to the first molars, and if the interproximal space appears limited then diverge the second premolar and first molar roots by adding mesial tip to the premolar bracket at bond-up. This causes the premolar root to move mesially during initial alignment (and the tip can readily be corrected at the treatment finishing stage).
6) Level and align either the whole maxillary dentition or only the posterior teeth adjacent to the mini-implant insertion sites using sectional fixed appliances. This decision depends on the extent of the vertical discrepancy between the anterior and posterior teeth, where a

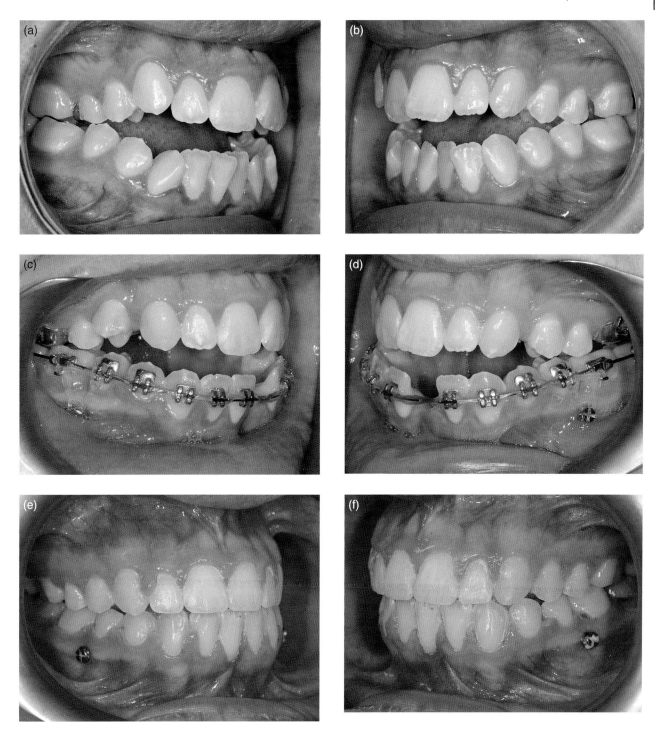

Figure 10.11 (a,b).Pretreatment photographs of an adult female patient who presented with an AOB and obvious reverse curve of Spee in the mandibular arch. (c,d) Maxillary arch expansion, a lower incisor extraction and lower fixed arch alignment have been performed, prior to this stage when both palatal alveolar and mandibular buccal mini-implants were inserted. Elastomeric traction can be seen between the lower first molar, mini-implant and second premolar teeth. (e,f) Debond photographs showing that the AOB has been corrected by a combination of maxillary molar intrusion and levelling of the mandibular curve of Spee.

large step favours segmental mechanics, whilst the risk of occlusal interferences from displaced anterior teeth necessitates full arch alignment.

7) Once a 0.019×0.025 in. sectional or full NiTi archwire has been inserted (assuming use of 0.022 slot brackets) then book two clinical appointments.

8) At the preparatory appointment, take an alginate impression or scan for fabrication of an intrusion TPA (leaving the original molar bands *in situ*) if one is required, and for guidance stent fabrication. New molar bands are placed in the impression for TPA fabrication rather than removing these from the teeth and/or expander appliance.

9) Evaluate the positions of the molars' palatal roots on the dental model and ideally with periapical radiographs or a sectional CBCT.

10.2.7.2 Intrusion TPA Fabrication (Figure 10.12)

10) Create working models – one with bands on the first molars if needed for TPA fabrication, and one for guidance stent fabrication.

11) A 1.0 mm diameter stainless steel wire is used to ensure that the TPA is sufficiently rigid. Its lateral ends are curved posteriorly to form a short hook extending 3 mm distal to the molar band (Figure 10.12a). The wire is soldered to the *mesiopalatal* corner of the first molar bands, rather than the standard midband position. This allows easy access between the TPA and the mini-implant heads.

12) Conversely, if the mini-implants are to be inserted mesial to the first molars, then the mesiodistal offset position of the TPA bar is reversed (as shown in Figure 10.8b).

13) Bilateral short (3 mm) anterior hooks are added to the TPA by soldering 1.0 mm wire onto the mesiopalatal aspect of the molar bands (Figure 10.12b).

14) The palatal bar must be offset from the palate, for example by 5 mm in the midline, to allow for its gradual vertical displacement during treatment. It must also have adequate clearance from the lateral aspects of the palatal alveolar tissues (Figure 10.12b).

15) The midpalatal loop should be wider than usual to provide a broader area of tongue contact, and hence reduce tissue discomfort.

10.2.7.3 Mini-implant Selection

16) Maxilla: use a long neck version to allow for the relatively thick mucosal tissue; for example, for Infinitas use a 1.5 mm diameter, 9 mm length, long neck one. If the palatal tissues are particularly thick or have a spongy texture, or the patient is still undergoing considerable somatic growth, then a 2 mm diameter version may be indicated to give maximum primary stability without full-depth intrabony insertion.

17) Mandible: body length selection depends on the anticipated cortical depth and density such that a long length (9 mm) version is preferable for adolescent patients, where the cortical support is reduced. An Infinitas 1.5 mm diameter, 6 mm length, short neck version may be used in an adult if strong cortical support and a perpendicular insertion are predicted.

10.2.7.4 Insertion

18) Superficial anaesthesia of the insertion sites; blanch the area overlying the first and second molar interproximal space. Topical anaesthetic may be applied

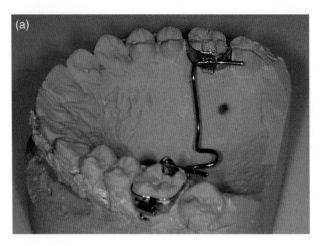
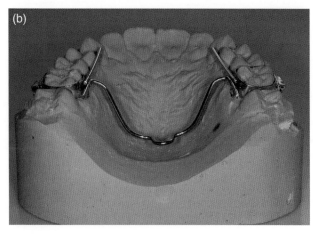

Figure 10.12   (a) Fabrication of a customised intrusion TPA where the wire is mesially offset to be clear of the mini-implant site (indicated by a red mark). (b) 5 mm palatal clearance of the middle TPA section, plus of the TPA flanks (from the palatal alveolus).

prior to local anaesthesia, but it is probably insufficiently effective on its own for such thick soft tissue.

19) Fit the stent (if available).

20) Use a mucosal punch to remove a circular section of the thick gingival tissue. After the surface has been marked with the stent *in situ*, temporarily remove it so that the mucotome can be applied perpendicular to the surface, providing a clean cut of the tissue. If necessary, then remove the mucosal tissue with either a mosquito forceps or Mitchell's trimmer.

21) In adults, use a cortical bone punch to perforate the relatively dense thick palatal cortex.

22) Insert bilateral mini-implants on the palatal side of the alveolus, using a speed-reducing (e.g. 128:1 ratio) contra-angle handpiece at less than 100 rpm.

23) Take an intraoral radiograph if close root proximity is clinically suspected, especially if an adjacent tooth is tender on percussion.

24) Complete insertion to the point where the mini-implant neck is partially submerged but the head is fully accessible.

10.2.7.5 Postinsertion

25) Cement the intrusion TPA on the first molars.

26) Traction is applied from the mini-implants to the TPA, as either an 'L' or 'V' configuration (Figure 10.13). The latter is more difficult to pass around (under) the TPA but is less prone to occlusal interferences.

27) Apply approximately 50 g (elastomeric chain) traction to the TPA hooks for the first 4–6 weeks, with the tendency to a longer period in adolescent patients. Subsequently use a stronger (150–200 g) elastomeric or NiTi closing coil auxiliary.

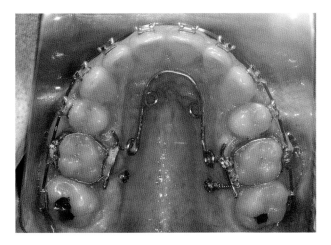

Figure 10.13 Palatal view showing an 'L' shape configuration of NiTi coil traction from the mini-implant. The coil spring passed *over* the distal end of this intrusion quadhelix and its end connected onto the mesial hook.

28) Monitor treatment progress by recording the following features at the start of intrusion and at subsequent appointments: overjet, AOB/overbite, canine relationship, upper incisor display (at rest and on full smiling), any molar openbite, and the TPA's proximity to the palate.

29) Monitor the periodontal condition (probing depth) of the terminal molars.

30) If appropriate, add a curve of Spee to the 0.019 × 0.025 in. stainless steel archwire to minimise incisor extrusion (as the maxillary occlusal plane rotates clockwise).

31) If necessary, in a large AOB case, replace the TPA when it contacts the palatal mucosa (although fortunately in my experience patients don't complain of pain when this occurs).

32) Overcorrect the AOB changes to allow for possible molar relapse.

33) After the main intrusion phase, either section the TPA or remove it altogether and bond buccal molar tubes. Consider the use of double tube attachments since this provides the option of adding an auxiliary buccal archwire (e.g. 019 × 025 in. steel) for molar expansion (Figure 10.10). This may be particularly beneficial if the main archwire needs to be a flexible NiTi one for alignment purposes; or occasionally if a TPA is not well tolerated at the outset (as occurred in the case shown in Figure 10.10, where the palatal gingival tissues were prone to a hyperplastic response).

34) Keep the mini-implants *in situ* until it is clear that further anchorage is not required. If later vertical control is needed then run traction to attachments bonded to the molar palatal surfaces (Figure 10.9b). Notably, the constrictive side-effects would need to be balanced by generous archwire expansion (hence the benefit in double molar tubes).

35) Consider an initially intensive retention regimen, for example three months full-time wear of plastic retainers with whole arch occlusal coverage. These should prevent early molar extrusion after debond.

> If appropriate, add a curve of Spee to the 0.019 × 0.025 in. stainless steel archwire to minimise incisor extrusion (as the maxillary occlusal plane rotates clockwise).

10.2.8 Case Examples

1) **Molar intrusion: adolescent patient (Figure 10.14)**
   - A 16-year-old female presented with a Class II division 1 malocclusion on a moderate skeletal II base with a 38° MMPA (Figure 10.14a–h). She had incompetent lips with overactive mentalis activity to achieve

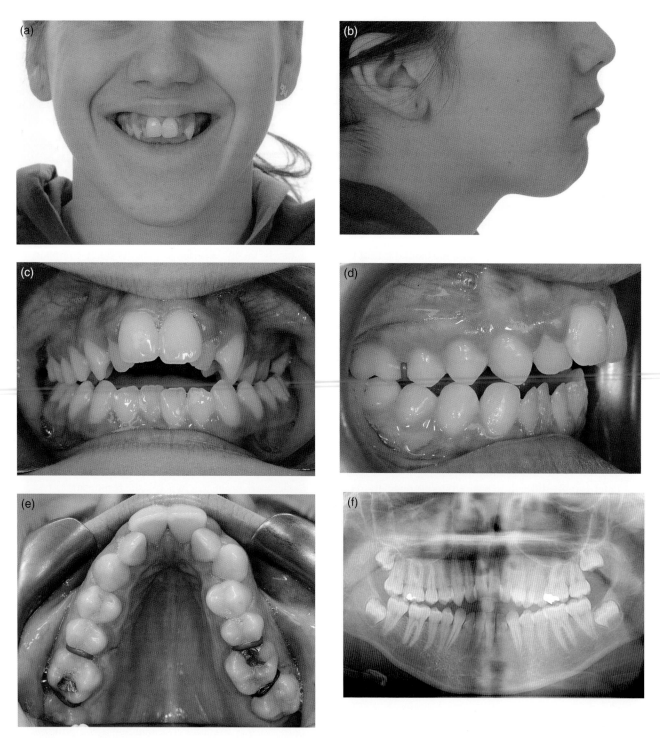

Figure 10.14 (a–e) Pretreatment photographs showing a Class II division 1 malocclusion on a moderate skeletal II base with an increased maxillomandibular planes angle. The patient had incompetent lips with excessive mentalis activity required to achieve lip closure. There was an 8 mm overjet and 5 mm AOB, with reduced upper incisor display at rest. The maxillary arch was narrow, with an associated left buccal cross-bite and functional displacement of the mandible to the left side. Orthodontic separators can be seen, mesial and distal to the upper first molars. (f,g) Pretreatment radiographs, confirming the presence of all permanent teeth. (h) The pretreatment cephalometric tracing confirms the Class II and vertical skeletal aspects, with retroclined lower incisors. (i–l) Views taken when the palatal mini-implants and lower plastic retainer were fitted, seven months into treatment. A full upper fixed appliance is seen, including tubes on the second molars. A 0.019 × 0.025 in. steel archwire has been inserted at this stage. (m,n) Lateral cephalograms taken at the start and end of the molar intrusion. (o) A cephalometric tracing showing the dental and skeletal parameters at the end of intrusion and the superimposition in (p) shows the changes during the 13 months molar intrusion phase. The main changes have been upper molar intrusion, some clockwise rotation of the maxillary arch and relative extrusion of the upper incisors, and counter-clockwise rotation of the mandible. (q–s) Photographs taken at the end of the intrusion phase, with the quadhelix having been removed. (t) A panoramic radiograph taken at the end of the intrusion phase, where the roots of the maxillary molar teeth appear superior to the sinus floor than the original OPG. (u–x) Debond photographs showing the mild Class facial profile, aesthetically pleasing exposure of the maxillary dentition, and a Class I occlusion.

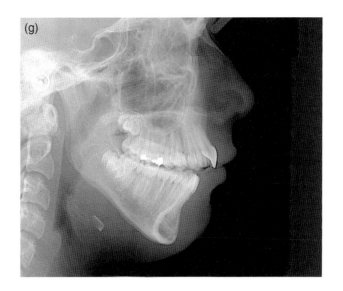

(g)

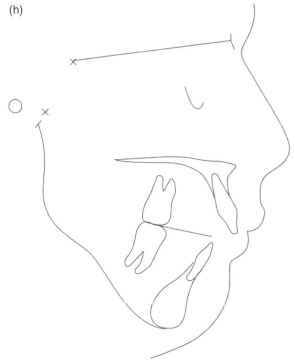

(h)

SKELETAL			SOFT TISSUES		
SNA	°	81.5	Lip Sep	mm	−0.0
SNB	°	73.5	Exp UI	mm	1.5
ANB	°	8.0	LS-E	mm	1.5
SN/MxP	°	10.0	LI-E	mm	−0.5
MxP/MnP	°	38.5	NLA	°	149.5
LAFH	mm	65.0	LLA	°	138.5
UAFH	mm	49.0	Holdaway	°	22.0
LAFH/TAFH	%	57.0			
LPFH	mm	34.5	NOSE PROMINENCE		
UPFH	mm	42.5			
PFH	mm	61.0	Nose tip	mm	19.5
Wits	mm	6.5	Nose angle	°	27.0

TEETH			CHIN PROMINENCE		
Overjet	mm	8.0	Chin tip	mm	−5.5
Overbite	mm	−5.0	B-NPo	mm	0.0
UI/MxP	°	112.5	LADH	mm	34.0
LI/MnP	°	83.5			
Ilangle	°	125.5			
LI-APo	mm	2.0			
LI-NPo	mm	6.5			

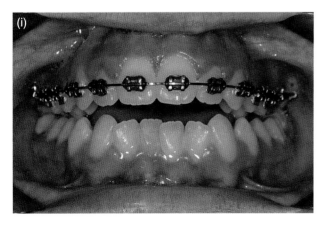

(i)

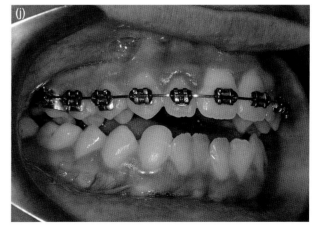

(j)

Figure 10.14 (Continued)

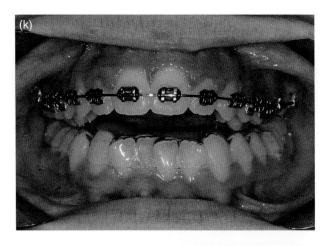

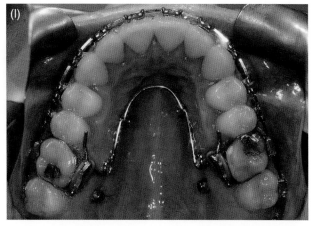

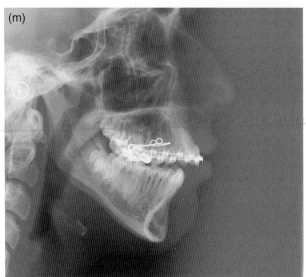

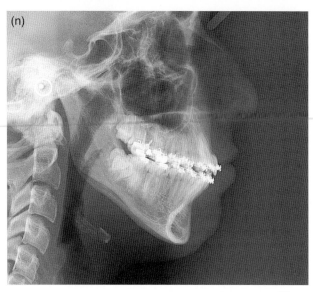

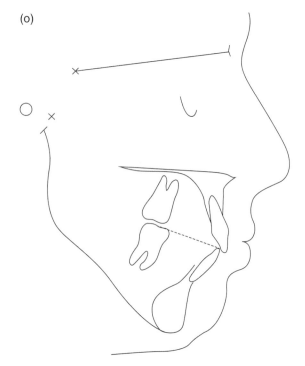

SKELETAL			SOFT TISSUES		
SNA	°	80.5	Lip Sep	mm	0.0
SNB	°	73.0	Exp UI	mm	5.5
ANB	°	7.0	LS-E	mm	−1.0
SN/MxP	°	12.0	LI-E	mm	1.5
MxP/MnP	°	37.0	NLA	°	139.5
LAFH	mm	66.0	LLA	°	137.0
UAFH	mm	51.5	Holdaway	°	19.0
LAFH/TAFH	%	56.0			
LPFH	mm	35.5	**NOSE PROMINENCE**		
UPFH	mm	43.5			
PFH	mm	62.0	Nose tip	mm	20.5
Wits	mm	0.0	Nose angle	°	26.0

TEETH			CHIN PROMINENCE		
Overjet	mm	2.5	Chin tip	mm	−7.5
Overbite	mm	1.5	B-NPo	mm	1.0
UI/MxP	°	108.0	LADH	mm	34.5
LI/MnP	°	92.0			
Ilangle	°	123.0			
LI-APo	mm	5.5			
LI-NPo	mm	10.5			

Figure 10.14 (Continued)

(p)

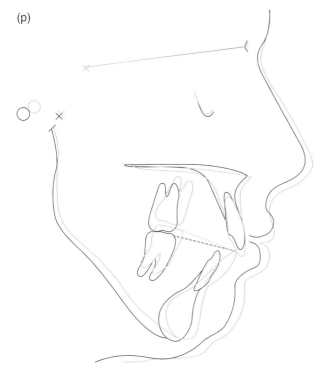

SKELETAL			SOFT TISSUES		
SNA	°	1.5	Lip Sep	mm	−2.0
SNB	°	1.5	Exp UI	mm	−0.0
ANB	°	−0.0	LS-E	mm	−0.0
SN/MxP	°	0.5	LI-E	mm	1.0
MxP/MnP	°	−2.5	NLA	°	10.5
LAFH	mm	−2.0	LLA	°	−9.5
UAFH	mm	1.0	Holdaway	°	−1.0
LAFH/TAFH	%	−1.0			
LPFH	mm	0.0	NOSE PROMINENCE		
UPFH	mm	2.0			
PFH	mm	−1.0	Nose tip	mm	2.0
Wits	mm	−6.0	Nose angle	°	3.5

TEETH			CHIN PROMINENCE		
Overjet	mm	−5.5	Chin tip	mm	3.0
Overbite	mm	4.0	B-NPo	mm	0.5
UI/MxP	°	−1.5	LADH	mm	−0.5
LI/MnP	°	11.5			
Iiangle	°	−7.5			
LI-APo	mm	3.5			
LI-NPo	mm	4.0			

(q)

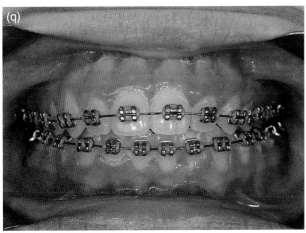

(r)

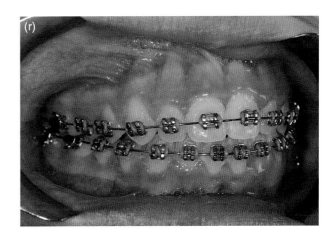

(s)

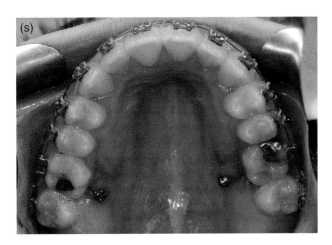

(t)

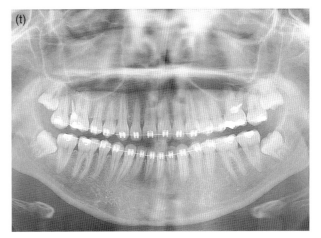

Figure 10.14 (Continued)

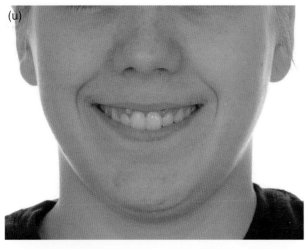

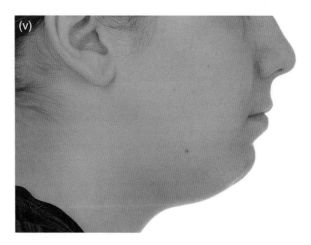

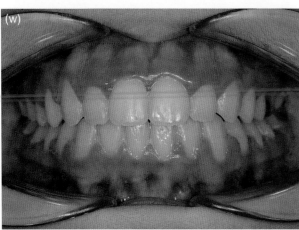

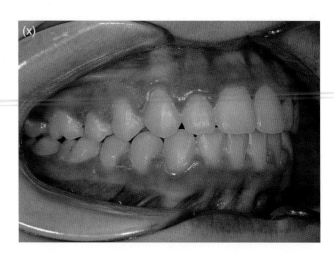

Figure 10.14 (Continued)

lip closure. There was an 8 mm overjet and 5 mm AOB, with reduced upper incisor display. The maxillary arch was narrow, with an associated left buccal cross-bite and functional displacement of the mandible to the left side.

- The maxillary arch was expanded with a modified removable quadhelix and aligned with a full fixed appliance, resulting in a 2 mm reduction in the AOB and increase in the upper incisor display.
- Mini-implants were inserted distal to the first molars and elastomeric traction applied to the quadhelix (Figure 10.14i–l).
- A full arch plastic retainer was worn on the lower teeth, from the start of intrusion until the lower arch was bonded.
- A bite-opening curve was added to the upper 0.019×0.025 in. steel archwire to counter the rotational effect on the whole arch of posterior intrusion biomechanics, and this also assisted incisor torque improvements. The amount of archwire curvature

was judged by monitoring the passive and active upper incisor display levels.

- The quadhelix was removed once a sufficient OB was present and bracket rebonding performed as the finishing stage (Figure 10.14n–t).
- Treatment was completed with an aesthetic level of incisor display, a reduction in lower face height, easier achievement of lip competence and an improvement in the chin–neck soft tissue contour (Figure u–x). These changes were primarily due to maxillary molar intrusion and counter-clockwise mandibular rotation (Figure 10.14p).
- Vacuum-formed removable retainers were fitted, and the patient instructed to wear them full-time (excluding meals) for the first three months, followed by night-time wear.

2) **Molar intrusion: adult patient (Figure 10.15)**
   - A 27-year-old female presented with a history of previous orthodontic treatment and absent upper right lateral incisor, first premolars in the other three

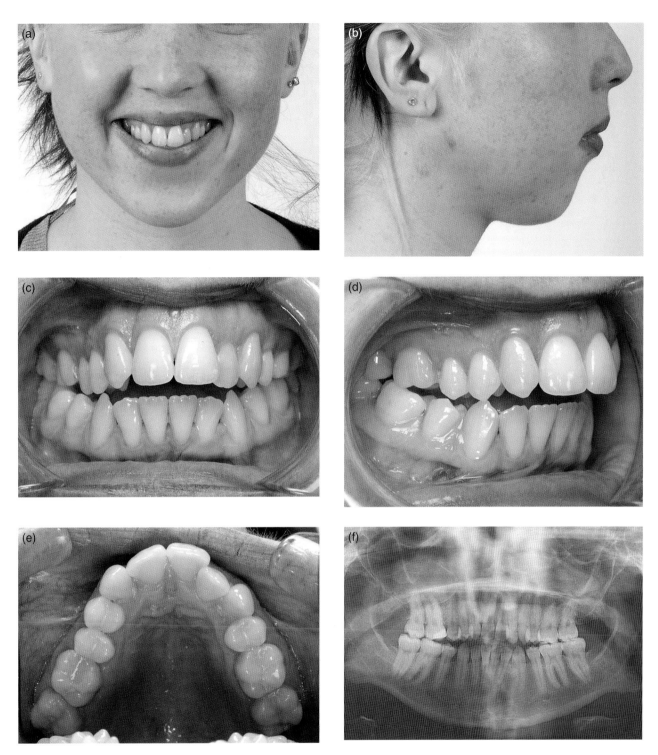

Figure 10.15 (a–e) Pretreatment photographs showing a Class II division 1 malocclusion on a moderate skeletal II base with an increased maxillomandibular planes angle. There was a 9 mm overjet and 3 mm AOB, with normal upper incisor vertical display. The upper right lateral incisor and the first premolars from the other three quadrants were absent. (f,g) Pretreatment radiographs, confirming the absence of the upper right lateral incisor, three first premolar teeth and third molar teeth. The lateral cephalogram confirms the Class II and vertical skeletal aspects. (h–j) Views taken when the palatal mini-implants were inserted, distal to the first molars. The sectional upper fixed appliances can be seen, with 0.019 × 0.025 in. steel archwires in place. (k) A lateral cephalogram taken at the start of the molar intrusion phase. (l–n) Photographs after 10 months of the intrusion phase, when there were anterior occlusal contacts and the upper anterior teeth had just been bonded. (o,p) A lateral cephalogram and panoramic radiographs taken after 17 months of the intrusion phase, where the roots of the maxillary molar teeth appear superior compared to the sinus floor than the original OPG. The incisor relationship has been corrected although the mandibular plane angle is still increased. (q–t) Debond photographs showing the mild Class facial profile, aesthetically pleasing exposure of the maxillary dentition, and a Class I occlusion. (u,v) Views of the dentition after 18 months of retention. (w,x) A lateral cephalogram taken 18 months after debond and its tracing superimposition onto the cephalogram taken at the start of intrusion. This shows that the long-term upper molar intrusion and counter-clockwise mandibular rotation treatment changes have remained stable. The extent of upper molar root projection above the palatal plane is evident. (y,z) Photographs taken six years after debond, showing a aesthetically pleasing smile, with normal upper incisor display, and a stable Class I occlusion and overbite.

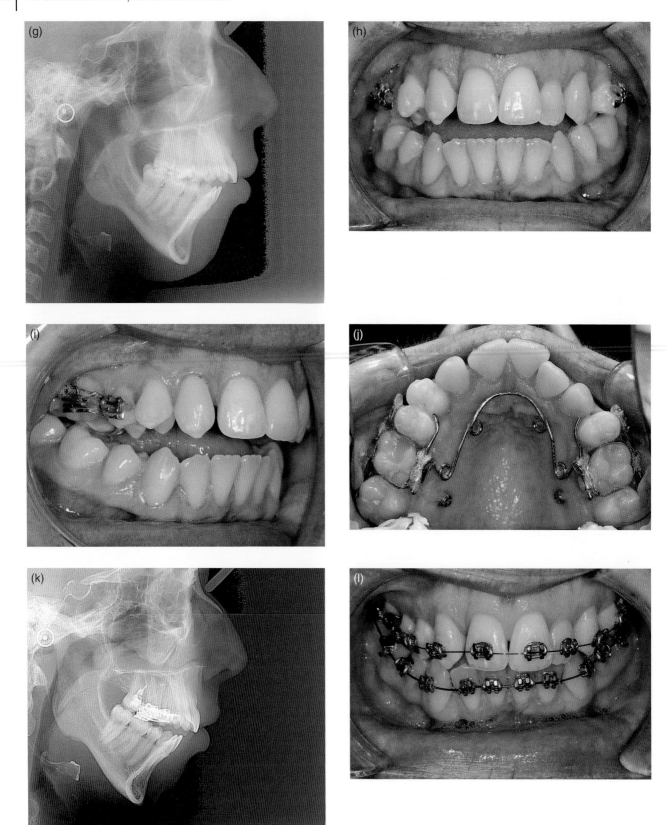

Figure 10.15 (Continued)

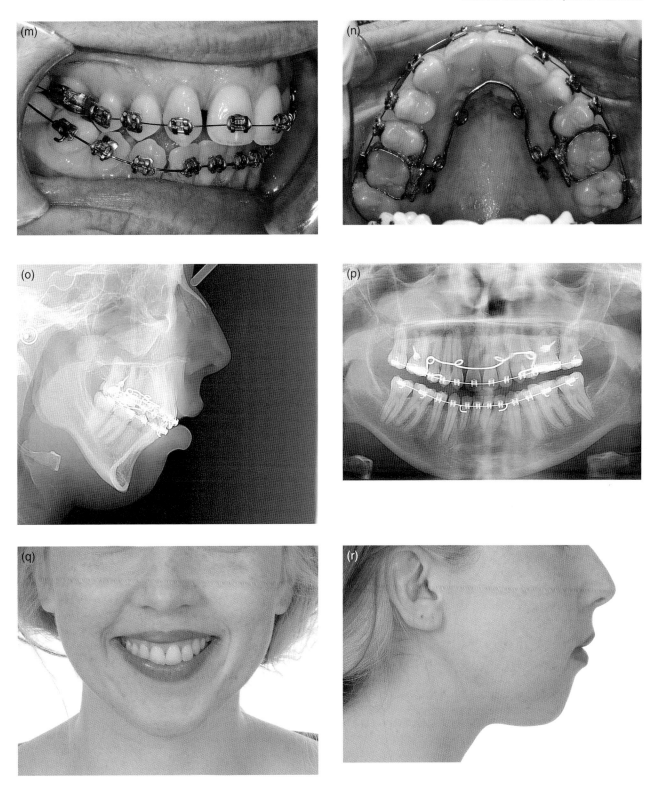

Figure 10.15 (Continued)

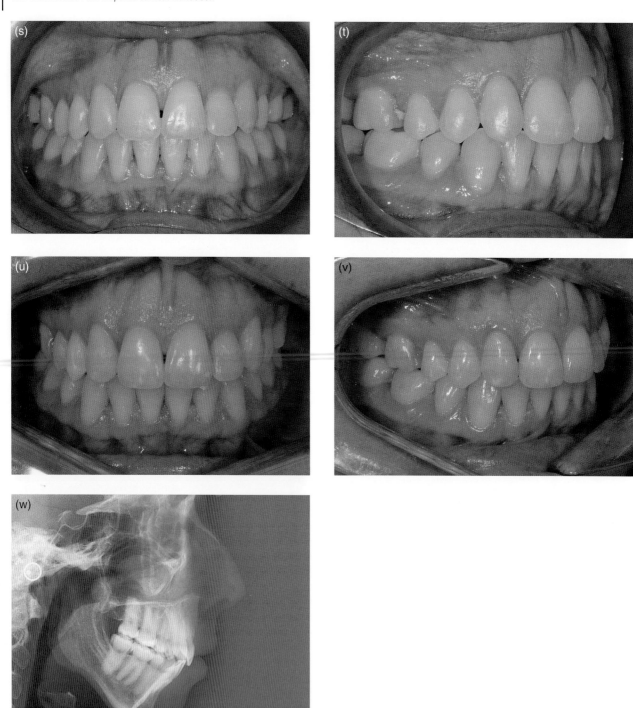

Figure 10.15 (Continued)

(x)

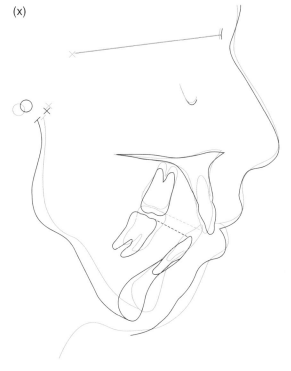

SKELETAL			SOFT TISSUES		
SNA	°	1.4	Lip Sep	mm	−0.3
SNB	°	3.4	Exp UI	mm	1.9
ANB	°	−2.0	LS-E	mm	−2.1
SN/MxP	°	−1.0	LI-E	mm	−3.5
MxP/MnP	°	−2.7	NLA	°	6.0
LAFH	mm	−3.8	LLA	°	1.3
UAFH	mm	−0.6	Holdaway	°	−2.8
LAFH/TAFH	%	−1.1			
LPFH	mm	−4.3	NOSE PROMINENCE		
UPFH	mm	0.2			
PFH	mm	−0.3	Nose tip	mm	−1.1
Wits	mm	−0.1	Nose angle	°	−2.0

TEETH			CHIN PROMINENCE		
			Chin tip	mm	6.1
Overjet	mm	−3.7	B-NPo	mm	0.9
Overbite	mm	6.9	LADH	mm	0.6
UI/MxP	°	−6.7			
LI/MnP	°	1.2			
Ilangle	°	8.2			
LI-APo	mm	−0.4			
LI-NPo	mm	−0.3			

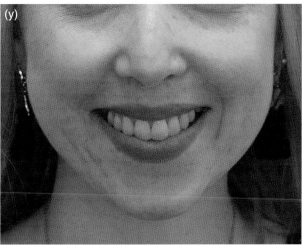

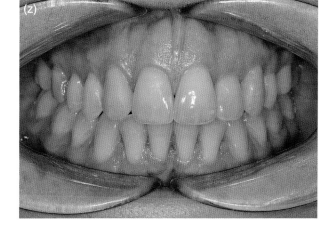

Figure 10.15 (Continued)

quadrants and all third molar teeth. She had a Class II malocclusion on a moderate skeletal II base with an increased MMPA (Figure 10.15a–g). There was a short chin–neck distance, but a reasonable upper incisor vertical display. The overjet was 9 mm and there was a 3 mm AOB.

- Treatment commenced with a sectional upper fixed appliance on the second premolar and molar teeth. The premolars were bonded because of the potential interference from their large palatal cusps. A modified (intrusion) quadhelix was used for expansion, and archwire sequence progressed to 0.019 × 0.025 in. steel archwires.

- Mini-implants were inserted distal to the upper first molars and elastomeric traction applied to the quadhelix (Figure 10.15h–k).

- The lower fixed appliance was bonded, then the rest of the upper teeth bonded after 10 months of intrusion, once anterior tooth contacts occurred (Figure 10.15l–o).

- Treatment continued for a further 12 months, without the need for any intermaxillary elastic traction.

- At debond (Figure 10.15q–v), vacuum-formed removable retainers were fitted, and the patient instructed to wear them full-time (excluding meals) for the first three months, followed by night-time wear.
- The patient declined an advancement genioplasty since she was very happy with her residual Class II facial profile (she had sought treatment to correct her Class II and AOB malocclusion features rather than facial features).
- There were no signs of relapse during the initial 18 months retention review period (Figure 10.15u–w), nor when the patient reattended six years after debond (Figure 10.15y,z).

3) **Molar intrusion: premolar extraction (Figure 10.16)**
- A 19-year-old male presented with a Class 1 malocclusion on a skeletal I base with an increased mandibular plane angle (Figure 10.16a–j). He had absence of the upper right lateral incisor and short upper and lower incisor root lengths. There was a 3 mm overjet, a 4 mm AOB and a satisfactory level of upper incisor display. The upper and lower centrelines were displaced to the right and left sides, respectively (Figure 10.16d,e).
- The extraction pattern decision was delayed until the AOB had been reduced, to allow for any mandibular autorotation effects on the overjet and buccal segment relationships.

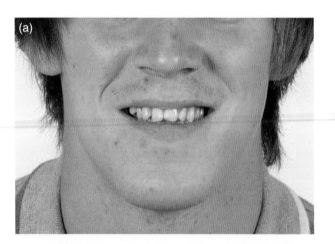
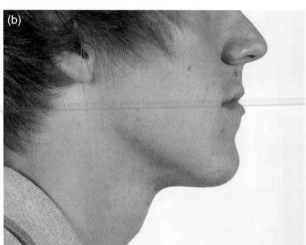
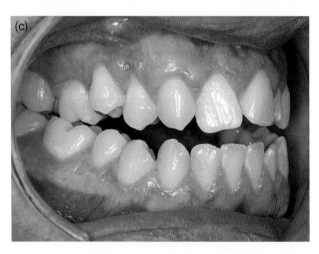
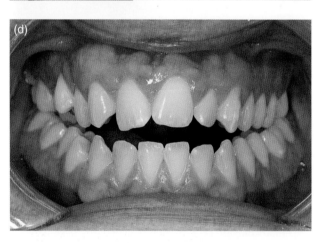

Figure 10.16 (a–g) Pretreatment photographs showing the Class I malocclusion and borderline Class III facial profile, the 4 mm AOB, absent upper right lateral incisor and centreline discrepancies. (h,i) Pretreatment radiographs and (j) the pretreatment cephalometric tracing. (k,l) Start of molar intrusion, after levelling and alignment of the premolar and molar teeth, and insertion of an intrusion TPA and palatal mini-implants (distal to the first molars). (m,n) Full upper arch engagement, excluding the left second premolar since this was planned for extraction. (o–q) The accentuated Class III incisor relationship is seen at the start of lower arch space closure (following extraction of the first premolars for incisor retraction purposes). (r) A panoramic radiograph taken during the later stages of treatment, after removal of the TPA. (s–x) Debond views, showing AOB, Class III and centreline corrections. Overcorrections of the molar intrusive changes remain, with a view to these settling in retention. (y) Cephalometric superimposition showing total treatment changes, e.g. maxillary molar intrusion, mandibular rotation and incisor retroclinations. (z) Photograph taken two years after the debond stage.

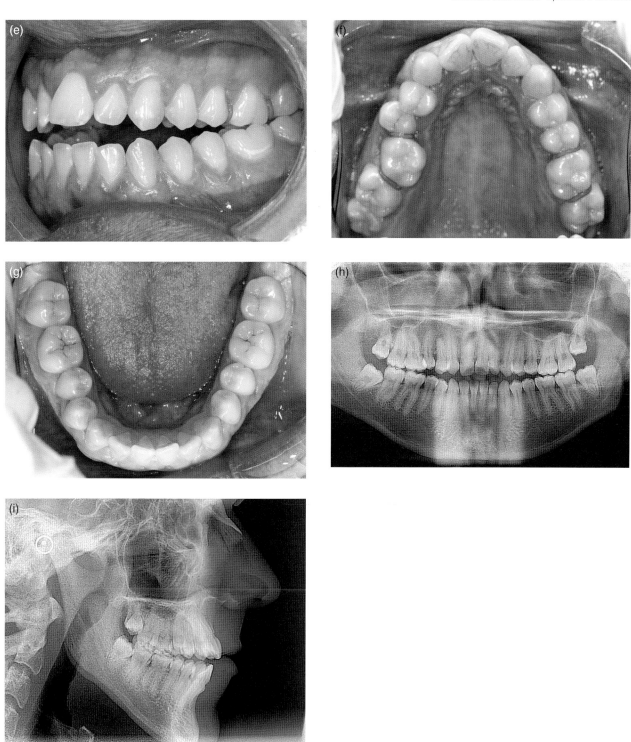

Figure 10.16 (Continued)

(j)

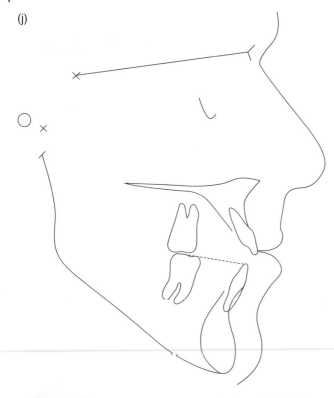

SKELETAL			SOFT TISSUES		
SNA	°	81.0	Lip Sep	mm	1.0
SNB	°	78.5	Exp UI	mm	2.0
ANB	°	2.5	LS-E	mm	−6.0
SN/MxP	°	6.0	LI-E	mm	−3.5
MxP/MnP	°	35.5	NLA	°	150.5
LAFH	mm	75.0	LLA	°	139.0
UAFH	mm	50.0	Holdaway	°	12.5
LAFH/TAFH	%	60.0			
LPFH	mm	39.5	**NOSE PROMINENCE**		
UPFH	mm	47.0			
PFH	mm	72.0	Nose tip	mm	26.5
Wits	mm	−2.0	Nose angle	°	34.0

TEETH			CHIN PROMINENCE		
Overjet	mm	3.0	Chin tip	mm	0.5
Overbite	mm	−4.0	B-NPo	mm	−3.5
UI/MxP	°	118.5	LADH	mm	43.0
LI/MnP	°	82.5			
IIangle	°	123.5			
LI-APo	mm	2.5			
LI-NPo	mm	3.0			

(k)

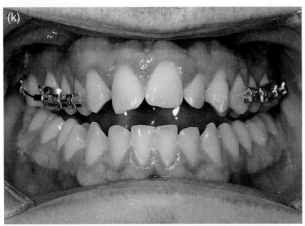

(l)

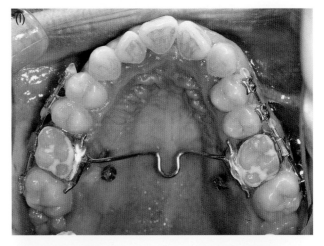

(m)

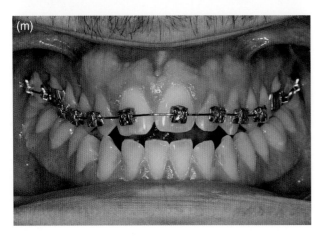

(n)

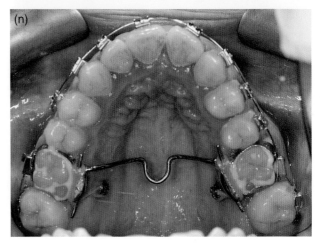

Figure 10.16 (Continued)

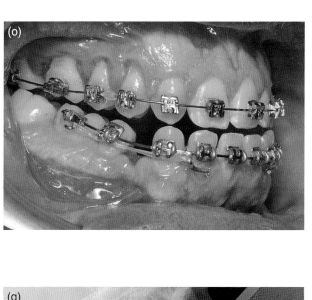

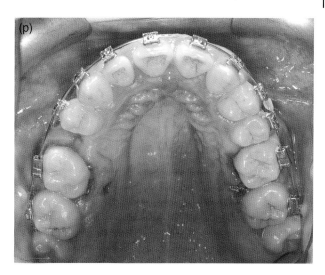

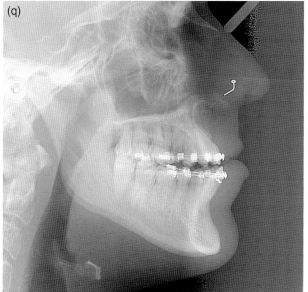

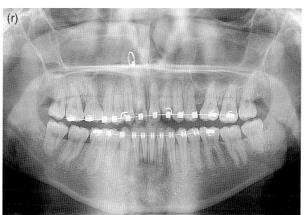

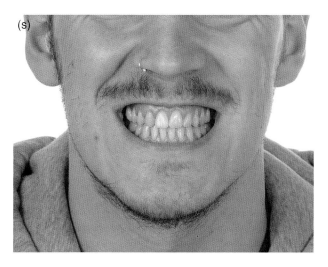

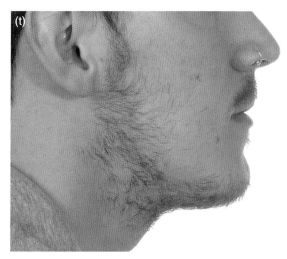

Figure 10.16 (Continued)

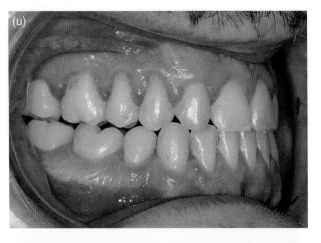

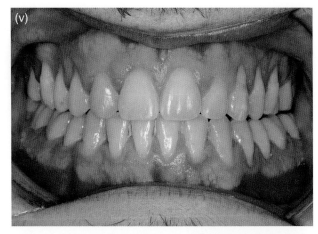

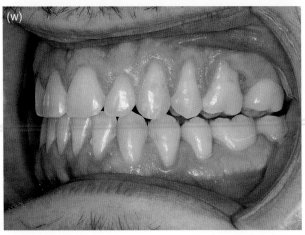

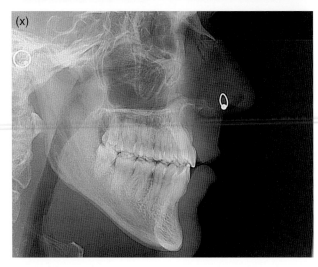

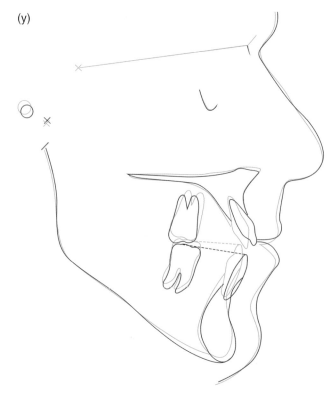

SKELETAL			SOFT TISSUES		
SNA	°	0.5	Lip Sep	mm	−1.0
SNB	°	−0.5	Exp UI	mm	−0.5
ANB	°	1.0	LS-E	mm	−2.0
SN/MxP	°	−2.0	LI-E	mm	−1.0
MxP/MnP	°	2.0	NLA	°	3.0
LAFH	mm	−1.5	LLA	°	−5.0
UAFH	mm	−1.0	Holdaway	°	−2.0
LAFH/TAFH	%	0.0			
LPFH	mm	0.5	NOSE PROMINENCE		
UPFH	mm	1.5			
PFH	mm	0.0	Nose tip	mm	−0.5
Wits	mm	4.0	Nose angle	°	−2.5

TEETH			CHIN PROMINENCE		
Overjet	mm	−0.5	Chin tip	mm	−2.0
Overbite	mm	5.5	B-NPo	mm	0.0
UI/MxP	°	−12.5	LADH	mm	1.5
LI/MnP	°	−6.5			
IIangle	°	17.0			
LI-APo	mm	−2.5			
LI-NPo	mm	−1.5			

Figure 10.16   (Continued)

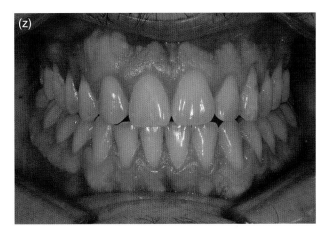

Figure 10.16 (Continued)

- The maxillary buccal segment was aligned, levelled and expanded using sectional fixed appliances and a quadhelix.
- Mini-implants were inserted distal to the first molars and an intrusion TPA fitted (Figure 10.16k,l). The TPA was replaced after it contacted the midpalatal mucosa, without eliciting pain (Figure 10.16m,n).
- Intrusion was stopped when the incisors had a −2 mm overjet and a 1 mm AOB (Figure 10.16o–q). The overbite correction then relapsed slightly when traction was discontinued for extraction of the upper left second premolar and lower right first premolar teeth. These extractions provided space for correction of the developing Class III incisor relationship and the centreline discrepancies.
- In hindsight, the lower second molars should have been banded early during the intrusion phase, for full molar control, rather than being omitted during space closure (Figure 10.16o and r).
- Conventional fixed appliance treatment continued in terms of space closure and right Class III elastic traction, then posterior box elastic settling for the final eight weeks.
- Treatment was completed with an aesthetic level of incisor display, a reduction in lower face height, easier achievement of lip competence and an improvement in the chin region's soft tissue contour (Figure 10.16s–x). These changes were primarily due to maxillary molar intrusion, mandibular autorotation and incisor retroclination (Figure 10.16y).
- The patient continued to have a positive overjet and overbite two years after debond, despite intermittent removable retainer wear (Figure 10.16z).

4) **Molar intrusion: lower incisor extraction in a Class II camouflage (Figure 10.17)**

- A 17-year-old male presented with a Class II division 1 malocclusion on a moderate skeletal II base with a normal mandibular planes angle. He had a 13 mm overjet and a minimal overbite. There was moderate lower anterior crowding with a risk of lower labial recession with non-extraction treatment (Figure 10.17a and g). Whilst there technically was a positive overbite in the retruded contact position, it was apparent that a mandibular advancement osteotomy (to correct the Class II features) would result in an AOB due to the downward trajectory of the mandibular movement.
- Therefore, the patient was planned for extraction of the lower right lateral incisor, upper molar intrusion (to reduce the AOB risk) and a mandibular advancement osteotomy.
- Treatment commenced with an 'intrusion' quadhelix and bilateral sectional fixed appliances on the molars. Palatal mini-implants were inserted distal to the first molars three months later and elastomeric traction applied to the first molars via the quadhelix. (Figure 10.17k–m).
- The rest of the maxillary dentition was bonded two months later (Figure 10.17n–p).
- Button attachments were bonded on the palatal surfaces of the second molars and 'V' configuration of traction applied from the mini-implants to the molars (Figure 10.17q).
- The molar intrusion phase was almost complete after 11 months (Figure 10.17r–u). The overbite was now deep, with considerable improvements in the Class II dental and skeletal features being noted. The maxillary molar root apices were much closer to the palatal plane in the panoramic radiograph (Figure 10.17u). The mandibular osteotomy was cancelled at this stage.

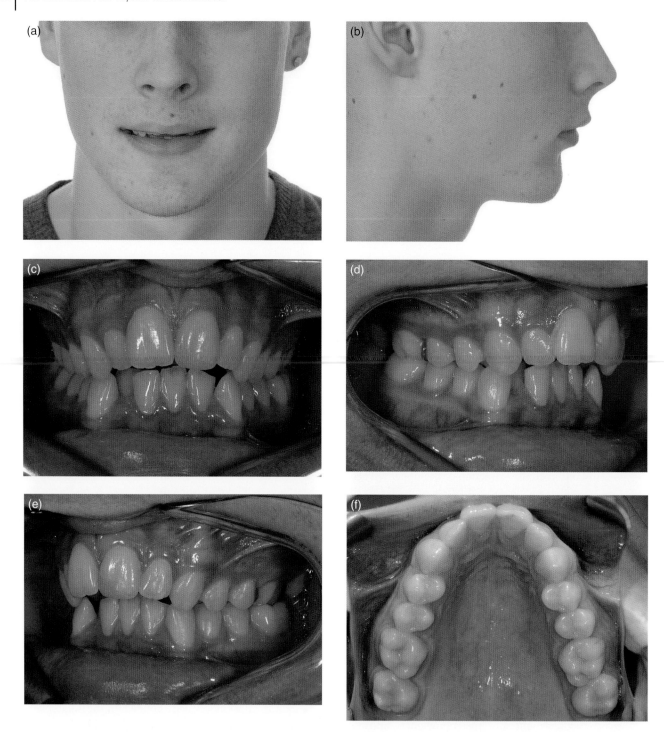

Figure 10.17 (a–g) Pretreatment photographs showing the Class II malocclusion and facial profile, small AOB, moderate lower arch crowding with lingual displacement of the lower right lateral incisor, and associated lower centreline discrepancy. (h,i) Pretreatment radiographs confirming the presence of all permanent teeth except the upper right third molar, the skeletal II features and the inferior level of the maxillary sinus floors. (j–l) Start of the molar intrusion phase, after initial expansion of the maxillary molars using a modified quadhelix. Bilateral palatal mini-implants have been inserted distal to the first molars and elastomeric traction applied. (m) Lateral cephalogram taken at time of mini-implant insertion. (n–p) The rest of the maxillary arch was bonded two months after molar intrusion commenced. (q) View of the maxillary arch four months after the bond-up, showing the addition of palatal button attachments on the upper second molars. This enabled direct traction to torque/intrude the palatal cusp of these teeth. (r,s) Photographs taken 11 months into the intrusion phase, where a deep overbite is evident. The palatal traction has resulted in an improvement in the vertical and transverse position of the upper second molars. (t,u) Radiographs taken at the end of the 15 month intrusion phase. These show considerable improvements in the Class II features and the closer proximity of the maxillary molar roots to the maxillary sinus. (v–z) Debond views, showing AOB, Class II and lower centreline corrections.

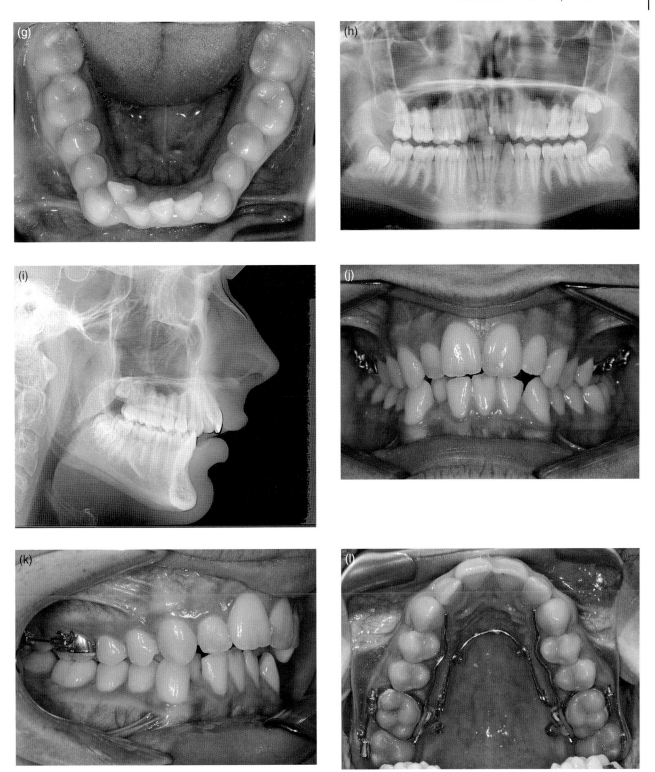

Figure 10.17 (Continued)

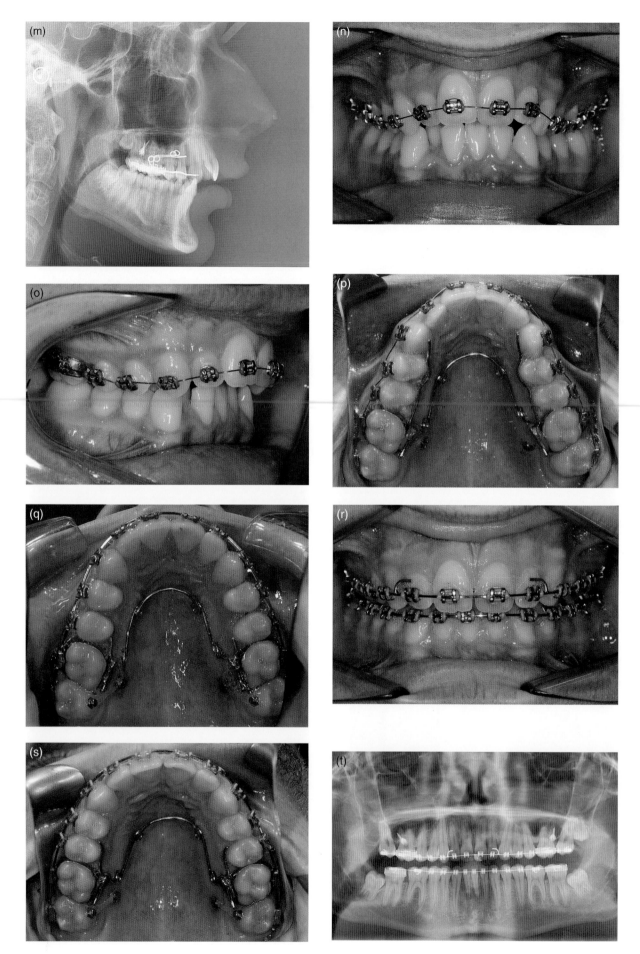

Figure 10.17 (Continued)

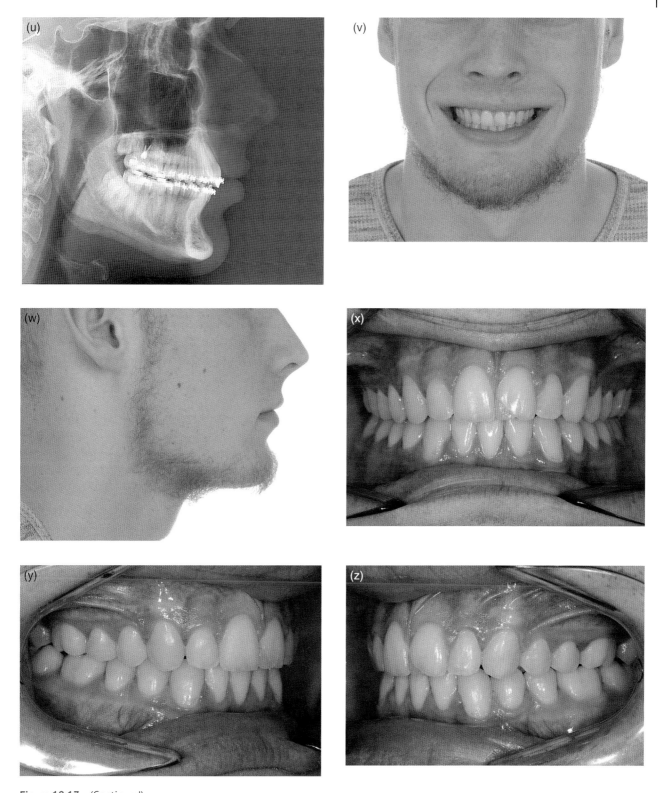

Figure 10.17 (Continued)

- Treatment was completed after a total of 26 months (Figure 10.17v–z). This had resulted in correction of the Class II and AOB features. In addition, the lower arch had been aligned, without a potential increase in

the overjet from this aspect. Removable plastic retainers were provided, with three months full-time wear and then night-time wear.

References

1 Hoppenreijs, T.J., Freihofer, H.P., Stoelinga, P.J. et al. (1997). Skeletal and dento-alveolar stability of Le Fort I intrusion osteotomies and bimaxillary osteotomies in anterior open bite deformities. *Oral Maxillofac. Surg.* 26: 161–175.

2 Teittinen, M., Tuovinen, V., Tammela, L. et al. (2012). Long-term stability of anterior open bite closure corrected by surgical-orthodontic treatment. *Eur. J. Orthod.* 34: 238–243.

3 Janson, G., Valarelli, F.P., Beltrão, R.T.S. et al. (2006). Stability of anterior open-bite extraction and nonextraction treatment in the permanent dentition. *Am. J. Orthod. Dentofac. Orthop.* 129: 760–774.

4 Gkantidis, N., Halazonetis, D., Alexandropoulos, E., and Haralabakis, N.B. (2011). Treatment strategies for patients with hyperdivergent class II division 1 malocclusion: is vertical dimension affected? *Am. J. Orthod. Dentofac. Orthop.* 140: 346–355.

5 Daimaruya, T., Takahashi, I., Nagasaka, H. et al. (2003). Effects of maxillary molar intrusion on the nasal floor and tooth root using the skeletal anchorage system in dogs. *Angle Orthod.* 73: 158–166.

6 Kanzaki, R., Daimaruya, T., Takahashi, I. et al. (2007). Remodeling of alveolar bone crest after molar intrusion with skeletal anchorage system in dogs. *Am. J. Orthod. Dentofac. Orthop.* 131: 343–351.

7 Sabuncuoglu, F.A. and Ersahan, S. (2014). Changes in maxillary molar pulp blood flow during orthodontic intrusion. *Aust. Orthod. J.* 30: 152–160.

8 Ramirez-Echave, J.I., Buschang, P.H., Carrillo, R. et al. (2011). Histological evaluation of root response to intrusion in mandibular in beagle dogs. *Am. J. Orthod. Dentofac. Orthop.* 139: 60–69.

9 Maeda, Y., Kuroda, S., Ganzorig, K. et al. (2015). Histomorphometric analysis of overloading on palatal tooth movement into the maxillary sinus. *Am. J. Orthod. Dentofac. Orthop.* 148: 423–430.

10 Carrillo, R., Rossouw, P.E., Franco, P.F. et al. (2007). Intrusion of multiradicular teeth and related root resorption with mini-screw implant anchorage: a radiographic evaluation. *Am. J. Orthod. Dentofac. Orthop.* 132: 647–655.

11 Al-Falahi, B., Hafez, A.M., and Fouda, M. (2018). Three-dimensional assessment of external apical root resorption after maxillary posterior teeth intrusion with miniscrews in anterior open bite patients. *Dental Press J. Orthod.* 23: 56–63.

12 Akan, S., Kocadereli, I., Aktas, A., and Taşar, F. (2013). Effects of maxillary molar intrusion with zygomatic anchorage on the stomatognathic system in anterior open bite patients. *Eur. J. Orthod.* 35: 93–102.

13 Gonzalez del Castillo McGrath, M., Araujo-Monsalvo, V.M., Murayama, N. et al. (2018). Mandibular anterior intrusion using miniscrews for skeletal anchorage: a 3-dimensional finite element analysis. *Am. J. Orthod. Dentofac. Orthop.* 54: 469–476.

14 Wilmes, B., Nienkemper, M., and Drescher, D. (2018). Upper-molar intrusion using anterior palatal anchorage and the 'mini-mousetrap' appliance. *Aust. Orthod. J.* 34: 263–267.

15 Senışık, N.E. and Turkkahraman, H. (2012). Treatment effects of intrusion arches and mini-implant systems in deepbite patients. *Am. J. Orthod. Dentofac. Orthop.* 141: 723–733.

16 Remmers, D., Van't Hullenaar, R.W.G.J., Bronkhorst, E.M. et al. (2008). Treatment results and long-term stability of anterior open bite malocclusion. *Orthod. Craniofac. Res.* 11: 32–42.

17 Kuroda, S., Saki, Y., Tamamura, N. et al. (2007). Treatment of severe anterior open bite with skeletal anchorage in adults: comparison with orthognathic surgery outcomes. *Am. J. Orthod. Dentofac. Orthop.* 132: 599–605.

18 Xun, C., Zeng, X., and Wang, X. (2007). Microscrew anchorage in skeletal anterior open-bite treatment. *Angle Orthod.* 77: 47–56.

19 Chaffee, M.P., Kim, S., and Schudy, G.F. (2009). Skeletal anchorage for vertical control in extraction treatment of dolichofacial patients. *J. Clin. Orthod.* 43: 749–762.

20 Baek, M., Choi, Y., Yu, H. et al. (2010). Long-term stability of anterior open-bite treatment by intrusion of maxillary posterior teeth. *Am. J. Orthod. Dentofac. Orthop.* 138: 396e1–396e9.

21 Buschang, P.H., Carrillo, R., and Rossouw, P.E. (2011). Orthopedic correction of growing hyperdivergent, retrognathic patients with miniscrew implants. *J. Oral Maxillofac. Surg.* 69: 754–762.

22 Scheffler, N.R., Proffit, W.R., and Phillips, C. (2014). Outcomes and stability in patients with anterior open

bite and long anterior face height treated with temporary anchorage devices and a maxillary intrusion splint. *Am. J. Orthod. Dentofac. Orthop.* 146: 594–602.

23 Hart, T.R., Cousley, R.R.J., Fishman, L.S., and Tallents, R.H. (2015). Dentoskeletal changes following mini-implant molar intrusion in anterior open bite patients. *Angle Orthod.* 85: 941–948.

24 Rice, A.J., Carrillo, R., Campbell, P.M. et al. (2019). Do orthopedic corrections of growing retrognathic hyperdivergent patients produce stable results? *Angle Orthod.* 89: 552–558.

25 Choi, Y.J., Kim, D.J., Nam, J. et al. (2012). Cephalometric configuration of the occlusal plane in patients with anterior open bite. *Am. J. Orthod. Dentofac. Orthop.* 141: 391–400.

26 Deguchi, T., Kurosaka, H., Oikawa, H. et al. (2011). Comparison of orthodontic treatment outcomes in adults with skeletal open bite between conventional edgewise treatment and implant-anchored orthodontics. *Am. J. Orthod. Dentofac. Orthop.* 139: S60–S68.

27 Marzouk, E.S. and Kassem, H.E. (2016). Evaluation of long-term stability of skeletal anterior open bite correction in adults treated with maxillary posterior segment intrusion using zygomatic miniplates. *Am. J. Orthod. Dentofac. Orthop.* 150: 78–88.

28 Cousley, R.R.J. (2010). A clinical strategy for maxillary molar intrusion using orthodontic mini-implants and a customised palatal arch. *J. Orthod.* 37: 197–203.

29 Horner, K.A., Behrents, R.G., Kim, K., and Buschang, P.H. (2012). Cortical bone and ridge thickness of hyperdivergent and hypodivergent adults. *Am. J. Orthod. Dentofac. Orthop.* 142: 170–178.

30 Ozdemir, F., Tozlu, M., and Germec-Cakan, D. (2013). Cortical bone thickness of the alveolar process measured with cone beam computed tomography in patients with different facial types. *Am. J. Orthod. Dentofac. Orthop.* 143: 190–196.

31 Veli, I., Uysal, T., Baysal, A., and Karadede, I. (2014). Buccal cortical bone thickness at miniscrew placement sites in patients with different vertical skeletal patterns. *J. Orofac. Orthop.* 74: 417–429.

32 Corbacho de Melo, M.M., Cardoso, M.G., Faber, J., and Sobral, A. (2012). Risk factors for periodontal changes in adult patients with banded second molars during orthodontic treatment. *Angle Orthod.* 82: 224–228.

33 Arriola-Guillena, L.E. and Flores-Mir, C. (2014). Molar heights and incisor inclinations in adults with class II and class III skeletal open-bite malocclusions. *Am. J. Orthod. Dentofac. Orthop.* 45: 325–332.

11

Transverse and Asymmetry Corrections

11.1 Asymmetry Problems

Mini-implant anchorage is invaluable for the correction of substantial asymmetry problems in all three planes of space, in both orthodontic and orthognathic cases. Asymmetrical anchorage reinforcement most obviously involves correction of large centreline discrepancies, but notably it is also now feasible to alter vertical dentofacial asymmetries which would otherwise be accepted in conventional treatment plans or deemed to require orthognathic surgery. This involves asymmetrical molar intrusion, typically to level a maxillary occlusal cant, followed by secondary orthodontic or surgical levelling of the mandibular plane. The latter will be discussed in more detail in Chapter 14 which focuses on orthognathic applications.

Conventional anteroposterior anchorage reinforcement involves connections on both sides of the arch (e.g. a transpalatal arch [TPA]), which may be unnecessary, and even contraindicated when fundamentally different movements are required in each quadrant. In comparison, mini-implant usage means that anchorage is only reinforced in the specific quadrant and direction(s) indicated for optimal treatment changes. This may involve posterior anchorage reinforcement to control asymmetrical incisor movements (Figure 11.1) or anterior anchorage to assist with molar protraction as part of centreline correction (Figure 11.2). For example, full correction of a substantial dental centreline displacement to the right side of the facial midline requires a unilateral mini-implant inserted mesial to the upper left first molar. In addition to the provision of maximum anchorage in such cases, unilateral mini-implant anchorage helps with bodily movements of the target teeth (by the use of powerarms) and increased treatment efficiency by enabling 'multitasking'. An example of the latter scenario is alignment of a palatally displaced lateral incisor at the same time as fully active bodily retraction of the contralateral canine (Figure 11.3) or space closure in the contralateral quadrant. This chapter describes unilateral mini-implant usage for the following applications:

- centreline (transverse) correction
- unilateral intrusion (vertical asymmetry correction).

> Mini-implant usage means that anchorage is only reinforced in the specific quadrant and direction(s) indicated for optimal treatment changes.

11.2 Dental Centreline Correction

11.2.1 Clinical Objective

Asymmetrical anchorage reinforcement to facilitate unilateral retraction of the incisor teeth or unilateral molar protraction.

11.2.2 Treatment Options

- Unilateral direct mini-implant anchorage and powerarm combination.
- Indirect mini-implant anchorage where the mini-implant stabilises an anchor tooth (for conventional traction application).
- Indirect palatal mini-implant anchorage of a TPA or Nance palatal button so that unilateral traction can be applied from a molar band (essentially a unilateral version of the technique described for bilateral traction in Chapter 7). This is particularly relevant in young adolescent patients where the maxillary alveolar bone is immature.
- Midpalatal anchored appliance for unilateral distalisation, or unilateral molar protraction, or a combined mesialiser-distaliser appliance (Figure 11.4).
- Conventional anchorage involving bilateral intraoral reinforcement or asymmetrical headgear.
- Asymmetrical intermaxillary elastic traction (but with the risk of unfavourable movement of the secondary arch centreline).
- Asymmetrically activated functional (orthopaedic) appliances.

The Orthodontic Mini-Implant Clinical Handbook, Second Edition. Richard Cousley.
© 2020 John Wiley & Sons Ltd. Published 2020 by John Wiley & Sons Ltd.

11.2.3 Relevant Clinical Details

- Many patients display asymmetry in several dimensions rather than just one, although one plane may predominate. Therefore, the diagnostic process should determine both the extent and nature of the transverse and vertical contributions to the whole asymmetry. In particular, is the asymmetry panfacial or localised, dental or skeletal, and is a functional mandibular displacement present? A frontal posteroanterior cephalometric view or cone beam computed tomography (CBCT) scan may be useful.
- The incisor (overjet, overbite) and canine relationships.
- The dental centrelines relative to the facial midline and (the lower one) to the mandibular midline.

11.2.4 Biomechanical Principles

- Determine the ideal traction vector prior to mini-implant insertion. For example, if there is sufficient height of attached gingiva then the mini-implant may be sited at a relatively apical ('high' vertical) level. This provides the option of supplementary vertical intrusive traction, although a powerarm may be required to prevent unwanted vertical side-effects due to an oblique vector of anteroposterior traction. Conversely, if there is only a narrow band of attached gingiva then the mini-implant is limited to a coronal insertion level, resulting in closer proximity to the archwire plane and a relatively horizontal line of traction, but little scope for intrusive effects.
- Indirect (midpalate) anchorage of a Nance palatal button involves force application from the molar's buccal hook. This means that the biomechanical effects are similar to conventional straight wire treatment.
- Transverse centreline correction involves either *en masse* incisor movements on a rigid (0.019×0.025 in.) steel archwire or the use of canine powerarm to enable movements on 'lighter' (e.g. 0.018 in.) archwires (Figure 11.3).

11.2.5 Clinical Tips and Technicalities

- Growing patients with reduced maxillary bone support (due to low density/thickness of the cortical plate) may be best treated with indirect palatal anchorage since the mid-palate cortex provides adequate stability in adolescents.

11.2.6 Midtreatment Problems and Solutions

- Vertical side-effects such as a lateral openbite and excessive incisor retroclination.
  - Avoid the application of traction with a flexible archwire *in situ* or when a working steel archwire (e.g. 0.019×0.025 in.) has not fully levelled the arch.
  - Accept any lateral openbite side-effect until anchorage is no longer required, then remove the mini-implant, bond the second molar in the affected quadrant, and use a flexible archwire to level the arch. Although most lateral openbites readily settle once traction has ceased and the archwire changes are expressed, it is also acceptable to add vertical elastic traction as necessary.
  - Vertical settling elastics may also be added during molar protraction, to counteract the effects of archwire binding in the molar tube and hence incisor proclination and intrusion. This can be done by a combination of methods such as adding a unilateral bite-closing curve (reverse curve of Spee) to the working archwire on the traction side or adding supplementary traction to the labial segment or a posted archwire, ideally from a lingual attachment on the molar. Further information on this is discussed in Chapter 9.

11.2.7 Clinical Steps for Centreline Correction

11.2.7.1 Preinsertion

1) Increase the interproximal space available at the insertion site by bonding the attachments on the teeth at altered tips; for example, for an insertion distal to the second premolar, add mesial tip to its bracket, causing the root to move mesially during alignment.
2) If canine retraction is indicated prior to centreline correction, then align most of the arch (except for substantially displaced incisors) to prepare for a 0.018 in. steel working archwire and add a powerarm to the canine. Otherwise, for *en masse* incisor movement, align and level the whole arch to be ready to accommodate a 0.019×0.025 in. steel archwire. A powerarm can then be crimped to this archwire.
3) If desired, fabricate a stent by taking an impression of the arch 1–2 weeks before insertion. Avoid waxing out brackets and the buccal sulcus near the insertion site and record the clinical level of the mucogingival junction (to transfer to the working model).

11.2.7.2 Mini-implant Selection

4) Maxilla: use a narrow, long body, short neck mini-implant (e.g. 1.5 mm diameter, 9 mm length, short neck Infinitas™ version).
5) Mandible: use a narrow, short neck mini-implant (e.g. Infinitas 1.5 mm diameter, 6 or 9 mm length, short neck version). The length selection largely depends on the height of attached gingiva and alveolar width at the insertion site; for example, a 9 mm length may be preferable where a limitation in one or both of these factors indicates the need for an oblique insertion angle.

11.2.7.3 Insertion

6) Identify the ideal buccal alveolar insertion point through attached gingiva (which does not require a soft tissue punch step).

7) Superficial anaesthesia of the insertion site.

8) Determine the angles of insertion. All mini-implants are inserted into the interproximal space and are perpendicular to the surface in the horizontal plane. Maxillary and posterior mandibular mini-implants may be inserted at either 90° (perpendicular to the surface) or angled obliquely by up to 30°, by inclining the screwdriver in an apical direction. Anterior mandibular insertions are inclined at 80–90° to the surface because of limitations due to the sloping shape of the alveolus.

9) Manual insertion is recommended where there is sufficient physical access (e.g. ease of stretching the cheek and buccal sulcus). Otherwise, contra-angle handpiece insertion may be performed, but with resultant loss of full tactile control.

10) A cortical bone punch is recommended as the first step for posterior mandibular alveolar and buccal shelf sites (except in young teenage patients with less dense cortex).

11) Complete the insertion to the point where the mini-implant neck is partially submerged but the head is fully accessible. This is best performed gradually and with intermittent release of the screwdriver during the final turns, so that overinsertion is avoided.

12) Percuss the adjacent teeth to gauge root proximity and take an intraoral radiograph if a problem is suspected.

11.2.7.4 Postinsertion

13) For initial canine retraction, apply traction directly from the mini-implant head to the canine bracket/powerarm (Figure 11.3).

14) For *en masse* labial retraction, crimp a powerarm to the archwire mesial to the canine bracket (Figure 11.1). If necessary, adjust the level of traction on the powerarm to create a horizontal line of traction (parallel to the occlusal plane).

15) Immediately load the mini-implant with *light* traction for the first 5–6 weeks, for example with a lightly stretched powerchain. Subsequently apply normal levels of traction using a NiTi closing spring or elastomeric.

16) Discontinue the traction and possibly explant the mini-implant once the anchorage requirements have been met, for example Class I canines and centred incisors.

17) If a lateral openbite has developed then (after explantation) bond the ipsilateral upper second molar and level the arch using a flexible NiTi archwire. Vertical or box elastics may also be used to settle the buccal occlusion.

11.2.8 Case Examples

1) Centreline correction involving incisor retraction (Figure 11.1)

- A 22-year-old female presented with a Class II division 2 malocclusion on a mild skeletal II base (Figure 11.1a–g). She had absence of both premolars from the upper right quadrant and a single premolar in the other three quadrants. The third molars were present and unerupted except in the upper right quadrant (Figure 11.1f). There was an associated large displacement of the maxillary dental centreline to the right side and a Class II relationship of the left canine teeth.

- There was a marked indentation in the palatal aspect of the alveolus mesial to the first molar (Figure 11.1e). Consequently, this site was not ideal for direct anchorage purposes. A midpalate anchored appliance was considered, but its reliance on conventional traction would have been suboptimal in terms of correction of the retroclined upper incisors and deep overbite (Figure 11.1h). Therefore, the combination of direct buccal anchorage and an anterior powerarm was deemed most appropriate for this case, accepting the limited interproximal space available mesiobuccal to the upper left first molar.

- The upper arch was initially levelled and aligned, until a 0.019 × 0.025 in. steel archwire could be inserted.

- Asymmetrical buccal anchorage was created by insertion of a 9 mm length mini-implant mesial to the upper left first molar (Figure 11.1i–l). Direct elastomeric traction was applied to a powerarm, which was crimped on the archwire mesial to the upper left lateral incisor.

- Mini-implant traction continued for 10 months, initially to move the upper incisors into the small upper left quadrant space available and then continued to distalise the whole upper left quadrant. This was manifest radiographically as distal movement of the upper left second molar relative to the posterior sinus wall (Figure 11.1o).

- The upper incisors were successfully torqued, due to palatal root movement, and intruded during the asymmetric traction phase (Figure 11.1p,q). This is pleasantly surprising given that the traction and powerarm were unilateral.

- The patient was debonded four months later, after a total treatment time of two years (Figure 11.1r–v).

2) Centreline correction involving molar protraction (Figure 11.2)

- This 27-year-old female presented with a Class II division 2 malocclusion on a mild skeletal II base (Figure 11.2a–g). She had transverse skeletal asymmetry with the chin point displaced to the left side (without a functional displacement) and a subtle degree of vertical asymmetry (occlusal cant slightly higher on the left side). The upper incisor–lip relationship was aesthetically satisfactory. The upper right canine and the first premolars from the other three quadrants were absent. The upper and lower dental centrelines were displaced to the right and left sides, respectively, and the buccal segments exhibited similar asymmetry, including a three-quarter unit Class II relationship of the left canines.

- Both arches were initially levelled and aligned. The left Class II canine relationship, deep overbite and lower centreline problems were additionally corrected by the use of pushcoil to reopen the lower left first premolar space. This meant that the lower arch anchorage reinforcement site would be mesial to the lower left canine.
- Asymmetrical anchorage was reinforced using 6 and 9 mm length mini-implants inserted mesial to the lower left canine and upper left first molar, respectively (Figure 11.2h–n). Direct traction was applied to pull the maxillary incisors towards the left, whilst indirect anchorage was utilised in the mandibular arch, since the insertion site was anterior to the canine. This involved a 0.019 × 0.025 in. steel auxiliary wire and a cross-tube connecting the mini-implant and the main archwire. Elastomeric traction was used to protract the lower left molars.
- The patient declined to correct the vertical asymmetry, so the mini-implants were removed once the left molar relationship had been overcorrected so that finishing alignment could be performed (Figure 11.2p–t). This was followed by asymmetrical traction, predominantly Class III elastics on the right side, although a small residual centreline discrepancy was accepted due to tooth size discrepancies (Figure 11.2u–z).

3) Centreline correction utilising powerarm control (Figure 11.3)

- A 23-year-old male presented with a Class III malocclusion and skeletal deformity, requiring orthognathic surgery. The upper right lateral incisor was palatally excluded and the upper dental centreline was severely displaced to the right side (Figure 11.3a–f).
- It was decided to extract the upper left first premolar tooth to provide space for relief of crowding and preoperative correction of the upper centreline correction. Movement of the upper anterior teeth towards the left side required maximum anchorage reinforcement.
- The upper arch was initially levelled and aligned to the stage of insertion of an upper 0.019 × 0.025 in. steel archwire. A buccal mini-implant (1.5 × 9.0 mm, short neck version) was inserted mesial to the upper left first molar. A powerarm was crimped onto the archwire, distal to the left lateral incisor, and elastomeric traction applied to it. On the right side, lightly activated pushcoil was placed across the right lateral incisor site (Figure 11.3g–j).
- The upper right lateral incisor was bonded eight weeks later. An auxiliary 0.012 in. NiTi wire engaged

this tooth and the base archwire was reduced to a 0.018 in. steel one. Consequently, the crimpable powerarm was replaced with a single-tooth powerarm on the upper left canine (Figure 11.3k–n).
- Traction continued to the left canine powerarm during alignment of the upper right lateral incisor, to continue upper centreline correction. The powerarm enabled controlled canine retraction despite NiTi alignment archwires being used (Figure 11.3o–r).
- The mini-implant and powerarm were removed (after eight months) once the upper centreline had been slightly overcorrected, and the patient proceeded to bimaxillary orthognathic surgery.

4) Centreline correction involving simultaneous molar distalisation and protraction (Figure 11.4)

- A 10-year-old boy presented with absence of the left maxillary central incisor and ectopic eruption of the left canine towards the central incisor space (Figure 11.4a). He presented with a Class I malocclusion with asymmetrical features in terms of upper centreline displacement to the left side, and right Class II/left Class III buccal segment relationships (Figure 11.4b–f).
- The treatment plan accepted eruption of the upper left canine into the central incisor space and closure of the edentulous left canine space. This, coupled with upper centreline correction, required a combination of right molar distalisation and left molar protraction. The latter was going to be especially challenging due to the alveolar deficiency/severe necking in the left canine region.
- The maxillary arch was first aligned and then pushcoil was placed between the upper right central incisor and upper left lateral incisor teeth to create sufficient space for the erupting left canine. Two paramedian mini-implants were inserted and a mesialiser-distaliser appliance fitted onto these and first molar bands (Figure 11.4g–j). Pushcoil was used on the right side of the 1 mm wire frame, for molar distalisation. Elastomeric traction was applied on the left side, to protract the molar and premolar teeth.
- The mesialiser-distaliser phase of treatment was completed once the upper left canine space had been substantially reduced by mesial movement of the buccal teeth and sufficient distalisation achieved on the right side to allow for space allocation anteriorly (Figure 11.4k–o).
- The left maxillary canine crown was provisionally restored to mimic a central incisor. The patient's upper centreline was correct at this stage, but the lower dental centreline was displaced to the right side. Therefore, treatment was to be concluded with the use of asymmetrical elastics, to both correct the lower centreline and complete closure of the residual maxillary arch spaces (Figure 11.4p–r).

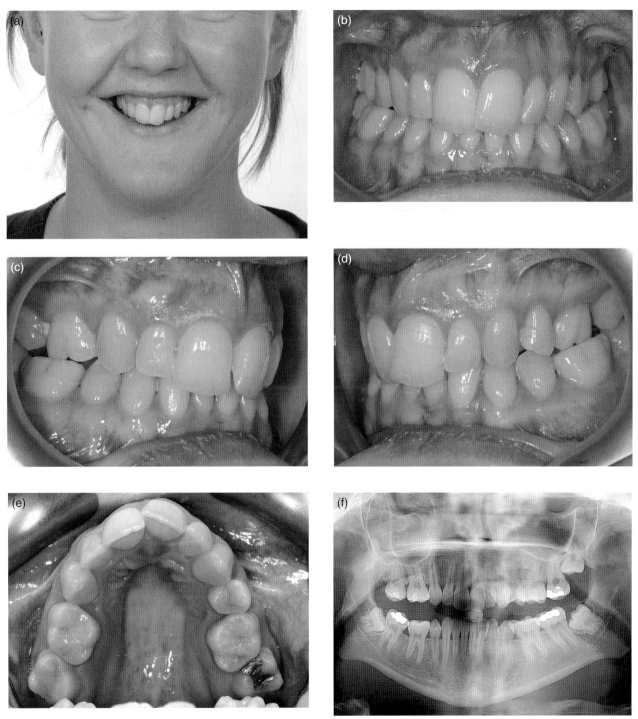

Figure 11.1 (a–e) Pretreatment photographs showing this Class II division 2 malocclusion with absence of the five premolars, including both in the upper right quadrants, and a significant shift of the upper centreline to the right side. The upper incisors are overerupted and there is increased gingival display on smiling. (f) Pretreatment panoramic radiograph showing the absence of both upper right premolars and a premolar tooth from the other three quadrants, plus three of the third molars. (g,h) Pretreatment lateral cephalogram and tracing which highlight the mild skeletal II relationship and bimaxillary retroclination. (i–l) Views taken after insertion of the buccal mini-implant, mesial to the upper left first molar, and placement of a powerarm on the 0.019 × 0.025 in. steel archwire. There is a small space distal to the upper left lateral incisor, and the mini-implant has been inserted close to the first molar to provide some clearance for distal movement of the adjacent premolar. (m,n) The upper centreline has almost been corrected after nine months of traction. Some mucosal inflammation is evident where the traction elastomeric has been in contact with it, due to the inward tilt of the powerarm. (o,p) Midtreatment radiographs showing the distal movement of the upper left molars, relative to the maxillary sinus boundaries, a Class I incisor relationship and normal incisor inclinations. (q) Cephalometric superimposition of the pretreatment and midtreatment cephalograms showing the 11° improvement in upper incisor torque, palatal root movement and intrusion. Some of the upper molar distalisation is evident, and lower incisor proclination. (r–v) Debond photographs showing the Class I occlusion, significantly improved upper dental centreline and reduction in gingival display on smiling.

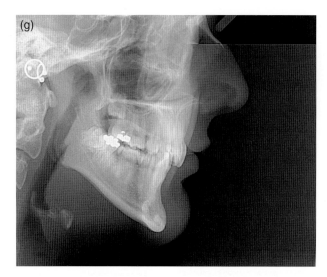

(h)

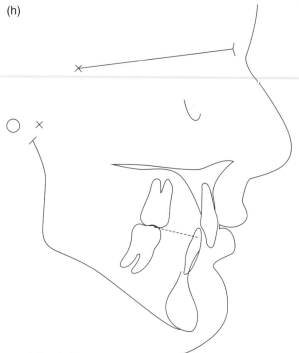

SKELETAL			SOFT TISSUES		
SNA	°	74.5	Lip Sep	mm	0.5
SNB	°	72.0	Exp UI	mm	8.0
ANB	°	3.0	LS-E	mm	−7.0
SN/MxP	°	5.5	LI-E	mm	−7.5
MxP/MnP	°	33.0	NLA	°	138.5
LAFH	mm	67.0	LLA	°	114.5
UAFH	mm	44.5	Holdaway	°	8.0
LAFH/TAFH	%	60.0			
LPFH	mm	40.5	**NOSE PROMINENCE**		
UPFH	mm	40.5			
PFH	mm	70.5	Nose tip	mm	19.0
Wits	mm	2.0	Nose angle	°	28.0

TEETH			CHIN PROMINENCE		
Overjet	mm	6.0	Chin tip	mm	−7.5
Overbite	mm	6.5	B-NPo	mm	−5.5
UI/MxP	°	94.5	LADH	mm	41.0
LI/MnP	°	77.0			
Ilangle	°	155.5			
LI-APo	mm	−3.5			
LI-NPo	mm	−3.5			

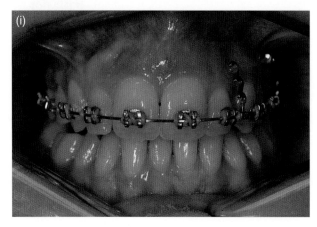

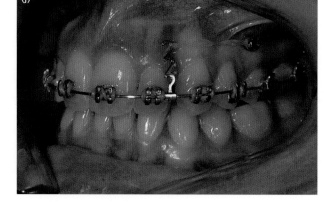

Figure 11.1 (Continued)

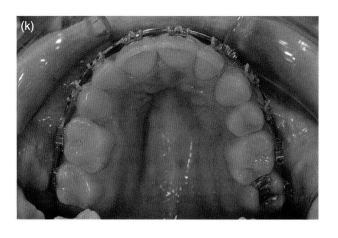

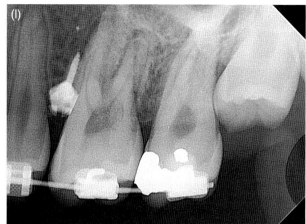

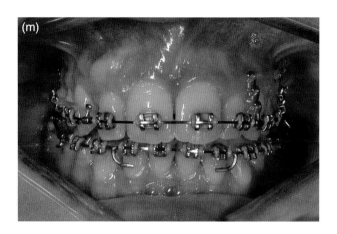

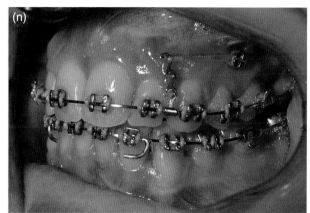

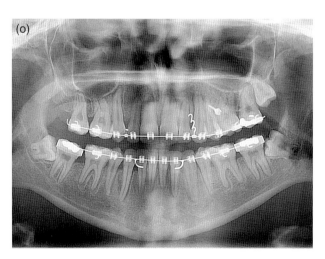

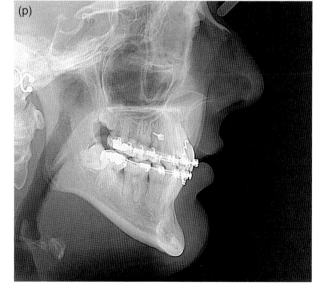

Figure 11.1 (Continued)

(q)

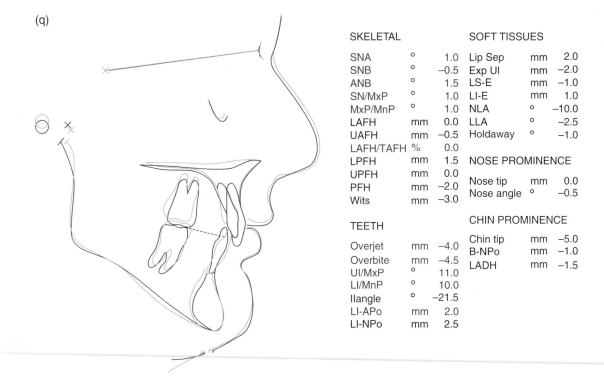

SKELETAL			SOFT TISSUES		
SNA	°	1.0	Lip Sep	mm	2.0
SNB	°	−0.5	Exp UI	mm	−2.0
ANB	°	1.5	LS-E	mm	−1.0
SN/MxP	°	1.0	LI-E	mm	1.0
MxP/MnP	°	1.0	NLA	°	−10.0
LAFH	mm	0.0	LLA	°	−2.5
UAFH	mm	−0.5	Holdaway	°	−1.0
LAFH/TAFH	%	0.0			
LPFH	mm	1.5	NOSE PROMINENCE		
UPFH	mm	0.0			
PFH	mm	−2.0	Nose tip	mm	0.0
Wits	mm	−3.0	Nose angle	°	−0.5

TEETH			CHIN PROMINENCE		
			Chin tip	mm	−5.0
Overjet	mm	−4.0	B-NPo	mm	−1.0
Overbite	mm	−4.5	LADH	mm	−1.5
UI/MxP	°	11.0			
LI/MnP	°	10.0			
Iiangle	°	−21.5			
LI-APo	mm	2.0			
LI-NPo	mm	2.5			

(r)

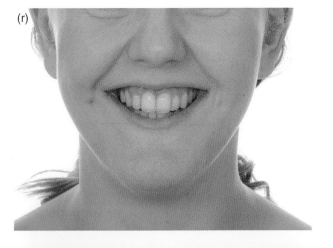

(s)

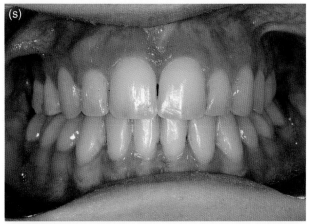

(t)

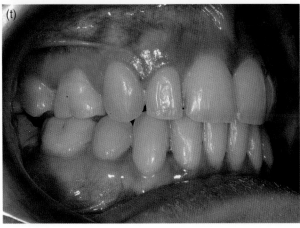

(u)

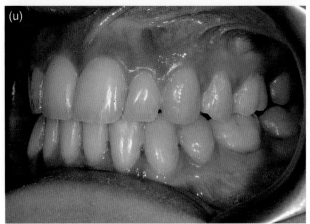

Figure 11.1 (Continued)

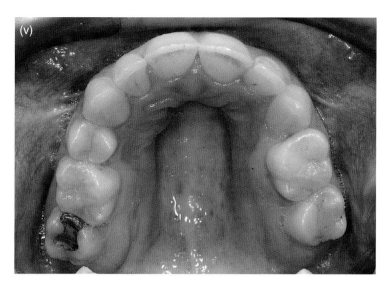

Figure 11.1 (Continued)

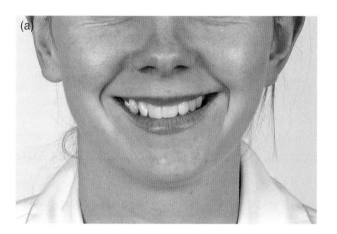

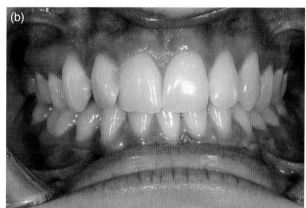

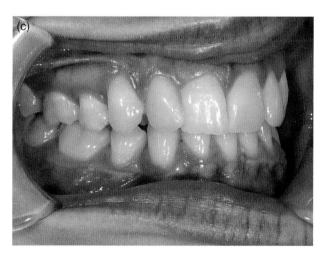

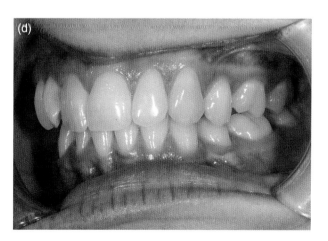

Figure 11.2 (a–g) Pretreatment views showing this Class II division 2 malocclusion with absence of the upper right canine and first premolars in the other three quadrants, asymmetrical buccal segment relationships and centreline discrepancies (upper displaced to the right, lower to the left sides). (h–n) The lower left premolar space has been reopened during alignment and as part of the lower centreline correction. Upper posterior and lower anterior mini-implants have been inserted for direct elastomeric traction to the upper anterior teeth and lower molar protraction, respectively. The latter involved indirect anchorage using a piece of 0.019 × 0.025 in. steel archwire and cross-tube to link the mini-implant to the archwire. Horizontal elastomeric traction was then applied from this vertical wire strut to the lower left molar hook. (o) Panoramic radiograph taken prior to removal of the mini-implants. (p–t) Photographs showing the finishing alignment stage, after removal of the mini-implants and prior to the use of asymmetrical settling elastics. (u–z) Debond views.

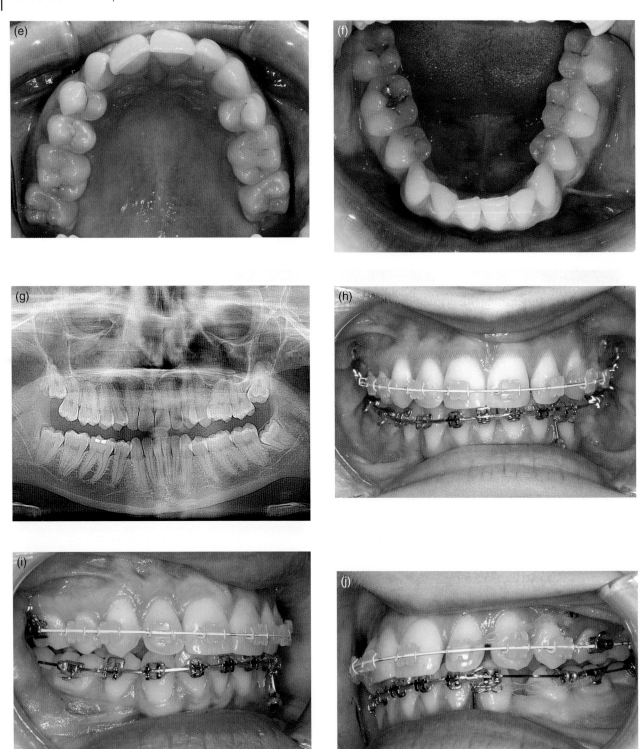

Figure 11.2 (Continued)

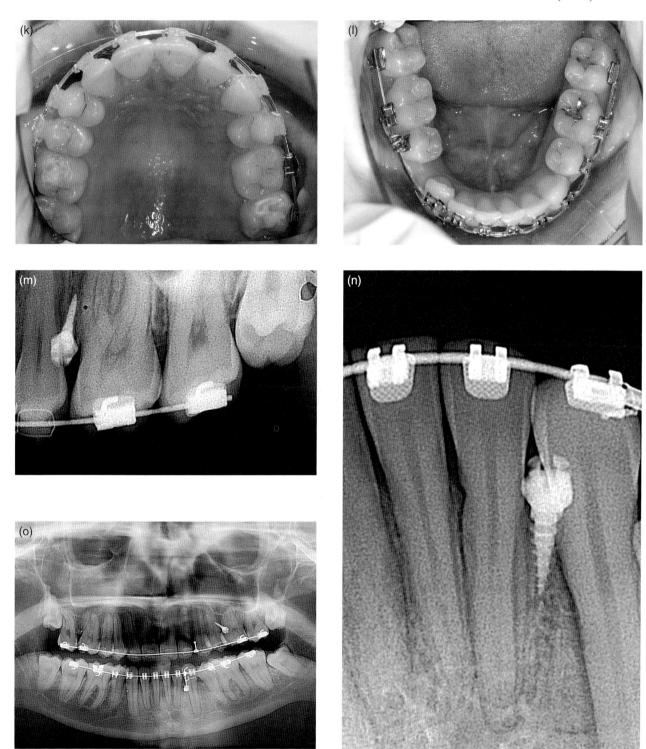

Figure 11.2 (Continued)

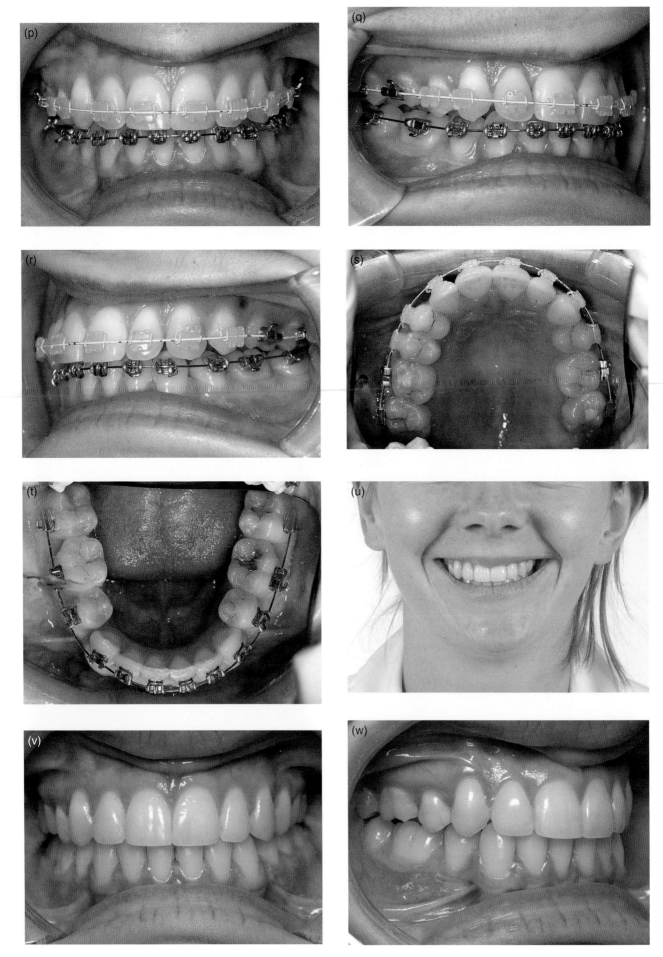

Figure 11.2 (Continued)

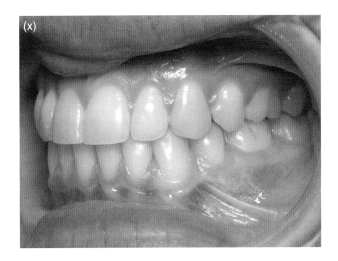
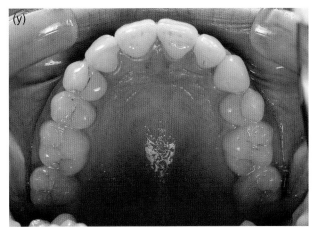
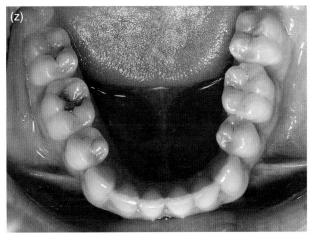

Figure 11.2 (Continued)

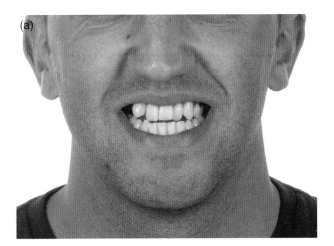
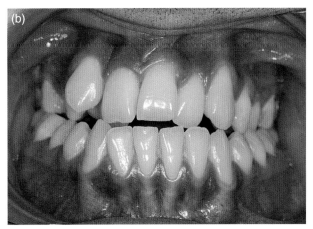

Figure 11.3 (a–e) Pretreatment views showing the Class III malocclusion, palatal exclusion of the upper right lateral incisor, severe displacement of the upper centreline to the right side and the Class II left canine relationship. (f–i) Elastomeric traction was applied from a mini-implant (inserted mesial and buccal to the upper left first molar) to a crimpable powerarm. (j) A lateral cephalogram, taken after mini-implant insertion, shows Class III dentoskeletal features, plus the relative mini-implant and powerarm heights. (k–n) Photographs taken eight weeks later when the upper right lateral incisor was bonded and a 'piggyback' 0.012 NiTi wire engaged. Arch support was provided by a 0.018 steel archwire. This required replacement of the crimpable powerarm with a single-tooth powerarm bonded on the upper left canine crown. Simultaneous alignment of the right lateral incisor commences, with a combination of 0.018 steel base archwire and 0.012 piggyback sectional NiTi. (o–r) Bodily retraction of the left canine is seen to continue with a 0.018 NiTi archwire *in situ*. (s–w) Photographs taken after eight months of mini-implant usage. The mini-implant and powerarm were removed, and the upper centreline appears to be slightly displaced to the left side. (x–z) Photographs taken after surgery and debond stages.

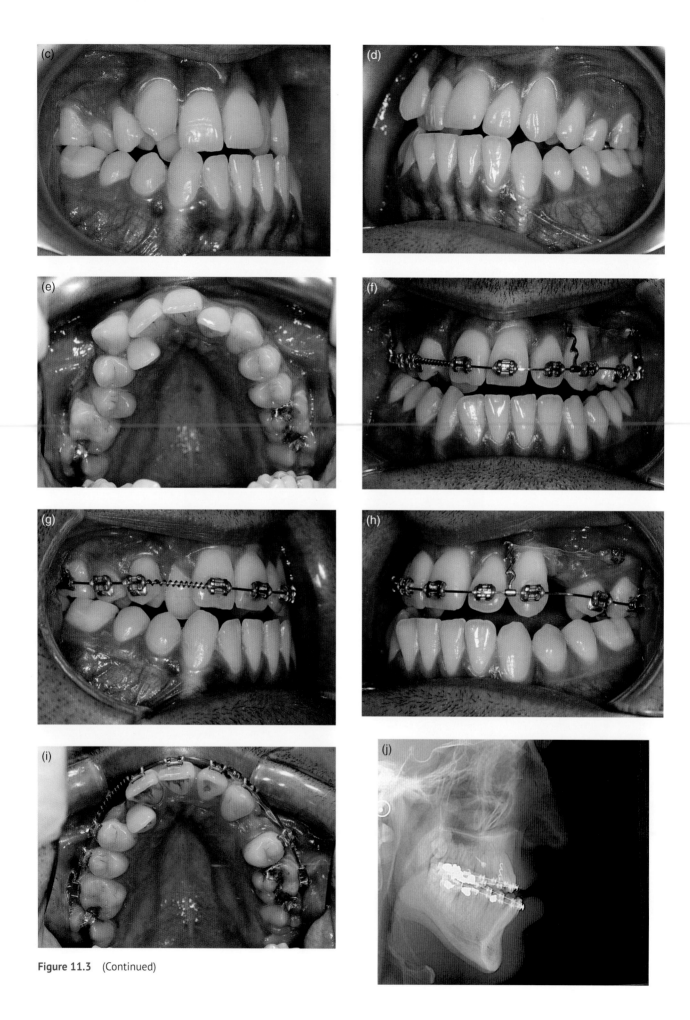

Figure 11.3 (Continued)

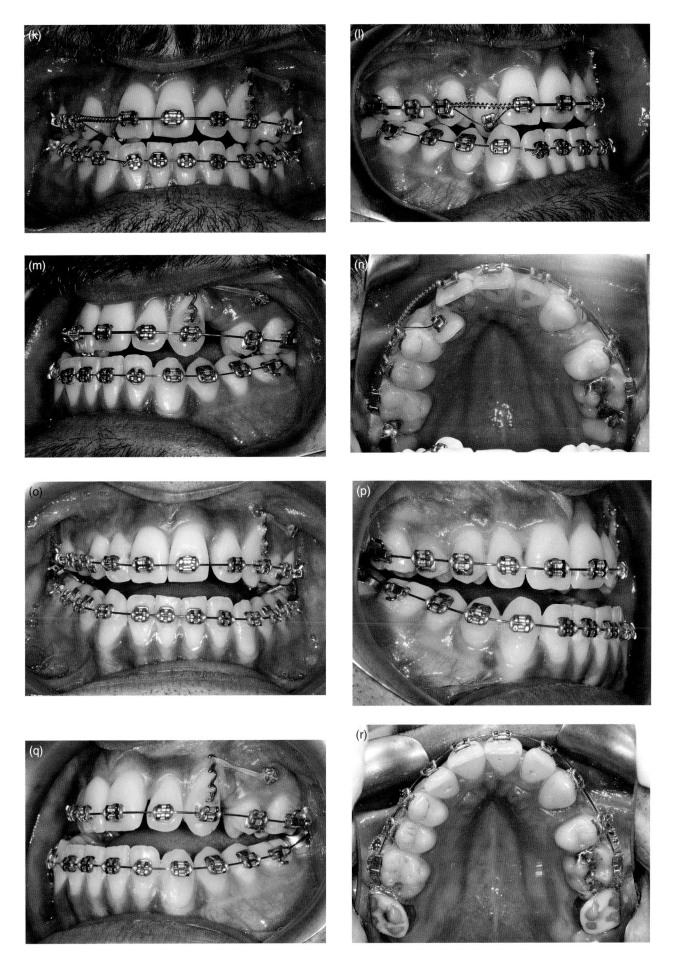

Figure 11.3 (Continued)

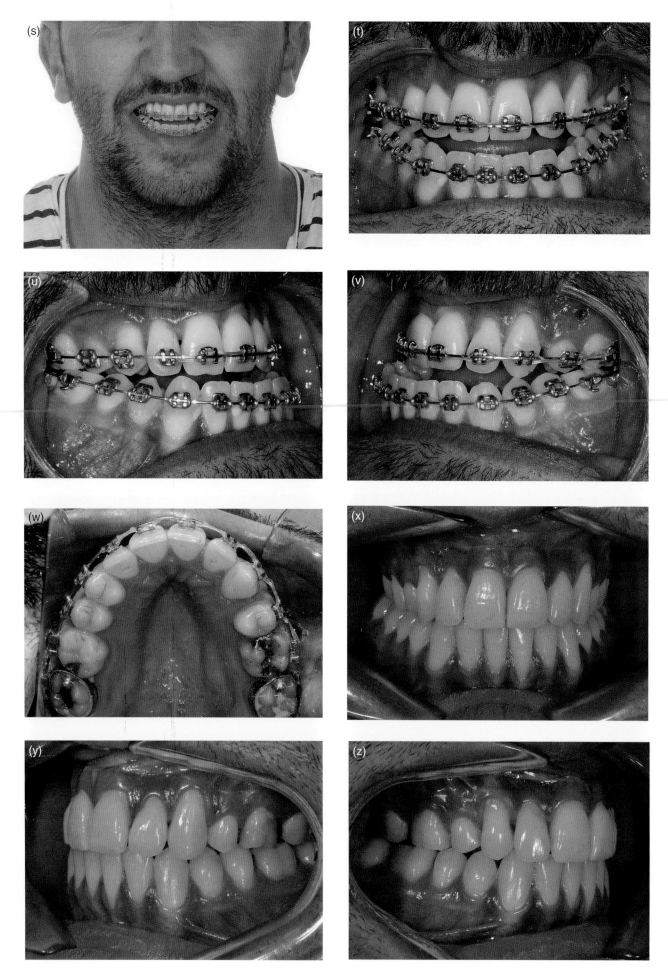

Figure 11.3 (Continued)

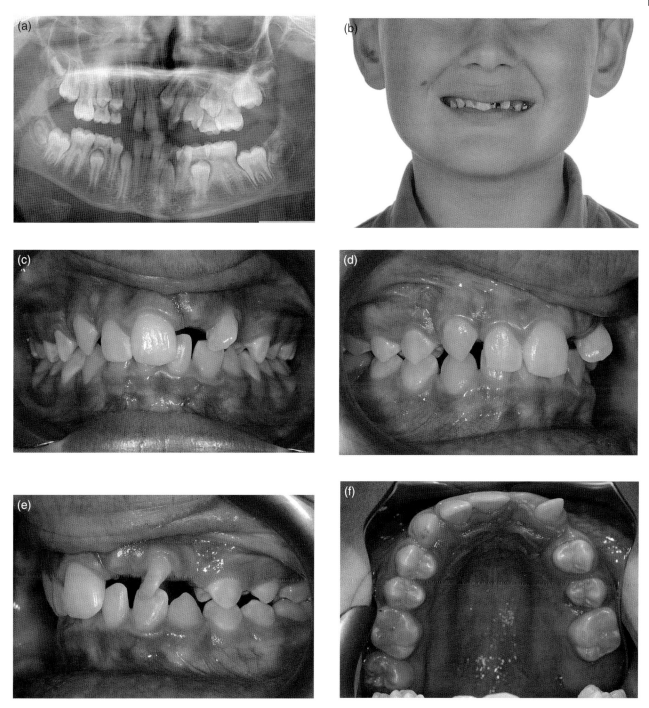

Figure 11.4 (a) A panoramic radiograph showing absence of the left maxillary central incisor and mesially ectopic eruption of the left canine into the central incisor space. (b–f) Photographs showing the Class I malocclusion with a deep overbite and asymmetrical buccal segment relationships. The upper centreline is displaced to the left side and there is a severe alveolar deficiency in the left canine region. (g–j) Photographs taken following initial alignment of the maxillary arch and showing pushcoil placed between the upper right central incisor and upper left lateral incisor teeth. Two paramedian mini-implants have been inserted and a mesialiser-distaliser appliance fitted onto these and the first molar bands. The mini-implant heads have been covered with composite resin. Pushcoil is seen on the right side of the 1 mm wire frame, and elastomeric traction on the left side. (k–n) Views showing the maxillary arch following 12 months with the mesialiser-distaliser in place. The alveolus in the left canine region appears normal with the first premolar in this site. The length of wire projecting distal to the left molar's (palatal) extraoral traction tube indicates the amount of canine space closure achieved through molar protraction, whilst the contralateral quadrant was simultaneously being distalised. (o) A midtreatment panoramic radiograph shows the upright position of the upper right first molar, but mild mesial tip of the upper left first molar tooth. (p–r) The left maxillary canine crown was provisionally restored to mimic a central incisor, following removal of the mesialiser-distaliser appliance and mini-implants. The patient's upper centreline was correct at this stage, but the lower dental centreline's displacement to the right side was still to be corrected.

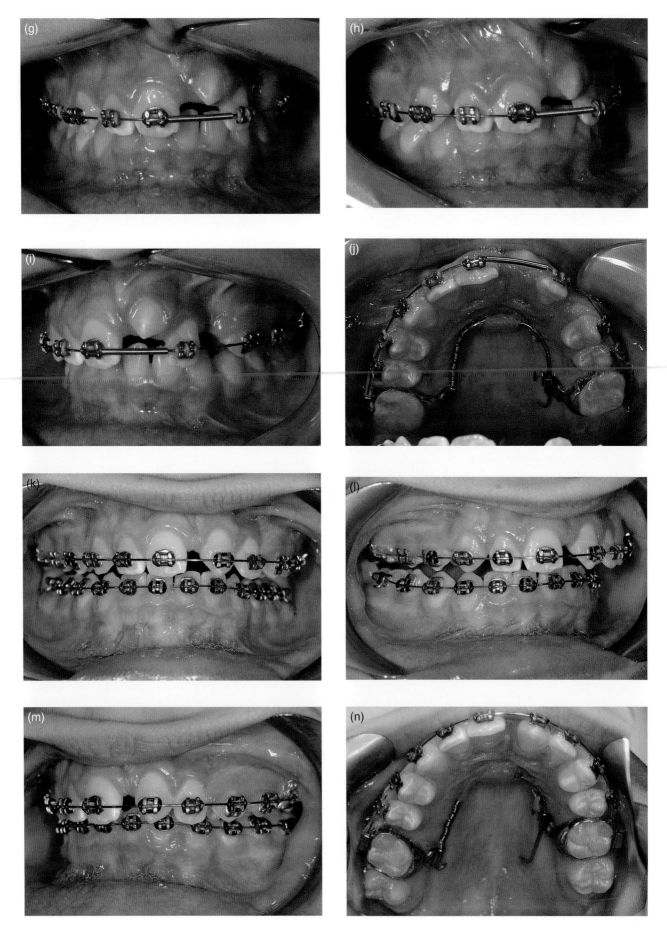

Figure 11.4 (Continued)

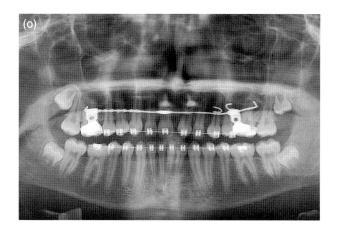

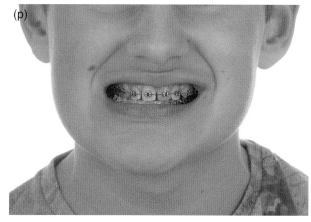

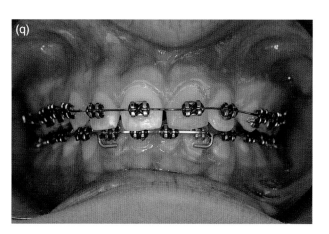

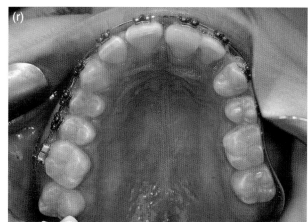

Figure 11.4 (Continued)

11.3 Unilateral Intrusion (Vertical Asymmetry Correction)

11.3.1 Clinical Objective

- Asymmetrical intrusion of the maxillary or mandibular teeth to level the occlusal plane and smile line.

11.3.2 Treatment Options

- Unilateral mini-implant intrusion, except where contraindicated in patients with a Class III skeletal pattern or reduced lower anterior face height.
- Conventional anchorage involving asymmetrical headgear.
- Hybrid functional (orthopaedic) appliance, but with a reliance on asymmetrical extrusive changes.
- Asymmetrical orthognathic surgical movements.

11.3.3 Relevant Clinical Details

- The anteroposterior focus of unilateral intrusion depends on the patient's facial height and overbite. For example, anterior intrusion is appropriate when the overbite is increased (Figure 11.5) whereas asymmetrical molar intrusion is ideal when the overbite is reduced or open.
- Asymmetrical bilateral intrusion is ideal for patients with vertical asymmetry accompanied by an increased maxillomandibular planes angle (MMPA) and Class II features.
- Active bilateral treatment may require intrusion of teeth in diagonally opposite quadrants (e.g. upper right and lower left quadrants).
- The incisor relationship (overjet, overbite).
- The maxillary and mandibular occlusal planes and whether an occlusal cant is present.
- The upper incisors' vertical display (on both passive and smiling exposure) and the smile arc.

11.3.3.1 Unilateral Intrusion, to Correct a Scissors Bite, and Centreline Correction (Figure 11.5)

- A 38-year-old female complained of a painful bite on the right side of her mouth and a tilt of her upper teeth. She gave a history of premature extraction of the upper right first molar.

- She presented with a Class II division 1 malocclusion on a skeletal I base with an average MMPA (Figure 11.5a–g). She had insignificant facial asymmetry but a downwards cant of the maxillary plane on the right side. There was a very deep, traumatic scissors bite with associated overeruption of the right maxillary canine and premolar teeth. The upper right first molar was absent with a significant displacement of the upper centreline to the right side. Both archforms displayed transverse midarch constriction, especially on the right side.
- The right second molars and upper right third molar teeth were partially impacted and the mandibular third molars were impacted (Figure 11.5h).
- Treatment commenced with a combination of a lower fixed appliance and an upper removable appliance, with a flat anterior biteplane to free the occlusion. A sectional fixed appliance was then bonded on the right maxillary canine and premolar teeth.
- Two mini-implants were inserted in the buccal side of the alveolus, mesial and distal to the upper right canine and first premolar teeth, after four months of treatment (Figure 11.5i,j). Elastomeric traction was applied from these mini-implants to the two teeth between them.
- The upper removable appliance was replaced by a full arch upper fixed appliance after four months of intrusion (Figure 11.5k,l). Traction was discontinued whilst flexible upper NiTi archwires were *in situ*.
- The patient's vertical asymmetry and dental centrelines were then re-evaluated after 13 months of treatment (Figure 11.5m–r). There had been slight overcorrection of the right maxillary intrusion in terms of the maxillary plane. The cant of the mandibular occlusion was still evident, as seen by convergence of the archwires on the right side. The upper centreline was still displaced to the right side and the patient requested its full correction.
- The upper left first premolar was extracted to enable upper centreline and Class II corrections. Anchorage was reinforced by insertion of a right mandibular mini-implant (mesial to the first molar) and one mesial to the upper left first molar (Figure 11.5s–u). These provided vertical and anteroposterior anchorage, respectively.
- Treatment was completed after a further 21 months (Figure 11.5v–z). Both occlusal planes had been levelled, correcting the right scissors bite, and the upper centreline had been corrected (although the lower centreline was displaced to the left side). Small residual spaces remained distal to the microdont upper lateral incisors.

11.3.4 Biomechanical Principles

- Simultaneous buccal and palatal mini-implant anchorage in the maxillary arch provides scope for true vertical movements within a quadrant, and avoids transverse side-effects or the need for a modified TPA (where the design has been altered to allow differential molar movements). Since lingual insertion sites have a low success rate, mandibular intrusion utilises buccal mini-implants only and requires transverse control using a full fixed appliance.
- In vertical terms, the mini-implants should be positioned in relatively apical sites, with the buccal one close to the mucogingival junction. This provides an adequate distance for effective traction, especially as the adjacent teeth intrude towards the implant head.
- Unilateral intrusion forces should be applied with a rigid (0.019×0.025 in.) steel archwire in place.

> Simultaneous buccal and palatal mini-implant anchorage in the maxillary arch provides scope for true vertical movements within a quadrant, and minimises transverse side-effects.

11.3.5 Clinical Tips and Technicalities

- Consider removal of erupted third molars prior to orthodontics in the quadrant(s) where molar intrusion is required if it is deemed too demanding to manage third molar intrusion.
- Bond the second molar (if fully erupted) early in treatment in the quadrant requiring intrusion.
- In vertical correction cases, monitor the occlusal plane by measuring the overbite involving the incisors and canine teeth, and their vertical display relative to the lip level. Also, monitor lateral openbites and hence the need for extrusion of the opposing teeth or additional intrusion in the diagonally opposite quadrant.

11.3.6 Midtreatment Problems and Solutions

- Creation of a lateral openbite or 'rollercoaster' partial openbite during unilateral intrusion:
  - Ensure that terminal erupted molars are bonded in the intrusion quadrant. Otherwise there will be a partial lateral openbite leaving the terminal molars propping the occlusion open on that side.
  - Avoid the application of traction with a flexible archwire *in situ*.
  - Bond the teeth opposing the intrusion quadrant with their brackets more gingivally positioned to encourage their eruption into the lateral openbite space.

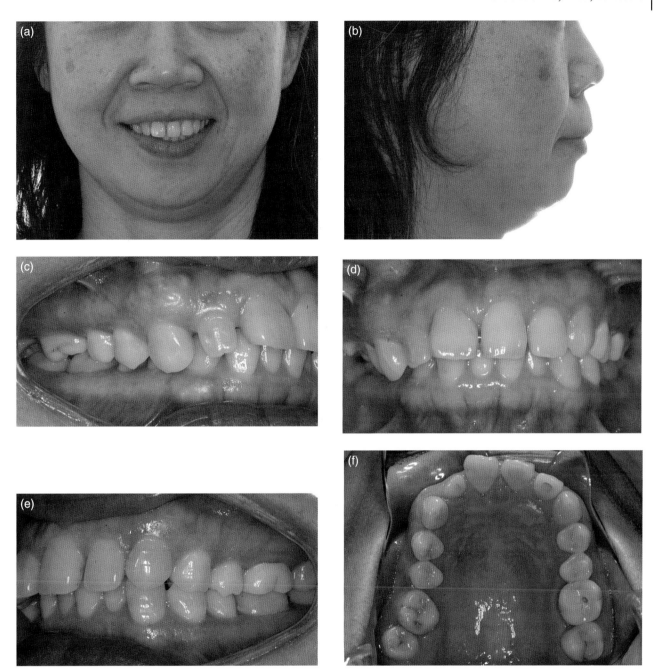

Figure 11.5 (a–g) Photographs taken at the start of treatment, showing the maxillary occlusal cant, upper centreline displacement, severe traumatic scissors bite and dysmorphic archforms. (h) Pretreatment panoramic radiograph showing the absent upper right first molar and multiple impacted molar teeth. (i,j) Photographs taken after four months of treatment with an upper removable appliance and lower fixed appliance. Two right maxillary buccal mini-implants had just been inserted and elastomeric traction applied to intrude the upper right canine and first premolar teeth. (k,l) Photographs taken after four months of intrusion, when the rest of the maxillary dentition was bonded. (m–r) Photographs taken after nine months of intrusion treatment, where the maxillary dentition had been levelled, the scissors bite improved and the archforms normalised. (s–u) Views taken after extraction of the left maxillary first premolar and insertion of a mini-implant in this quadrant for anteroposterior anchorage. A mini-implant had also been inserted, mesial to the lower right first molar, for intrusion in this quadrant and hence levelling of the mandibular occlusal plane. (v–z) Debond photographs showing the Class I features and slight overcorrection of the original maxillary occlusal cant.

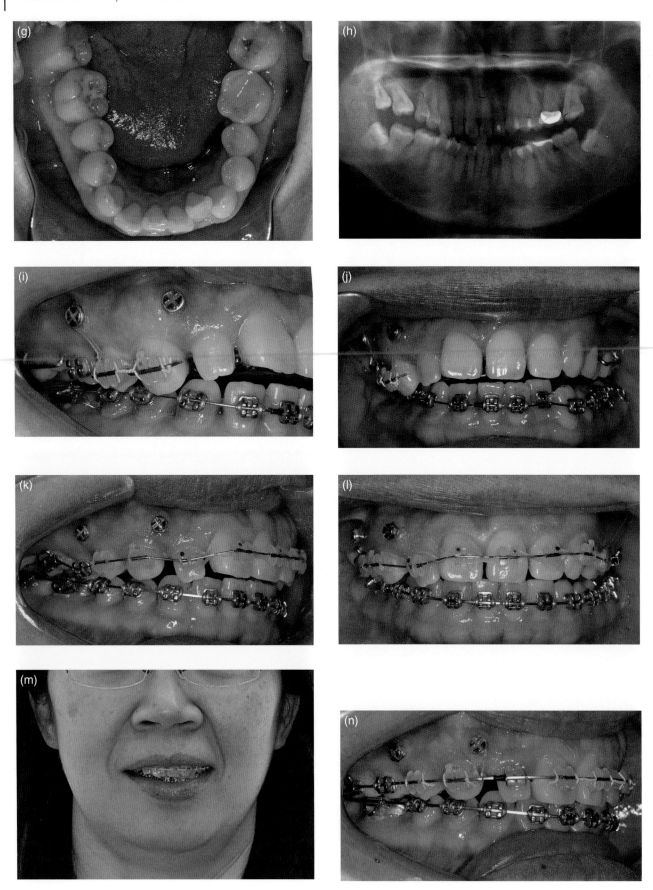

Figure 11.5 (Continued)

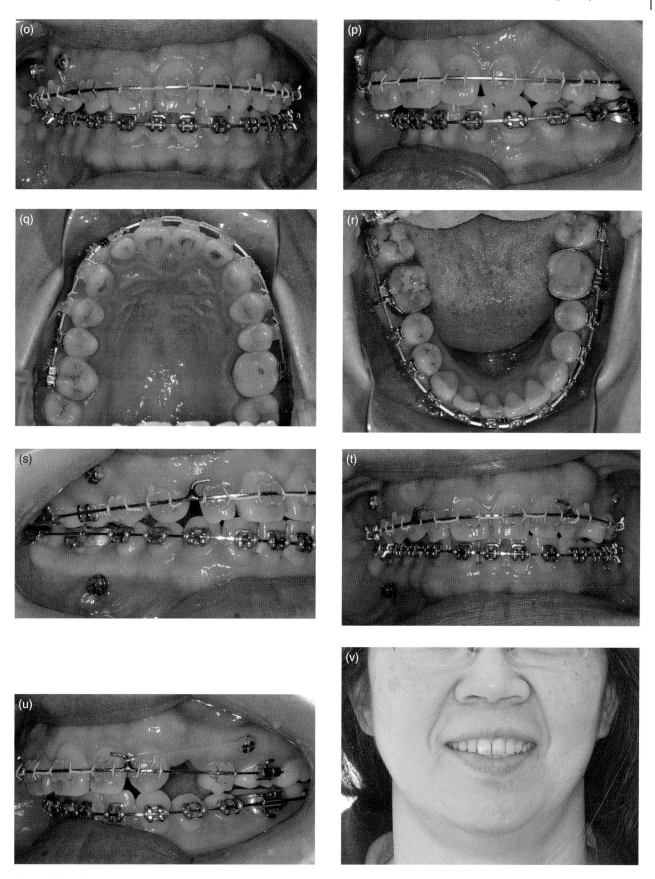

Figure 11.5 (Continued)

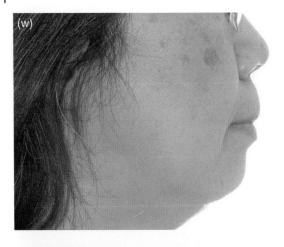
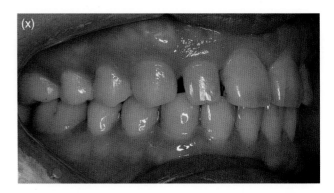
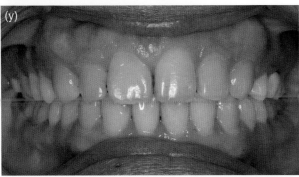
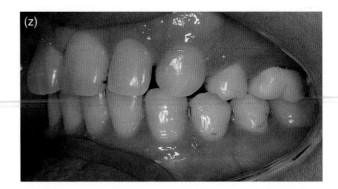

Figure 11.5   (Continued)

– Use vertical settling elastics to close a lateral open-bite by active extrusion of the opposing arch. The elastics may be connected either to the mini-implant anchored teeth (Figure 11.6) or directly to the mini-implant head. Crucially, anchorage must be maintained in the intruded quadrant to avoid any extrusive relapse of the intruded teeth.

11.3.7   Clinical Steps for Unilateral Intrusion

11.3.7.1   Preinsertion

1) Determine the mini-implant insertion sites prior to bond-up so that root divergence can be performed as necessary. Do not aim to insert buccal and palatal mini-implants in the same interproximal space. Instead, I tend to insert the palatal one more distally than the buccal one since there is more molar interproximal space available on the palatal aspect. For example, the buccal one is sited mesial or distal to the maxillary second premolars and the palatal one between the molars. However, if the overbite is increased then move both anchorage sites more mesially.

2) This preplanning enables active divergence of adjacent premolar roots to be undertaken, to allow for both ease of buccal mini-implant insertion and subsequent vertical tooth movements. For example, diverge the premo-lar roots by adding mesial and distal tip to the first and second premolar brackets, respectively. Remember that these tip alterations can readily be corrected at the treatment finishing stage.

3) Align and level the whole arch or initially only the segment due for intrusion. This depends on whether there is a vertical discrepancy between the anterior and posterior teeth, where a large step favours segmental mechanics, while the risk of occlusal interferences from displaced anterior teeth necessitates full arch alignment.

4) Expand the maxillary arch, to facilitate arch co-ordination, if an increase in overbite and mandibular autorotation are anticipated.

5) Include bonded tubes on the second molars, if fully erupted, early in treatment. If the second molars are not fully erupted then do not bond them during initial alignment. Remember to avoid molar bands in order to facilitate effective gingival hygiene at the posterior limit of the dental arch where a reduction in crown height may occur and toothbrush access is most limited.

6) Once a 0.019×0.025 in. NiTi archwire has been inserted then book two clinical appointments if a stent is to be fabricated (which is especially valuable for palatal site guidance).

7) At the preparatory appointment, take an alginate impression or intraoral scan for a guidance stent, if desired.

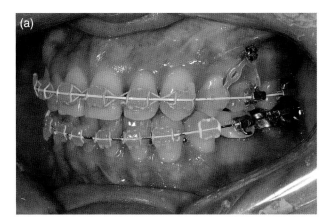 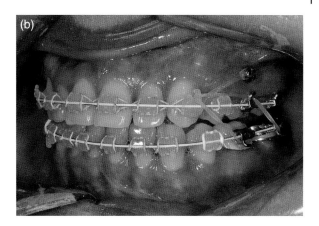

Figure 11.6 Photographs of the left side of an adult dentition where the upper left quadrant is being intruded by elastomeric traction from mini-implants on the buccal and palatal (not shown) sides of the alveolus. Initial intrusion shown in (a) leads to a lateral openbite seen in (b). A rhomboid (Class II/box) elastic has been added to level the lower left quadrant and simultaneously improve the Class II buccal segment contacts. Supportive traction continues from the mini-implants, although oblique buccal traction has been applied to the canine only at this stage.

Remember, for a dental impression, not to wax out the brackets adjacent to a buccal insertion site.

8) Take periapical radiographs or a sectional CBCT to evaluate the positions of the roots adjacent to the insertion sites, either at the preparatory stage (when stent usage is planned) or at the start of the insertion appointment.

11.3.7.2 Mini-implant Selection

9) Maxilla: use 1.5 mm diameter, 9 mm length mini-implants (for Infinitas), with short and long necks on the buccal and palatal alveolar sides, respectively. However, if the palatal tissues are particularly thick or the patient is still undergoing considerable somatic growth, then a 2 mm diameter version may be indicated to give maximum primary stability without relying on full depth intrabony insertion.

10) Mandible: body length selection depends on the anticipated cortical depth and density such that a long length (9 mm) version is preferable for adolescent patients, where the cortical bone is immature. An Infinitas 1.5 mm diameter, 6 mm length, short neck version may be used in an adult if there is sufficient height of attached gingiva.

11.3.7.3 Insertion

11) Superficial anaesthesia of the insertion sites; blanch the overlying mucosal area with a local anaesthetic injection. This may be preceded by topical anaesthesia.

12) Fit the stent (where applicable) after soaking it in chlorhexidine antiseptic.

13) Use a mucosal punch for palatal insertions. Temporarily remove any stent, after the surface has been marked with it *in situ*, so that the mucotome can be applied perpendicular to the surface, providing a clean cut of the tissue. If necessary, then remove the mucosal tissue with a mosquito forceps and/or Mitchell's trimmer.

14) In adults, use a cortical bone punch to perforate the relatively thick and dense palatal and mandibular cortex.

15) Insert buccal and palatal maxillary and buccal mandibular mini-implants, according to the treatment plan. Remember to use a speed-reducing (e.g. 128:1 ratio) contra-angle handpiece at less than 100 rpm for palatal sites.

16) The buccal insertion sites should be at or close to the mucogingival junction and the vertical angle of insertion should be perpendicular to the bone. These details enable reliable attachment of the traction and a maximum range of intrusion movement.

17) Take an intraoral radiograph if close root proximity is clinically suspected (due to pain on percussion of an adjacent tooth).

18) Complete insertion to the point where the mini-implant neck is partially submerged but the head is fully accessible.

11.3.7.4 Postinsertion

19) Insert a 0.019 × 0.025 in. steel archwire.

20) Bond attachments (buttons or cleats) to the palatal surfaces of the crowns adjacent to any palatal mini-implants.

21) Apply approximately 50 g (elastomeric chain) traction for the first 4–6 weeks. This utilises the palatal attachments and the simplest configuration is a 'V', where the traction component's ends are attached to the teeth and its midsection engages the mini-implant head. On the buccal side, the traction may be applied directly to the adjacent brackets or around the archwire. Following

the initial healing period, stronger (150–200 g) elastomeric or closing coil auxiliary traction should be used.

22) Monitor treatment progress by recording the following features at the start of intrusion and at subsequent appointments: overjet, anterior openbite/overbite, canine relationship, upper incisor display (at rest and on full smiling), occlusal cant and presence of any molar openbite.

23) Monitor the periodontal condition (probing depth) of the terminal molars.

24) Consider overcorrection of the intrusion changes to allow for possible relapse and/or keep the mini-implants *in situ* until it is clear that further anchorage is not required.

25) Consider an initially intensive retention regimen, for example three months full-time wear of plastic retainers with whole-arch occlusal coverage. These should prevent early molar extrusion after debond.

11.3.8   Case Example (Figure 11.7)

- A 28-year-old female complained of greater display of her upper teeth and gums on the left side than on the right. She had a history of congenital left facial haemangioma, which had been surgically removed. There had also been two unsuccessful episodes of surgical recontouring of the maxillary gingival margin. She presented with a Class II division 2 malocclusion on a skeletal I base with an average MMPA (Figure 11.7a–e). She had panfacial asymmetry with the maxillary plane canted downwards on the left side and more gingival display on this side on full smiling. The patient habitually camouflaged this by smiling to a limited extent. All first premolars plus a lower incisor were absent (Figure 11.7f).

- The left maxillary third molar was extracted prior to orthodontics, to eliminate its interference with intrusive treatment.

- The maxillary arch was levelled and aligned to accommodate a 0.019 × 0.025 in. steel archwire (Figure 11.7g–k). A 1.5 mm diameter, 9 mm length mini-implant was then inserted on both sides of the left maxillary alveolus, mesiobuccal and distopalatal to the first molar (Figure 11.7l). Elastomeric traction was applied buccally to the upper left premolar bracket and molar tube, and palatally to buttons on the palatal surfaces of the molars.

- Both the malocclusion and smile aesthetics were improved by five months of intrusion prior to bonding the lower fixed appliance (Figure 11.7m–p). Notably, there was more vertical clearance for the left molars, although it appeared that these had undergone some passive eruption.

- Intrusion continued for a further year, followed by four months of finishing prior to debond (Figure 11.7q–t).

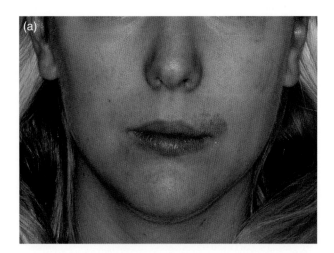 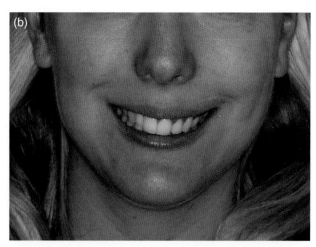

Figure 11.7   (a–e) Pretreatment views where the patient's habitual smile partly camouflages her vertical maxillary cant and asymmetrical gingival display. The Class II division 2 malocclusion is shown with absence of upper first premolars and a lower incisor. (f) A pretreatment panoramic radiograph showing absence of the upper first premolars, the lower left central incisor and the right third molars. (g–k) Photographs showing the upper fixed appliance with a 0.019 × 0.025 in. steel archwire *in situ*. Left-sided intrusion has commenced with elastomeric traction applied from the brackets and palatal buttons to mini-implants sited buccal and mesial to the maxillary left first molar, and palatal and distal to this first molar. (l) A periapical radiograph showing the buccal and palatal mini-implants mesial and distal to the first molar, respectively. (m–p) Photographs taken when the lower arch was bonded. The maxillary cant is levelling by this stage. The vertical position of the lower buccal brackets has been altered, with the lower left quadrant ones being bonded in relatively gingival positions, to assist with vertical compensation and overbite reduction. (q–t) Debond views showing the patient's natural/full smile, reduced overbite and improved symmetry. This was maintained two years later (u,v) after standard retainer wear.

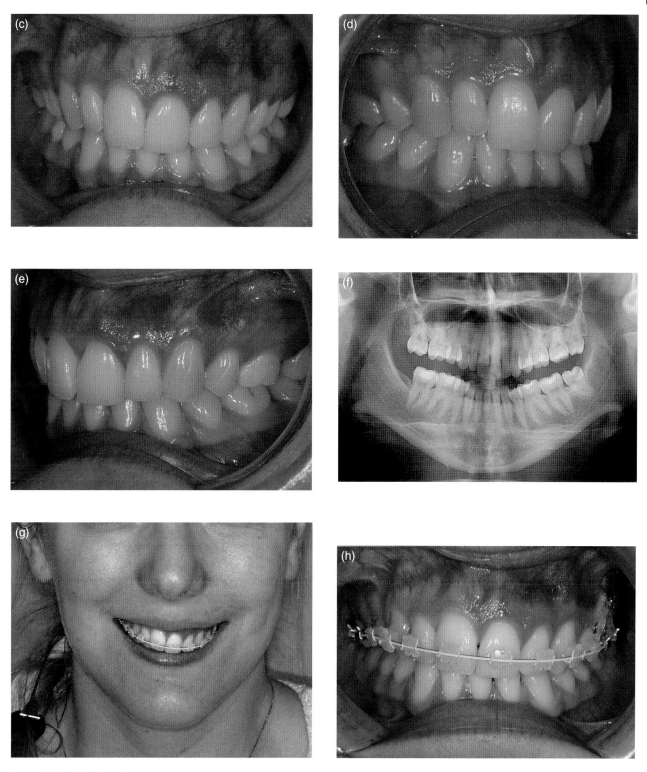

Figure 11.7 (Continued)

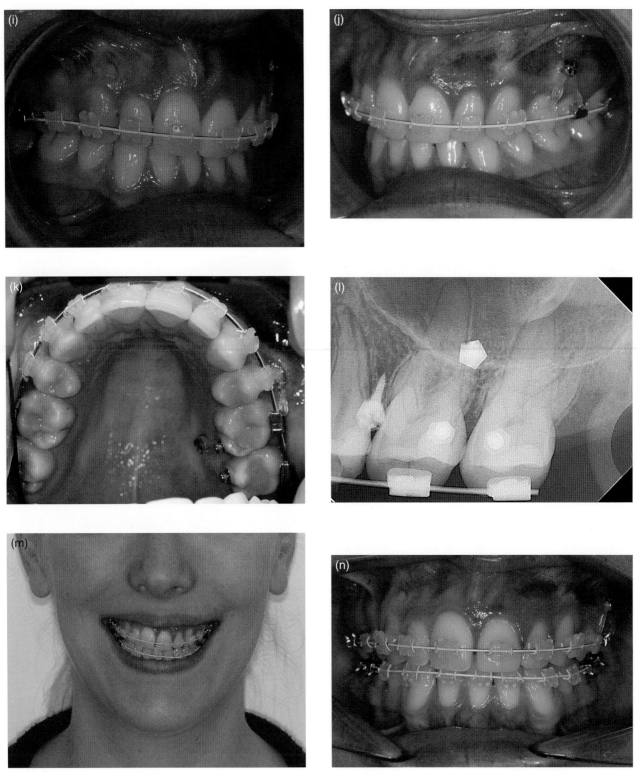

Figure 11.7   (Continued)

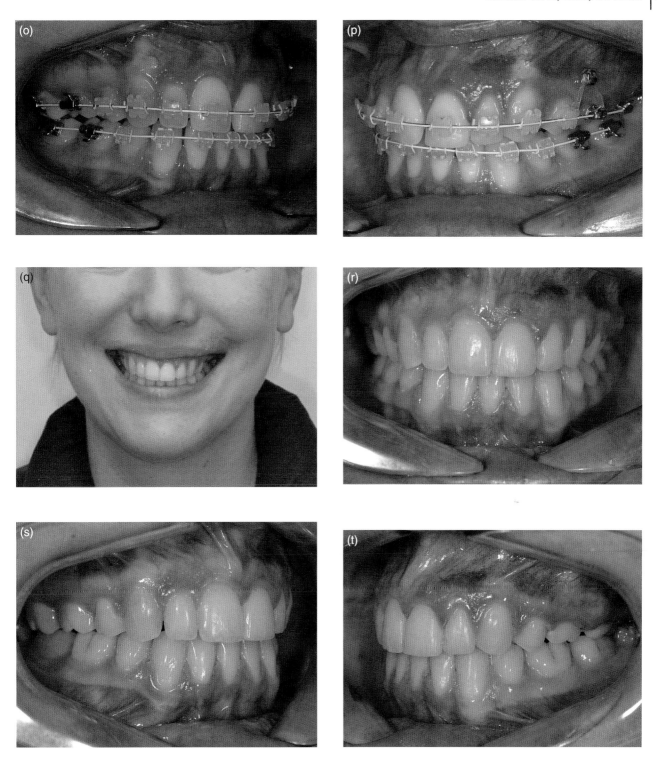

Figure 11.7 (Continued)

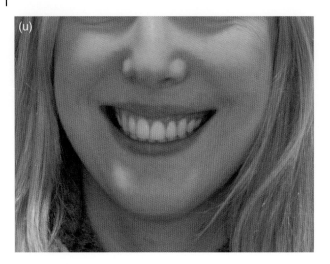

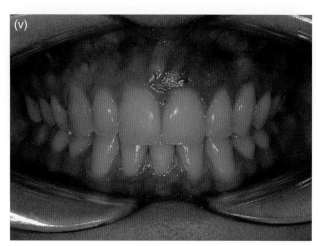

Figure 11.7 (Continued)

12

Ectopic Teeth Anchorage

Many of the orthodontic patients who present with ectopic or impacted teeth, such as maxillary canines and central incisors, can be successfully treated with conventional anchorage. Conventional anchorage reinforcement involves either the formation of dental anchor units or indirect reinforcement of an anchor tooth from the contralateral side of the arch. The latter requires molar bands on both sides of the arch for a transpalatal arch (TPA). However, TPA usage is often associated with anchorage loss as the anchored molar tooth tips mesially and may also be intruded. This is especially the case in adults where the ectopic tooth is fully developed and may be very resistant to movement (Figure 12.1), or when the target tooth has to move through cortical bone (such as a buccally impacted maxillary canine). Furthermore, a TPA may be contraindicated when fundamentally different movements are required in contralateral quadrants.

This leaves the conventional option of a full fixed appliance or a partial one. However, this may mean that the patient has a fixed appliance which is otherwise passive on many teeth for a protracted period of time. In addition, it may be difficult to achieve the optimum vector of traction and anchorage loss may cause unfavourable loading and movement of adjacent teeth, especially if they have reduced root or periodontal support.

The alternative is to use a mini-implant either to provide an anchorage point for direct traction to the ectopic tooth or to stabilise a dental anchor unit (indirect anchorage). In contrast to conventional options, mini-implant usage means that anchorage is only reinforced in the specific quadrant and direction(s) indicated for optimal treatment changes. It is particularly useful when either the potential anchor teeth are compromised (by root shortness or resorption by the ectopic tooth) or the patient has hypodontia. The key factor in deciding between direct and indirect anchorage depends on whether there is a suitable insertion site in an area of reliable bone support (in terms of quantity and quality), or if this would compromise movement of the target tooth towards the line of the arch. In effect, the biomechanics needs to be configured to provide the appropriate transverse, vertical (extrusive) and mesiodistal movement of the ectopic tooth, plus sufficient range of action to allow its progressive movement over time. Consequently, there are several different approaches to consider, and these will be outlined in this chapter.

> Mini-implant usage means that anchorage is only reinforced in the specific quadrant and direction(s) indicated for optimal treatment changes.

12.1 Clinical Objectives

Anchorage reinforcement to facilitate alignment (of at least the crown) of an impacted, ectopic or ankylosed tooth or teeth.

12.2 Treatment Options

- Conventional anchorage involving a full fixed appliance, or a sectional appliance supported by a TPA.
- Direct mini-implant traction using either a traction auxiliary or cantilever arm between the mini-implant and the target tooth.
- Indirect mini-implant anchorage, where either an anchor tooth or the archwire is stabilised.

12.3 Relevant Clinical Details

- The number and location of teeth to form a potential anchorage unit.
- The length and shape of the roots of teeth adjacent to the ectopic tooth, since these may be short due to microdontia

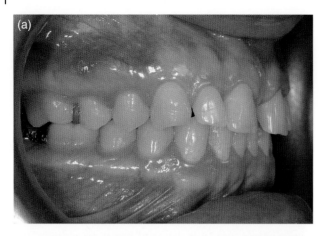
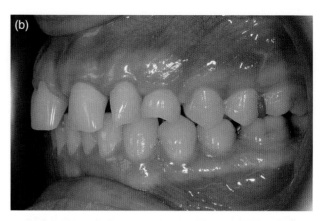
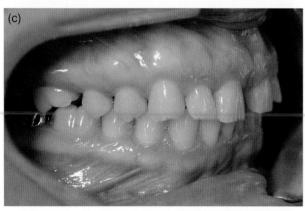
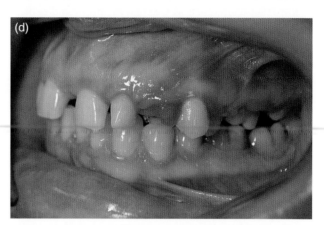

Figure 12.1 Example of an adult patient with a palatally ectopic left maxillary canine. (a,b) Photographs taken at the start of treatment. Cantilever traction was then applied from a TPA's molar band on the upper left first molar (after removal of the elastic separators shown in this photograph) to the left canine tooth. (c,d) The canine's resistance to movement caused severe mesial tipping and relative intrusion of both first molars, especially on the left side. The upper left premolars had also been forced out of alignment as the left molar lost anchorage.

and/or root resorption. A typical example of this is a microdont lateral incisor adjacent to an ectopic maxillary canine. Consequently, these adjacent teeth may be unable to tolerate the prolonged and relatively heavy force application associated with alignment of an ectopic tooth.

12.4 Biomechanical Principles

- Determine the direction of tooth movement and hence the ideal traction vector prior to mini-implant insertion. For example, does the ectopic tooth need to be moved distally as well as laterally? This helps to decide whether direct or indirect anchorage is appropriate.
- If there is not a suitable site for a mini-implant to provide direct traction then the orthodontist must decide on the optimum insertion site (in terms of anatomy) and the means of indirect anchorage connection to either an anchor tooth or the fixed appliance.

- The simplest form of direct traction involves insertion of a mini-implant near the final target position for the ectopic tooth (Figure 12.2). This is a relatively simple set-up, but requires several key features. First, there needs to be sufficient bone support (volume and cortical strength) at the insertion site. This may be problematic in the case of palatally ectopic canines since the canine eminence will not have formed, resulting in less potential bone support mesial to the adjacent first premolar. There then needs to be sufficient separation of the mini-implant and target tooth to provide effective traction and allow for the tooth's movement towards the mini-implant. It also requires adequate soft tissue clearance so that the traction auxiliary does not impinge on/dig into the adjacent mucosa.
- Direct traction may also be delivered from a more remote insertion site by the use of a cantilever arm (Figure 12.3). This is effective as a means of separating the anchorage site from the target site and the planned path of tooth movement. However, it requires two mini-implants in

series, such that the second mini-implant stabilises the first one from the rotational/torque effects of the cantilever arm. In addition, it is limited in practical terms by the difficulty of removing and replacing a cantilever arm (since it is fixed into the mini-implant heads).

- Alternatively, indirect anchorage also provides the means of separating the anchorage site from the target site and the planned path of tooth movement. It involves a rigid auxiliary wire linking the anchor tooth to a mini-implant (Figure 12.4). This enables traction to be applied from this anchor unit to the ectopic tooth, for example from a buccally anchored maxillary first premolar to a palatally ectopic canine. While there is a small risk of anchorage loss due to the wire connection, an indirect anchorage arrangement decouples the anchor and active components to the extent that the cantilever arm may be easily adjusted (extraorally) or changed without affecting the anchorage. Alternatively, the working archwire (of a fixed appliance which is already *in situ*) may be stabilised using a combination of an auxiliary wire and cross-tube (Figure 12.5).
- Indirect anchorage may also be gained from the opposing jaw, where anchorage reinforcement in the target jaw is not feasible or multiple teeth need to be aligned in the same arch (Figure 12.6).

> Indirect anchorage decouples the anchor and active components to the extent that the cantilever arm may be easily adjusted (extraorally) or changed without affecting the anchorage.

12.5 Clinical Tips and Technicalities

- If a cantilever arm is non-tooth borne then it should be attached to two mini-implants. This linkage minimises the rotational destabilising side-effects on a single mini-implant.
- Alternatively, a cantilever arm may be either attached to a single mini-implant which is (rotationally) stabilised by an adjacent tooth, or fitted to a molar tube/orthodontic bracket where this tooth is anchored by the mini-implant.
- Consider mini-implant insertion when the ectopic tooth is being surgically exposed, provided that the insertion site does not interfere with the access flap. Otherwise, delay insertion until the traction is required, especially if the deciduous tooth is also being retained prior to orthodontics.
- If a deciduous tooth is retained in the ideal insertion site then extract this and allow a minimum of two months

for alveolar bone healing. Even then, it is prudent to insert the mini-implant into interseptal bone since the buccal cortex may be deficient in a deciduous tooth site.

12.6 Midtreatment Problems and Solutions

- Close proximity of the ectopic tooth and mini-implant may render the traction ineffective. If so, either the mini-implant should be removed and replaced in a new location (which is favourable for the direction and distance of traction) or the treatment continued by conventional means.
- Anchorage loss may occur with indirect anchorage when the connecting wire distorts or slips (Figure 12.4).

12.7 Clinical Steps for Ectopic Tooth Alignment

12.7.1 Preinsertion

1) For alveolar sites, check whether there is sufficient interproximal space at the mini-implant insertion site(s). If not, then choose an alternative site (and possibly different biomechanics) or first increase the interproximal space by diverging the adjacent roots. This may be achieved with a sectional fixed appliance where the attachments are bonded on the adjacent teeth at altered tips; for example, add mesial and distal tip to the first and second premolar brackets, respectively, when an interpremolar insertion is required.
2) If desired, especially for palatal sites, prepare an insertion stent by taking a dental impression or intraoral scan of the arch 1–2 weeks before insertion. Avoid waxing out brackets and the buccal sulcus near a buccal insertion site (for an impression) and record the clinical level of the mucogingival junction.

12.7.2 Mini-implant Selection

3) Maxilla: use a narrow long body, short neck mini-implant (e.g. Infinitas 1.5 mm diameter, 9 mm length, short neck version).
4) Mandible: use a narrow, short neck mini-implant (e.g. Infinitas 1.5 mm diameter, 6 or 9 mm length, short neck version). The length selection largely depends on the height of attached gingiva and alveolar width at the insertion site; for example, a 9 mm length may be preferable where a limitation in one or both of these factors indicates the need for an oblique insertion angle.

12.7.3 Insertion

5) Identify the ideal buccal or palatal insertion point, through attached gingiva (which does not require a soft tissue punch step for buccal sites).

6) Superficial anaesthesia of the insertion site.

7) Determine the angles of insertion. Mini-implants inserted into the interproximal space are generally perpendicular to the surface in the horizontal plane. Maxillary and posterior mandibular mini-implants may be inserted at either 90° (perpendicular to the surface) or angled obliquely by up to 30° to the vertical plane, by inclining the screwdriver in a slightly apical direction. Anterior mandibular insertions are inclined at 80–90° to the surface because of limitations due to the sloping shape of the alveolus.

8) Manual insertion is recommended where there is sufficient physical access (e.g. stretching of the cheek and buccal sulcus). Otherwise, contra-angle handpiece insertion may be performed, but with resultant loss of full tactile control.

9) A cortical bone punch is recommended as the first step for posterior mandibular sites (except in young teenage patients with less dense cortex).

10) Complete the insertion to the point where the mini-implant neck is partially submerged but the head is fully accessible. This is best performed gradually and with intermittent release of the screwdriver during the final turns, so that overinsertion is avoided.

11) Percuss the adjacent teeth to gauge root proximity and take an intraoral radiograph or cone beam computed tomograph (CBCT) if close root proximity is suspected.

12.7.4 Postinsertion

12) For direct anchorage, either connect the traction auxiliary between the mini-implant and the ectopic tooth (Figure 12.2) or use a cantilever arm from the mini-implant(s).

13) For indirect anchorage, bond a 0.019×0.025 in. steel auxiliary wire from the mini-implant head, and connect it either to an anchor tooth's crown (Figure 12.4) or to a cross-tube on the working archwire (Figure 12.5).

14) Immediately load the mini-implant with *light* traction for the first 5–6 weeks, with a lightly stretched powerchain. Subsequently, apply normal levels of traction using a NiTi closing spring or elastomeric.

15) Discontinue the traction and explant the mini-implant once the anchorage requirements have been met or there is insufficient distance for continued effective traction.

12.7.5 Case Examples

1) **Direct anchorage and traction (Figure 12.2)**
   - This 31-year-old female presented with a Class II division 1 malocclusion on a Class I skeletal base with an ectopic upper right canine and retained deciduous canine (Figure 12.2a–c). She had a history of aggressive periodontal disease predominantly affecting the incisors and first molars, and requiring extraction of the upper left central incisor.
   - Since it was ideal to limit the time and periodontal side-effects of fixed appliance treatment, initial movement of the ectopic canine was planned with direct traction from a mini-implant.
   - Elastomeric traction was applied between the buccal mini-implant, inserted in the interseptal bone mesial to the upper right first premolar (Figure 12.2d,e). This enabled the patient to simultaneously wear a vacuum-formed appliance containing two incisor pontics for aesthetic purposes (Figure 12.2f).
   - The mini-implant was explanted when the canine crown approximated the alveolar crest and there was insufficient traction distance left (Figure 12.2g–i). Conventional fixed appliance treatment was commenced and supplemented with a removable partial denture (Figure 12.2j,k).
   - Treatment was completed after full arch alignment and space reduction (from 2 to 1 incisor space) had been achieved (Figure 12.2l–n).

2) **Direct anchorage involving a cantilever arm (Figure 12.3)**
   - This 14-year-old female presented with a Class II division 2 malocclusion on a Class I skeletal base with bilaterally ectopic maxillary canines (Figure 12.3a–d). Treatment was complicated by the severe shortness of the roots of multiple teeth, especially the premolars (Figure 12.3e,f). The upper left lateral incisor displayed severe root resorption and had a poor prognosis.
   - In order to minimise the amount of orthodontic treatment and hence risks of premolar root resorption, it was decided to surgically remove the upper right canine, extract the upper left lateral incisor and expose the upper left canine.
   - Initial anchorage support involved a TPA, but the upper left first molar became symptomatic after three months of cantilever traction. Since this tooth required endodontic treatment (due to previous caries), it was decided to use mini-implant anchorage for the cantilever traction.
   - Two (1.5 mm diameter, 9 mm length) mini-implants were inserted in the buccal aspect of the alveolus,

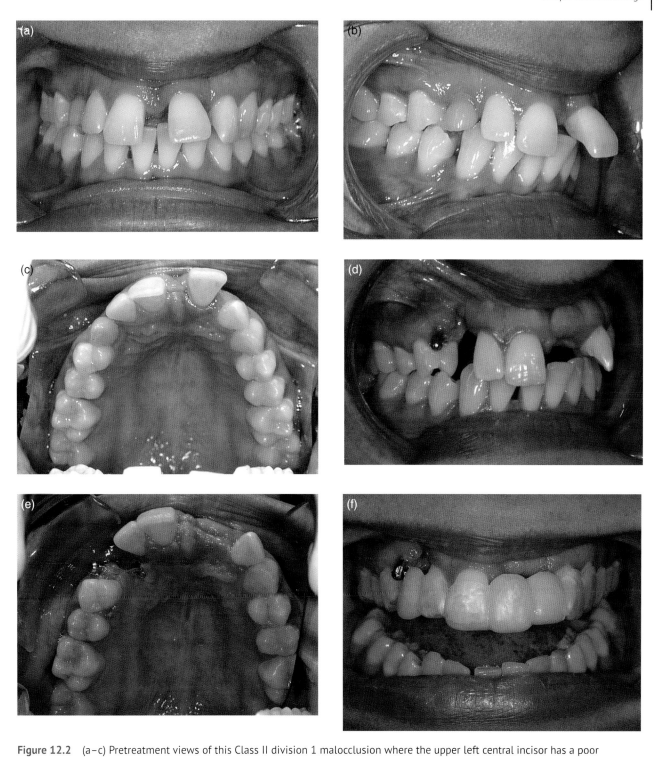

Figure 12.2 (a–c) Pretreatment views of this Class II division 1 malocclusion where the upper left central incisor has a poor prognosis and the upper right canine is ectopic. (d–f) Vertical and lateral traction applied to the exposed canine crown from a mini-implant sited in the interseptal bone on the mesial aspect of the right first premolar. A vacuum-formed appliance with two incisor pontics was worn at this time. (g–i) The mini-implant was removed when the canine crown approximated it, resulting in insufficient distance for traction. (j,k) Fixed appliance treatment involved relatively light forces, for changes such as upper right canine extrusion. (l–n) Debond views, including with a temporary incisor pontic in the retainer.

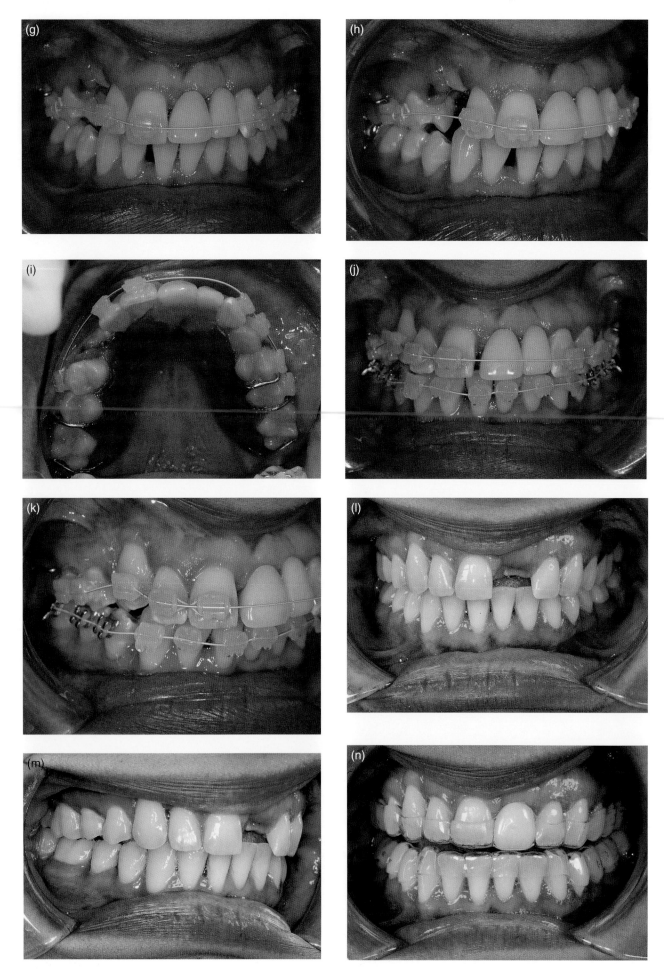

Figure 12.2 (Continued)

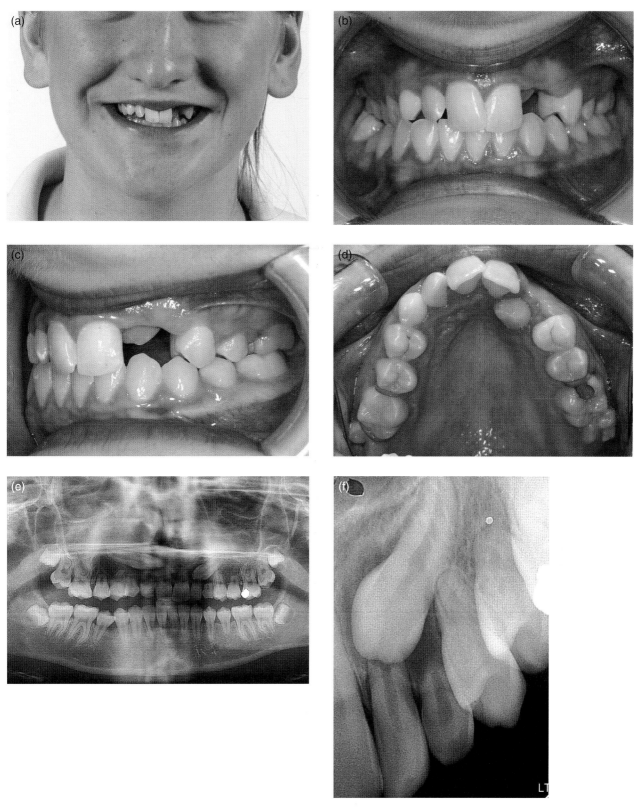

Figure 12.3 (a–d) Pretreatment photographs showing the absent upper left lateral incisor and recently exposed maxillary canine. Orthodontic separators have been placed for TPA preparation. (e,f) Pretreatment panoramic and intraoral radiographs showing the ectopic maxillary canines, severe root resorption of the upper left lateral incisor, and the generalised severe root shortness, especially of the premolar teeth. (g) An intraoral radiograph, taken after three months of treatment, showing the severity of the upper left premolar teeth roots and a molar band/cantilever wire *in situ*. (h–j) Photographs taken seven months into treatment, showing the cantilever traction to the canine crown using a 0.017 × 0.025 in. beta titanium wire from two buccal mini-implants, which have been inserted in series. Composite resin covers the mini-implant heads. (k–m) Progressive lateral movement of the canine tooth is seen after two months of mini-implant anchorage. (n–p) Photographs taken when the mini-implants were removed, after a total of five months, and when the upper fixed appliance was bonded. (q–t) Debond views showing the upper left canine aligned, after 18 months with fixed appliances. The upper right deciduous canine had been extracted during this phase.

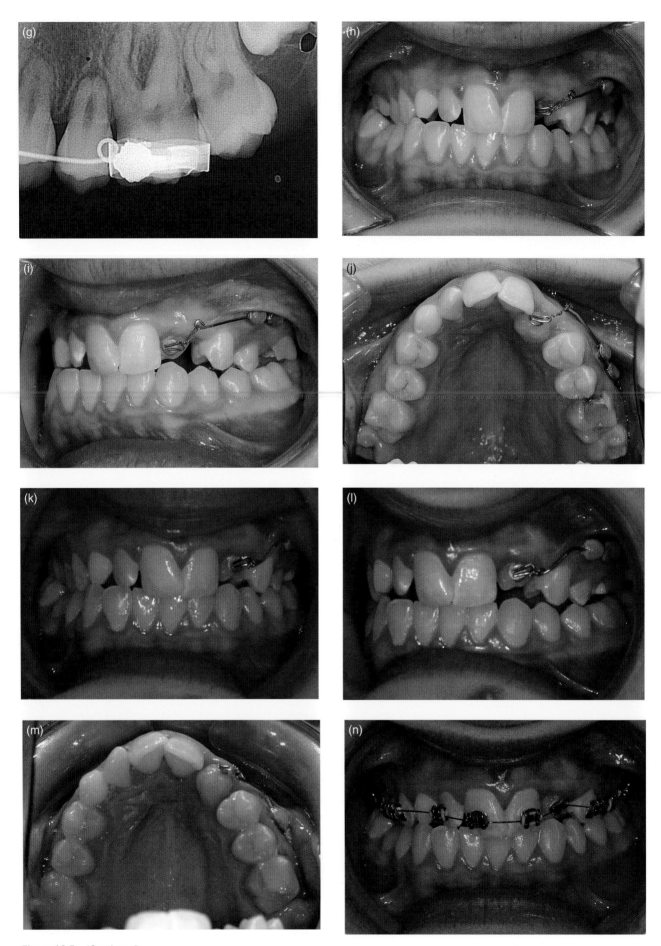

Figure 12.3 (Continued)

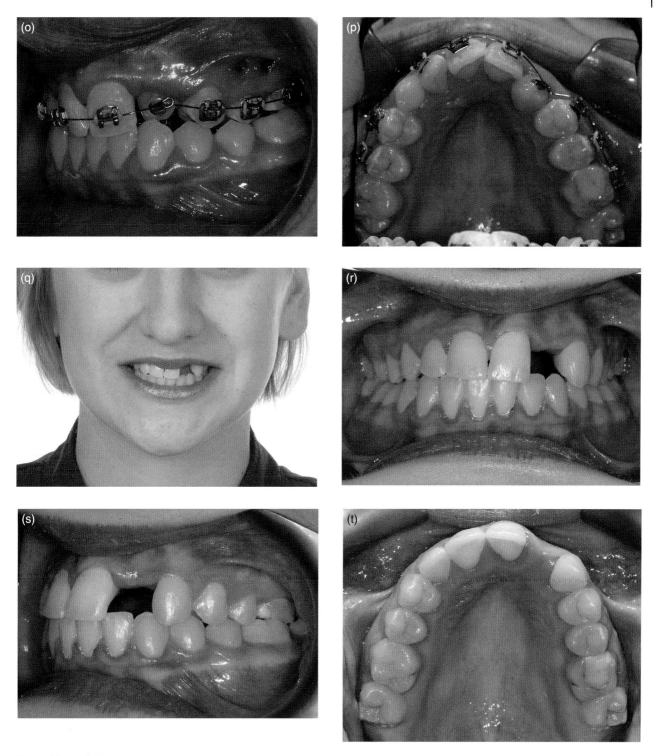

Figure 12.3 (Continued)

mesial and distal to the upper left second premolar (Figure 12.3h–j). A cantilever arm was fabricated from a 0.017×0.025 in. beta titanium wire, inserted into the paralleled slots of the mini-implant heads and secured with composite.

- The lever arm was adjusted *in situ* during alignment of the canine, e.g. to extrude the tooth after crossbite correction (Figure 12.3k–m). However, the amount of canine movement was limited by the single cantilever arm's range of activation and adjustability.

- Once the canine crown approximated the line of the arch it was feasible to complete treatment with a conventional fixed appliance treatment utilising light forces (Figure 12.3n–p). The upper right deciduous canine was extracted as part of this phase.

3) **Indirect anchorage of an anchor tooth and cantilever arm traction (Figure 12.4)**
    - A 17-year-old male presented with a Class II division 2 malocclusion on a Class I skeletal base with a palatally ectopic right maxillary canine (Figure 12.4a–d). The roots of the upper incisors were short, especially where the right lateral incisor root had been obliquely resorbed (Figure 12.4e). Therefore, it was ideal to align this canine without putting strain on the upper incisor teeth. In addition, the patient was concerned about the aesthetic prospect of prolonged fixed appliance treatment.
    - Treatment commenced with indirect anchorage of the right maxillary first molar. A mini-implant (1.5 mm diameter, 9 mm length) was inserted in the buccal aspect of the alveolus, mesial to the upper right first molar. This site was chosen since there was already adequate root divergence, without the need for a sectional fixed appliance (Figure 12.4f).
    - The mini-implant stabilised the first molar as the anchor tooth, using a piece of 0.019 × 0.025 in. steel wire inserted into the auxiliary tube of a double molar tube attachment (Figure 12.4g–i).
- A cantilever arm was fabricated from a 0.016 × 0.022 in. titanium molybdenum alloy (TMA) wire. This wire was inserted into the main tube of the right molar's double tube attachment (Figure 12.4g–i).
- The cantilever arm was adjusted monthly and then replaced after three months. It was used to align the canine and initially distalise it (away from the lateral incisor). The arm was then adjusted to move the canine buccally, and finally to extrude this tooth after cross-bite correction at seven months (Figure 12.4j–l). The anchor (molar) tooth remained stable throughout this time, displaying the same extent of mesial angulation as it had before treatment.
- Once the canine crown was in the line of the arch, after eight months, then it was feasible to complete treatment with a conventional fixed appliance treatment and only light forces (Figure 12.4m–p). The mini-implant was removed at the same time. In an attempt to avoid the right maxillary canine from approximating the adjacent lateral incisor, it had been overretracted with the cantilever arm. There has also been some distortion of the anchorage connecting steel wire, resulting in modest further mesial tipping of the anchor tooth (upper right first molar). Both molar and canine movements caused palatal displacement of the upper right second premolar, although this will readily be realigned in the fixed appliance phase (Figure 12.4p).

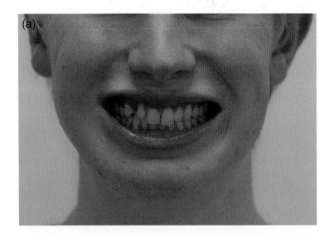
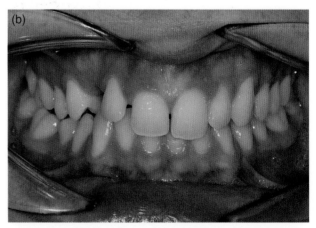

Figure 12.4 (a–d) Preorthodontic photographs showing the recently exposed right maxillary canine. (e,f) Pretreatment CBCT showing the palatally ectopic right maxillary canine, moderate root resorption of the upper right lateral incisor, and divergence of the upper right second premolar to first molar space. (g–i) Photographs taken at the time of mini-implant insertion. A steel archwire linked the mini-implant head to the auxiliary tube of a double tube bonded on the right first molar. A 0.016 × 0.022 TMA wire cantilever arm was then used to apply traction to the canine crown. Composite resin covers the mini-implant head. (j–l) Progressive lateral movement of the canine tooth is seen after seven months of mini-implant anchorage. A buccal swelling is evident in the canine eminence area, due to the underlying canine crown. An extrusive vector of traction was now being applied from the cantilever arm. The anchor (molar) tooth displays the same mesial angulation and vertical position as it had before treatment. (m–p) Photographs taken when the mini-implant was removed and the upper fixed appliance bonded, eight months into treatment. There had been a small increase in mesial tip of the upper right first molar and temporary palatal displacement of the upper right second premolar tooth.

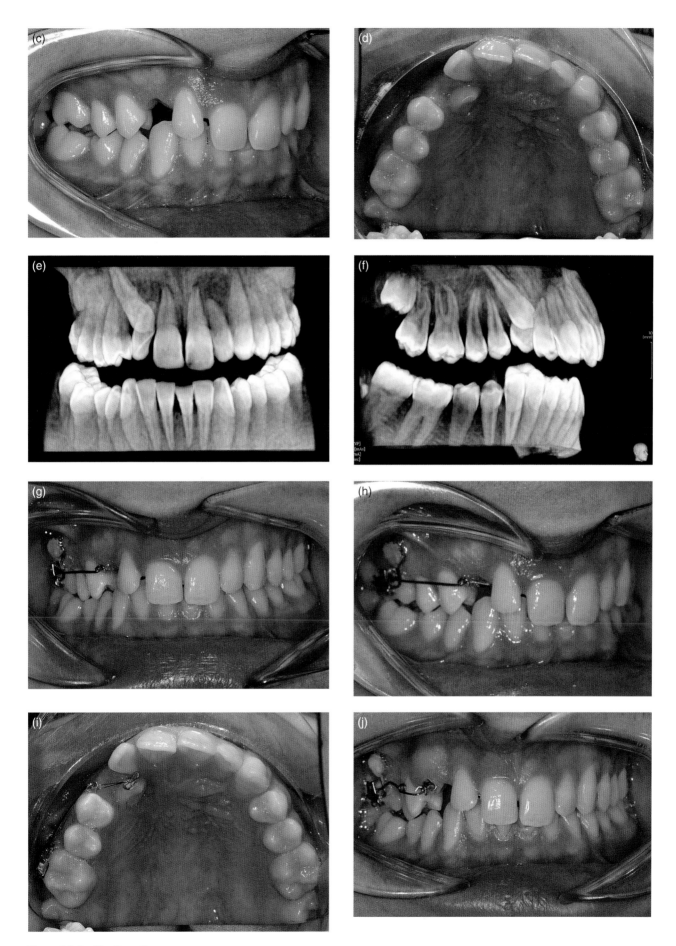

Figure 12.4 (Continued)

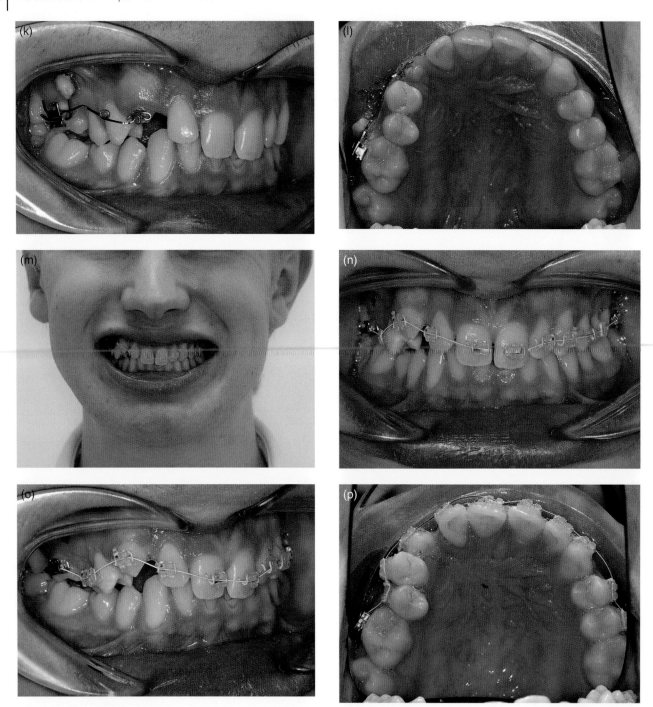

Figure 12.4 (Continued)

4) **Indirect anchorage of a fixed appliance archwire (Figure 12.5)**

- A 16-year-old girl presented with a Class I malocclusion on a Class I skeletal base with a history of traumatic avulsion of the right maxillary central incisor. This tooth was ankylosed and infraocclusal (Figure 12.5a,b). It also had signs of external root resorption and hence had a poor prognosis. Therefore, treatment aimed to align the dentition and attempt surgical extrusion of the ankylosed incisor in order to develop the alveolar bone height for future implant treatment.
- Both arches were aligned with fixed appliances, bypassing the upper right central incisor. Space was created mesial and distal to this tooth for surgical access.
- Bilateral mini-implants (1.5 mm diameter, 9 mm length) were inserted in the buccal aspect of the alveolus, distal to the upper lateral incisors (Figure 12.5c,d). These mini-implants stabilised the maxillary archwire using vertical struts of 0.019 × 0.025 in. steel wire inserted into the auxiliary cross-tubes on the main archwire.
- The patient had surgical corticotomies to create and mobilise a bone block around the upper right central incisor and immediate elastomeric traction was applied from the fixed appliance (Figure 12.2e). This was then changed to a 0.012 NiTi 'piggyback' after initial movement of the incisor block (Figure 12.5f–h).
- While the indirect anchorage configuration was effective, the bone cuts healed quicker than anticipated and the light traction force was insufficient to prevent this. The tooth was therefore only partly distracted and this position was accepted at debond (Figure 12.5i,j).

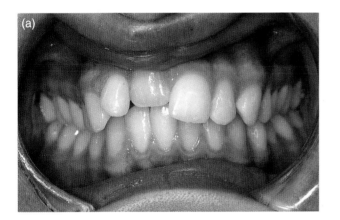
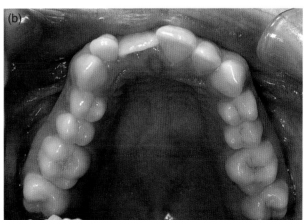
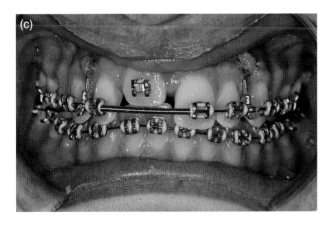
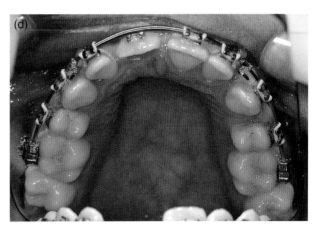

Figure 12.5 (a,b) Pretreatment photographs showing this girl's Class I malocclusion with severe infraocclusion of the right maxillary central incisor. (c,d) Dental views after alignment of the maxillary arch with a fixed appliance, bypassing the upper right central incisor. Space had been opened mesial and distal to this tooth for surgical access. Bilateral mini-implants had been inserted in the buccal aspect of the alveolus, distal to the upper lateral incisors. These mini-implants indirectly anchored the maxillary archwire using vertical struts of 0.019 × 0.025 in. steel wire inserted into the auxiliary cross-tubes on the main archwire. (e) Photograph taken five days after surgical corticotomies around the upper right central incisor and with elastomeric traction applied between this incisor and the adjacent teeth. (f–h) Photographs and a panoramic radiograph taken three weeks after surgery with a 0.012 NiTi piggyback *in situ*. (i,j) Debond views showing the corrected malocclusion but residual infraocclusion of the right maxillary incisor.

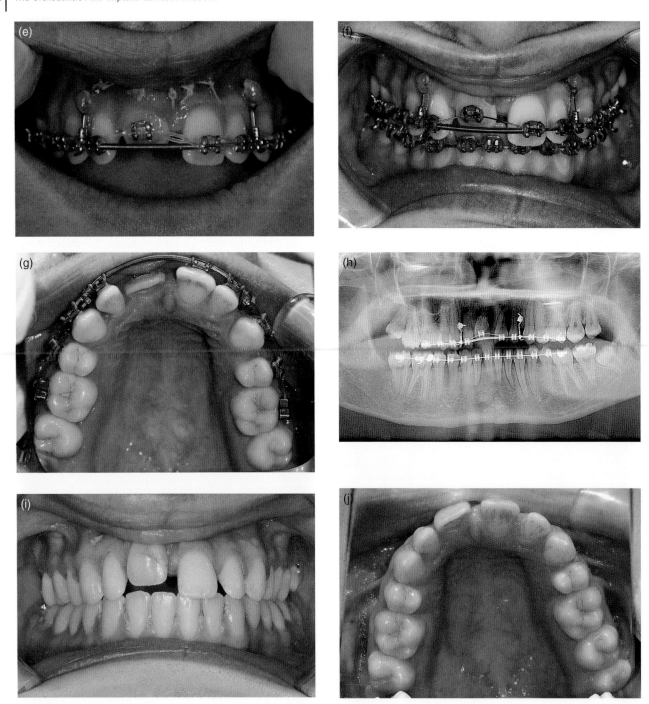

Figure 12.5 (Continued)

5) **Indirect anchorage from mini-implants in the opposing arch (Figure 12.6)**
   - A 15-year-old boy presented with a Class I malocclusion on a Class I skeletal base with failure of eruption of all upper left premolar and molar teeth, and premature loss of the lower left second molar (Figure 12.6a–e). The mesially tipped upper left first

premolar had a gold chain attachment bonded to it. There was an occlusal cant, higher on the left side, due to the left maxillary vertical alveolar deficiency combined with left mandibular height overgrowth.
   - Vertical traction was required to erupt these teeth, following further surgical exposures, but intraarch traction was not feasible, especially given the limited

occlusal clearance. Therefore, it was necessary to apply traction from the opposing mandibular arch. However, dental anchorage would have extruded the lower left quadrant teeth and hence worsened the occlusal cant.

- The lower left canine to first molar teeth were aligned with a sectional fixed appliance in order to level them and particularly diverge the roots. Adequate interproximal space was created for insertion of two mini-implants, mesial and distal to the lower left first premolar (Figure 12.6f–i). Infinitas IMT mini-implants were used since these have a mushroom head for elastic traction purposes (as discussed in more detail in Chapter 14 on orthognathic applications).

- Elastic intermaxillary traction was applied immediately to a connecting piece of steel wire attached to the upper left second premolar and first molar teeth. Direct traction from the mini-implants, rather than from the fixed appliance, avoided extrusion of the lower posterior teeth.

- The upper arch was bonded with a standard fixed appliance after seven months (Figure 12.6j–m). It was feasible to continue Class III/vertical elastic to the upper left first molar during initial alignment and then four months later when 0.012 in. piggyback NiTi traction was applied to the upper left first premolar tooth (Figure 12.6n–q).

- Use of the mini-implant anchorage was changed, after 29 months, to provide direct intrusive traction in the lower left quadrant. This was aimed at levelling the mandibular plane, in advance of further levelling of the maxillary plane (Figure 12.6r,s).

- The mini-implants were explanted after 35 months (Figure 12.6u,v). The previous six months of direct traction has created a left lateral openbite and divergence of the archwires on the left side.

- Treatment was completed five months after mini-implant removal. All the maxillary teeth were erupted, in occlusion, but accepting residual upper left quadrant spaces (Figure 12.6w–z).

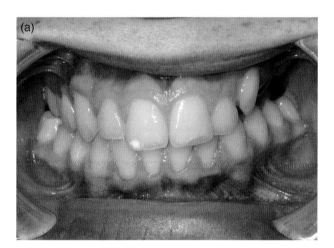
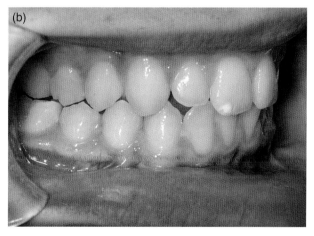

Figure 12.6 (a–d) Pretreatment photographs showing a Class I malocclusion where all of the upper left premolar and molar teeth were unerupted. Gold chain is seen emerging transmucosally on the distal aspect of the upper left canine. (e) A sectional panoramic radiograph shows the unerupted left maxillary buccal teeth and absent lower left second molar. There is severe mesial angulation of the upper left first premolar, with a gold chain attachment bonded on it. Vertical alveolar deficiency is present on the left side of the maxilla. (f,g) Intraoral views showing the sectional lower fixed appliance and IMT type of mini-implants in place. Intermaxillary elastic traction has been fitted between the mini-implants and a connecting bar on the upper left posterior teeth. (h,i) Radiographs showing the left mandibular mini-implants (1.5 mm diameter, 9 mm body length) and the connections on three of the upper left teeth. (j–m) Photographs taken when the upper arch was bonded, after seven months of traction. (n–q) A Class III/vertical configuration of intermaxillary elastic is being worn after a further four months, when 0.012 piggyback NiTi traction has been added to the upper left first premolar tooth. (r,s) These views, taken after 29 months with the mini-implant *in situ*, show direct elastomeric traction applied between the mini-implants and the lower left canine/premolar brackets. The convergence of the archwires can be seen on the left side of the dentition. (t) A panoramic radiograph taken after 32 months of mini-implant anchorage, showing the vertical improvements in both the left maxillary alveolar bone level and tooth positions. There is an incidental finding of a lower right second molar follicular cyst. (u,v) Photographs taken on removal of the mini-implants, after 35 months *in situ*. Divergence of the archwires on the left side and a small left lateral openbite are visible. (w–z) Debond views showing the Class I malocclusion result, with residual upper left quadrant spaces and a small centreline discrepancy. All of the left maxillary teeth are fully erupted.

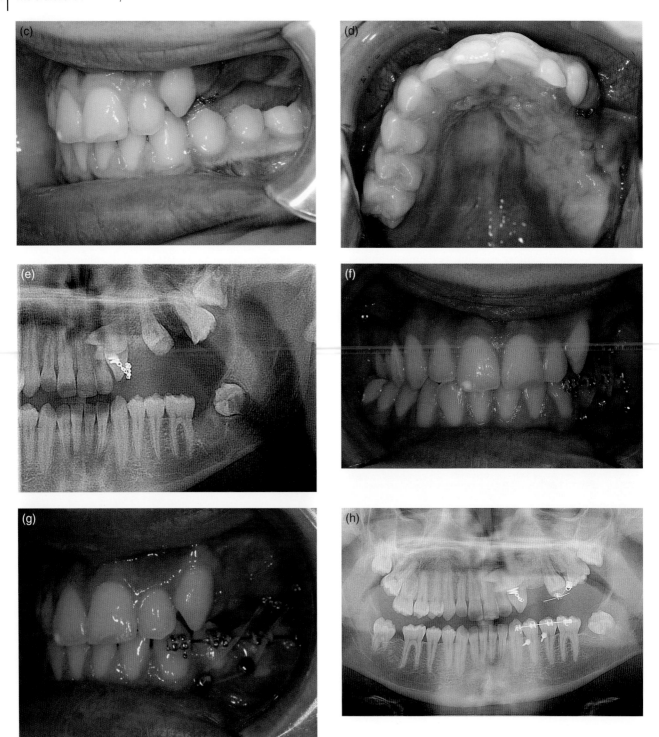

Figure 12.6 (Continued)

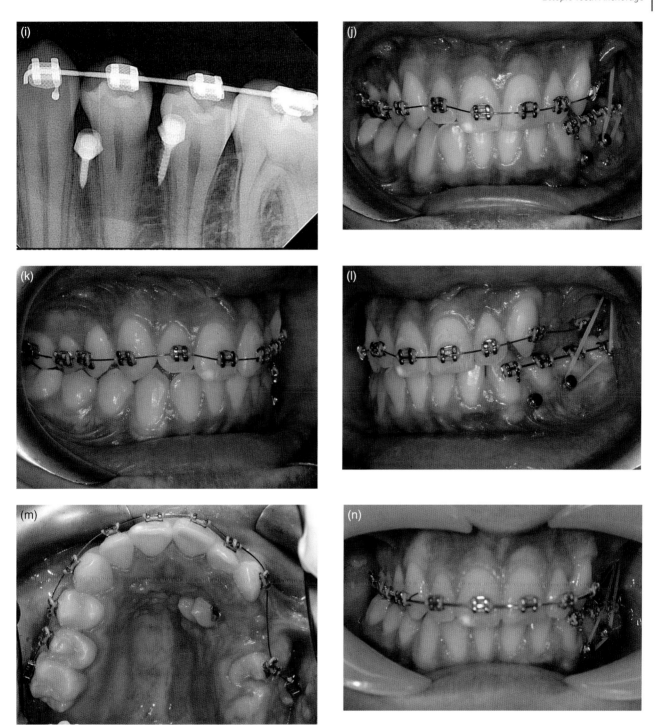

Figure 12.6 (Continued)

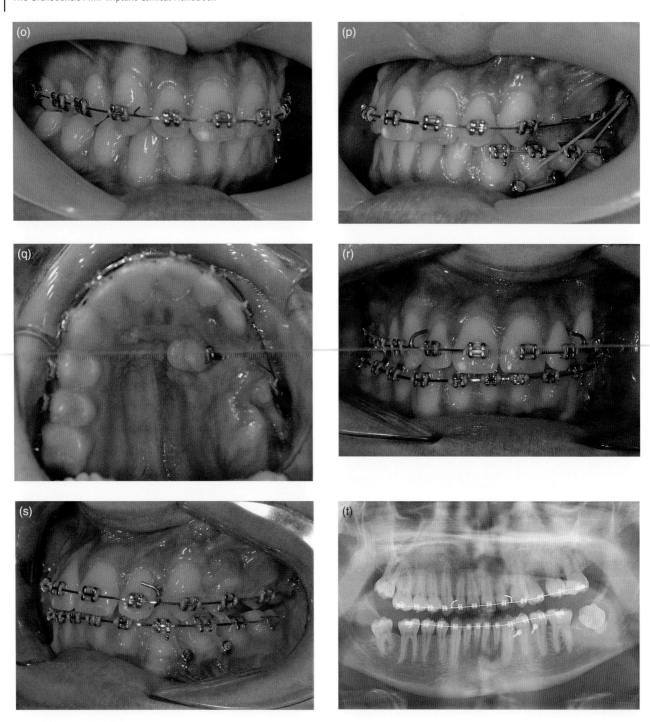

Figure 12.6 (Continued)

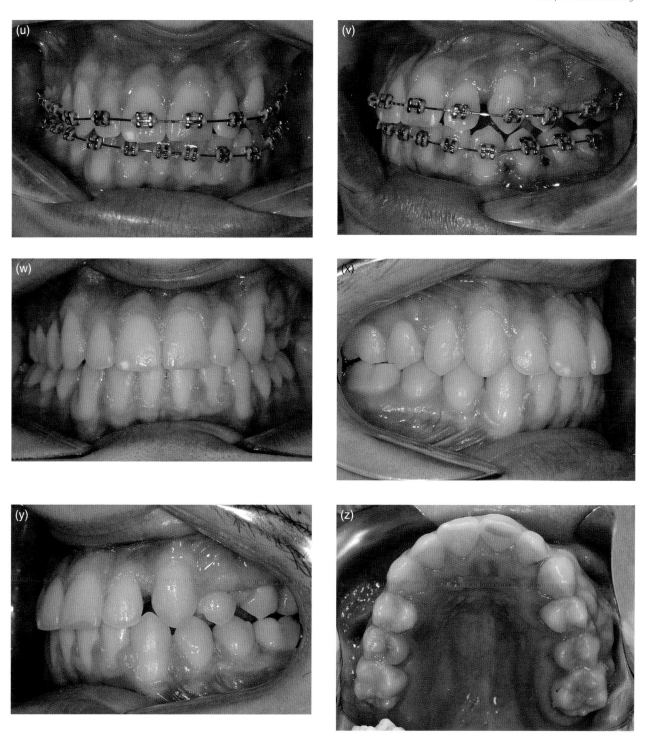

Figure 12.6 (Continued)

13

Bone-anchored Maxillary Expansion

13.1 Conventional Rapid Maxillary Expansion

The search for optimal correction of transverse maxillary deficiency (and the associated cross-bite malocclusion problems) has attracted a huge volume of published work over the last few decades. Conventional techniques involve a variety of orthodontic expansion appliances incorporating screw or active wire active components, such as rapid maxillary expansion (RME) and the quadhelix, respectively. RME appliances are either tooth-borne (fitted on the molar and premolar teeth) or mucosa-borne (resting on the palatal alveolar shelf mucosa and often referred to as a Haas expander). Their activation protocols may involve 'slow' (e.g. 0.25 mm every second day), 'rapid' (e.g. 0.2–0.5 mm per day), or alternating opening and closing activation cycles (known as Alt-RAMEC). However, a recent meta-analysis study has indicated that there is probably little clinically significant difference in outcome between slow and rapid expansion protocols, although gradual RME tends to cause more molar expansion and more dental movements than rapid RME [1].

All forms of RME treatment aim to produce skeletal (basal) expansion, rather than just dentoalveolar remodelling. This is typically characterised by the creation of a midline diastema (Figure 13.1). However, dental and alveolar changes are major side-effects of conventional nonsurgical expansion outcomes. These side-effects have been repeatedly documented in the literature in terms of buccal tilting (buccal crown inclination) of the anchor teeth, buccal root prominence, periodontal recession and bone dehiscence, root resorption, buccal tilting (divergence) of the alveolar complex, an opening of the occlusion (due to a shift to occlusal contacts on the 'hanging' palatal cusps) with clockwise rotation of the mandibular plane, and high relapse rates [2,3]. Notably, the side-effects are potentially more pronounced in patients with large expansion movements and/or when the patient is somatically mature. However, a reduction in the width of the buccal alveolar

bone even occurs in prepubertal patients treated with tooth-borne expanders [4]. Consequently, it is important to remember that gingival tissues may camouflage this loss of buccal bone thickness and height (of the anchor teeth) in the short term, but tooth-borne expansion may predispose to gingival recession in the long term in those patients with thin gingival biotypes [2]. Finally, the combination of buccal crown tipping and divergent alveolar bending (rather than true basal expansion) is especially unfavourable in patients requiring subsequent molar intrusion (for the correction of anterior openbite). This is because traction from palatal mini-implants to maxillary molars tends to upright/torque these teeth, with the consequential risk of excessive buccal root prominence beyond the alveolar bone width (Figure 13.2).

Consequently, many orthodontists refer postpubertal adolescent and adult patients for surgically assisted rapid maxillary expansion (SARME). This is a form of distraction osteogenesis, where the rationale is that the corticotomies circumvent the resistance caused by maturation (closure) of the circummaxillary and palatal sutures. In addition, provided that there has been pterygoid dysjunction then significant posterior midpalate suture expansion is achievable compared with non-surgical expansion in adults [5]. However, such surgical procedures have associated additional costs, morbidity and stability risks, and there is still no clarity on which surgical technique is optimal [6]. In addition, the age and expansion range thresholds between non-surgical and surgical approaches are unclear. For example, a recent cone beam computed tomography (CBCT) study of suture maturation in 11–15-year-old subjects indicates that conventional RME would probably successfully separate the midpalatal suture up until the age of 13 years [7]. A subsequent CBCT study in 16–20-year-old subjects demonstrated incomplete transitional ossification in many midpalate sutures, which indicates that there is likely to be interindividual variation in the proportion of skeletal expansion even when expanders are bone anchored [8]. Therefore, the authors concluded that CBCT of the

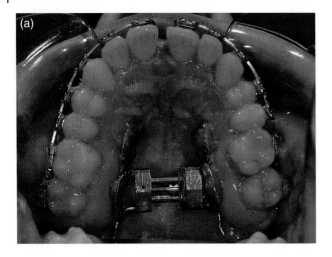

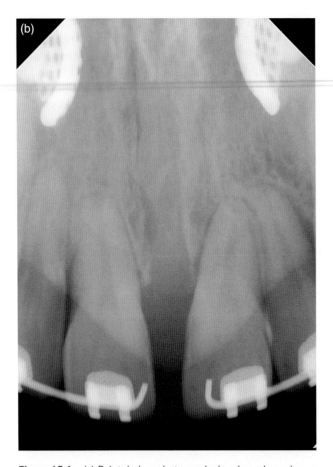

Figure 13.1 (a) Palatal view photograph showing a bone-borne RME appliance *in situ* in a 25-year-old female patient. There are four palatal alveolar mini-implants in place: two inserted bilaterally under the wire mesh pads. The RME screw has been expanded and there is a midline diastema, following recent surgical corticotomies. (b) Intraoral radiograph showing separation of the midpalatal suture in the patient shown in (a). The short root lengths of the central incisors are pre-existing.

maxilla is justified in postadolescent patients to determine if SARME is required or not.

Given the limitations of conventional expansion options, it is unsurprising that skeletal anchorage has been introduced to maxillary expansion techniques and that previously unthinkable levels of maxillary suture separation may be achieved. This approach originated in Belgium with the transpalatal distractor (TPD) [9,10]. However, this appliance requires both invasive surgical insertion and removal (via palatal flap elevations) of bilateral fixation plates and screws. In turn, this increases the level of morbidity and cost. Therefore, in a similar way that mini-implant anchorage is less invasive than miniplate techniques in other anchorage situations, the application of mini-implants in maxillary expansion ought to reduce patient morbidity and surgery costs.

13.2 Expansion Forces and Speed

The traditional viewpoint on RME is that the rate of expansion needs to be 'fast' (0.5–1 mm screw expansion per day) so that the resultant high force levels will maximise sutural expansion and minimise dental movements (by virtue of hyalinisation of the compressed periodontal tissues adjacent to the anchor teeth). However, this concept does not fully apply to mini-implant (only) supported expanders where no anchor teeth are involved. Therefore, the force level and rate of expansion may both be reduced, which is more practical for patients since fewer activation turns are required per day. This is particularly the case once the midpalatal suture has been opened (which is indicated by creation of a diastema), but a high frequency of expansion turns may still be required initially to split the suture.

Evidence to support gradual non-surgical bone-anchored expansion has been provided by Pulver et al. [11]. They observed slow and linear basal suture expansion in adult rabbits despite the mature status of their palatal suture. This was achieved with a light force (proportionate to the animal model's size), involving a 100 g compressed coil spring directly attached to two parasagittal mini-implants. Therefore, only 50 g applied directly to the palatal bone on each side was sufficient to open mature rabbit sutures by approximately 50% of the amount of mini-implant separation. This is at odds with the traditional concept of facial growth, but is explicable by more recent knowledge that facial sutures do not completely fuse until much later in life than early adulthood, and that even mature sutures contain the necessary cells for bone remodelling. The amount of suture separation observed by Pulver et al. [11]

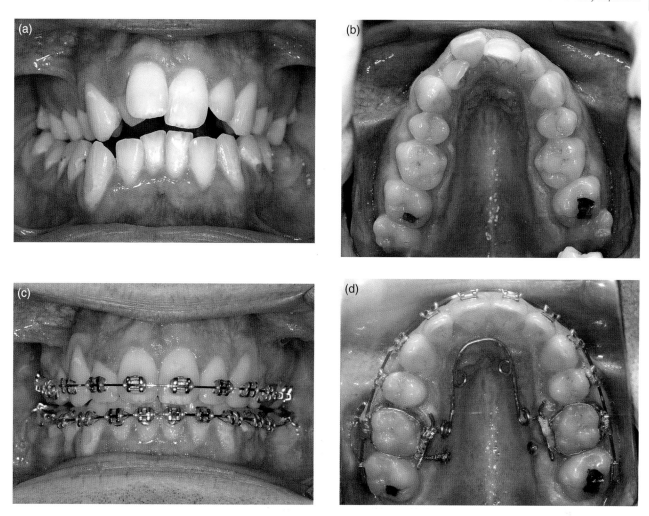

Figure 13.2 (a,b) Pretreatment photographs of a 27-year-old male with a narrow high-vaulted palate, buccal crossbites and an anterior openbite. (c,d) This patient's maxillary arch has been expanded with a modified quadhelix appliance. Palatal alveolar mini-implants are being used for molar intrusion and hence anterior openbite correction. However, the mesiobuccal root of the upper right first molar is now very prominent on the buccal aspect of the alveolus. This has occurred as the molars have been torqued as a side-effect of the (intrusive) palatal traction.

was less than in similar animal studies of adolescent subjects, because of the slower bone turnover rate and greater sutural complexity in their adult subjects. In addition, the gradual expansion process did not result in a midline diastema in this study, and consequently it is reasonable to assume that slow palatal expansion in adult humans may not produce a midline diastema. This concept supports the approach adopted by pioneering orthodontists such as Professor Moon in the USA, who recommend protocols with a high frequency of screw turns (e.g. 4–6 per day) until a midline diastema opens and then a slower rate of turns (e.g. twice per day) thereafter [12]. If this early rapid expansion is not undertaken then it is likely that the sutures will remain intact and that only alveolar expansion will result, as shown in Figure 13.3.

Slow expansion with lighter (e.g. 800 g), continuous forces may also be better for mini-implant success rates since the lower (e.g. 200 g) force applied per implant is unlikely to exceed its physiological stability threshold. Furthermore, low RME forces may cause less deformation of connecting wires between the expansion screw and mini-implants [13]. Such continuous, relatively low-force RME is facilitated by newer designs of RME screw where the screw activation is more gradually delivered to the target teeth and/or mini-implants via a nickel titanium intermediary such as an internal compression spring or leaf spring (Figure 13.1a) [14,15]. A study of a 'memory' screw in conventional RME demonstrated that 'slow' expansion may be achieved by gradual expression of the stored spring compression [14]. In effect, these studies highlight that

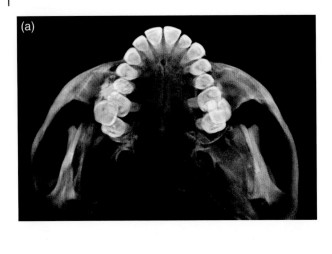

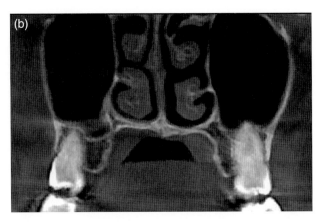

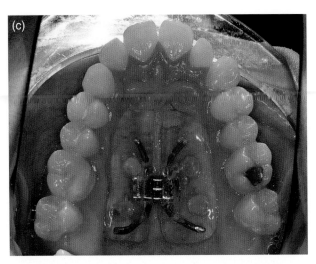

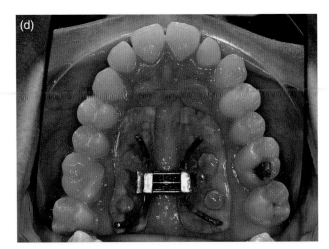

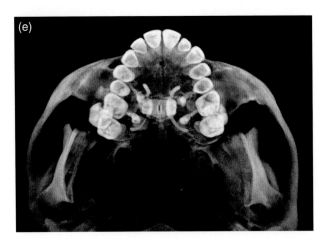

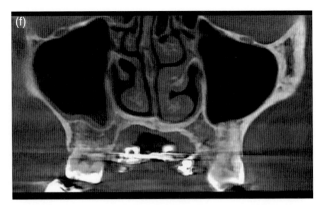

Figure 13.3 A 19-year-female patient had non-surgical RME with a Haas-type bone-borne RME appliance. (a,b) Pretreatment CBCT views showing the interdigitated midpalatal suture in 3D reformatted and coronal views. (c) Photograph of the RME appliance at the start of expansion and (d) after three weeks of expansion. There has been 2 mm and 4 mm expansion at the level of the first premolar and first molar crowns, but no diastema opening. (e,f) These postexpansion CBCT views show the intact midpalatal suture in 3D reformatted and coronal views. The four palatal alveolar mini-implants are also seen.

the final effects of expansion are a question of thresholds – whether the teeth, alveolus or basal bones expand most easily. In turn, this depends on the nature of the force application (teeth, mucosal, bone borne or a mixture of these), the screw force levels, and patient age and suture maturity.

In conclusion, memory screws are very useful for young and SARME patients where the sutural resistance is low and these patients (or their family) benefit from fewer activation requirements. However, it is my experience that currently available memory screws are not sufficiently 'powerful' to separate the suture in adolescent and non-surgical adult patients since the maximum force is not delivered at a single time to force the suture to open.

> Memory screws are not sufficiently 'powerful' to separate the suture in adolescent and non-surgical adult patients since the maximum force is not delivered at one time point to force the suture to open.

13.3 Potential Advantages of Mini-implant Anchored RME

In summary, mini-implant anchored RME appears to provide several key advantages over conventional (tooth-borne) RME techniques, as described here.

13.3.1 Greater Basal Skeletal Expansion

Direct skeletal engagement means that a higher proportion of the screw expansion is expressed in terms of midpalate suture opening. This was demonstrated in a finite element analysis (FEA) model where the addition of four palatal screws distributed the expansion force to the posterior palate and zygomatic areas, while reducing the stress in alveolar sites [16]. A subsequent CBCT analysis of the effects of a specific appliance, the Maxillary Skeletal Expander (MSE), showed that up to 71% of the screw opening was expressed as opening of the midpalatal suture [17]. In contrast, only 43% suture opening was observed in a study of tooth-borne RME [18]. A recent randomised controlled trial involving 40 adolescent patients (with a mean age of 14 years) treated with bone-only (palatal alveolar) anchored RME demonstrated similarly contrasting results: 26% and 68% of the molar expansion was due to suture opening in the conventional and orthodontic mini-implant (OMI)-RME groups, respectively [19]. In addition, more parallel suture opening and both minimal buccal bone loss and lingual crown inclination occurred in the OMI group in this study.

13.3.2 Basal Expansion in Older Aged Patients (Postpuberty)

This would be without the need for surgical corticotomies [17,20]. However, adults over the age of 30 years, with skeletal maturity, may still benefit from SARME according to several reasons highlighted by a FEA study [21]. In particular, an expander based on palatal alveolar mini-implants may exert excessive stress on peri-implant bone where there are high levels of skeletal resistance and it is more likely to cause maxillary deformation rather than midpalatal displacement in lieu of surgery. A possible exception to this may be the MSE appliance, where the forces are applied to the midpalate shelves, as discussed in a following section.

13.3.3 Greater Posterior Palatal Expansion

This will result in more linear opening of the midpalatal suture and possibly pterygopalatine suture opening. For example, Cantarella et al. [17] observed that the MSE appliance resulted in fairly similar amounts of anterior and posterior midpalatal suture opening: 71% at the anterior nasal spine (ANS) and 63% at the posterior nasal spine (PNS) [17]. In contrast, Lione et al. [18] reported 'V'-shaped expansion with only 43% and 16% of the conventional screw expansion expressed at the levels of the ANS and PNS, respectively [15]. Celenk-Koca et al. [19] observed greater anterior opening with RME anchored on four palatal alveolar mini-implants, but the pattern of suture opening appeared more parallel than the conventional RME group [19].

13.3.4 Increased Nasal Airflow

Greater proportions of palatal (skeletal) expansion result in a reduction in nasal resistance. This was demonstrated in a randomised controlled trial of conventional and hybrid RME appliances in 40 prepubescent children [22].

13.3.5 Fewer Dental and Periodontal Side-effects

Two retrospective studies and one prospective randomised controlled trial have compared different types of conventional and bone-anchored RME in adolescent [19,23] and postpubertal subjects [24]. All three studies found fewer side-effects in the mini-implant groups with less buccal tilting of the dentoalveolar complex and less buccal alveolar bone loss. Indeed, if there were no expander anchorage points on the teeth, then palatal (inwards) tipping of the upper first molars was observed [19,23].

13.4 Clinical Objective

Expansion of the maxillary dental arch, through a maximum amount of skeletal expansion and the limitation of unfavourable dental movements and side-effects.

13.5 Treatment Options

- Conventional approaches such as RME or quadhelix expansion.
- Surgically assisted RME (SARME), for either all postpubertal or only mature adult patients when associated with conventional RME and bone-anchored RME, respectively.
- Non-surgical RME using mini-implant anchorage within one of the following design options: a hybrid implant-tooth borne expander, an Haas-implant borne one, or a mini-implant (only) borne appliance.

13.6 Relevant Clinical Details

- Patient age and likely skeletal maturity (suture ossification).
- The transverse arch discrepancy, and extent of the posterior cross-bites and any functional mandibular displacement.
- Number of buccal teeth present and their relative buccopalatal positions and inclination.
- The periodontal status, especially the presence of gingival recession and/or a thin gingival biotype.
- The root proximity of teeth adjacent to any planned alveolar insertion sites.

13.7 Design Options for Mini-implant Expanders

Rapid maxillary expansion appliances involving mini-implant anchorage may be categorised as follows

1) Hybrid RME:
    - MARPE appliance
    - hybrid hyrax appliance
    - tooth and palatal alveolar RME
2) Mini-implant only RME
3) Haas-type (mucosa) and mini-implant borne RME

13.8 Hybrid RME

At first glance, the easiest way to integrate mini-implants with RME is to produce a hybrid appliance involving part tooth and part bone-derived anchorage. Two FEA studies have compared multiple types of conventional RME design options with adjunctive mini-implant versions [20,21]. These studies have shown that the addition of skeletal anchorage close to the palatal suture causes more effective distribution of the expansion forces along the whole (both anterior and posterior) length of the palatal suture and less buccal crown tipping of the anchor teeth. There are currently two principal versions of hybrid expanders, as described below.

13.8.1 Mini-implant Assisted Rapid Palatal Expansion (MARPE)

This appliance was introduced and popularised in South Korea [20]. It uses four palatal mini-implants connected to a modified version of the metal framework of a conventional RME appliance (featuring molar and first premolar bands). The mini-implants are vertically orientated, under the lateral nasal buttresses, rather than angled towards the palatal alveolus area. However, these mini-implant sites require adequate handpiece access to the palatal vault, which may be difficult in patients with narrow, high-arch palate morphology. In my experience, this excludes the use of the MARPE in many hyperdivergent and anterior openbite cases (Figure 13.4). Several studies have clarified the mechanism of action and final effects produced by MARPE. For example, a FEA study showed that MARPE causes a more uniform dissemination of the expansion forces, rather than concentrating high levels of force solely in either the buccal alveolar bone and teeth, or in the bone immediately around mini-implants (as occurs with tooth-borne or mini-implant only borne expanders, respectively) [25].

Choi et al. [26] reported a retrospective study of 20 young adults (with a mean age of 21 years) who had non-surgical hybrid RME using a MARPE device and a 47-month follow-up period [26]. Clinical opening of the midline diastema and radiological signs of suture opening were observed in 87% of patients (despite their postpubertal age). On average, 2 mm of skeletal and 4 mm of molar expansion appeared to be stable in the long term. Similarly, Lim et al. [27] undertook a retrospective clinical study of 24 young adult patients (mean age 22 years) where the midpalatal suture was opened non-surgically (notably in a sample of 38 cases where the suture remained closed in five other patients) [27]. The authors found excellent skeletal stability after an average of four months retention and then 14 months follow-up. The final percentage of expansion changes was 43% skeletal (basal), 15% alveolar and 42% dental. Broadly similar findings of the proportions of dental and skeletal expansion (37.0% skeletal, 22.2%, alveolar, 40.7% dental expansion, respectively) were reported in a CBCT study of 14 postpubertal patients who all exhibited midline diastema opening (out of 17 patients) following MARPE expansion [28]. The authors also observed modest levels of expansion as coronal as the zygoma level, but with alveolar bending and a loss of buccal plate coverage (of teeth) expressed as side-effects; that is, dentoalveolar changes still occurred despite the mini-implant support. Interestingly, the proportional results in these latter two MARPE studies are similar to those reported following SARME, yet the MARPE results were obtained non-surgically in somatically mature adults. This supports the concept that the addition of mini-implant anchorage to some

form of conventional RME appliance offers a similar long-term amount of skeletal expansion to that provided by surgical expansion techniques, although surgical assistance may still be indicated in more mature adult patients.

A recent modification of the MARPE appliance has been designed by Professor Won Moon in the USA, called the MSE (Figure 13.5). He has made several key changes to maximise the skeletal effects: the mini-implants are sited in the posterior midpalate area, their depth of insertion aims for bicortical engagement, and the metal connecting arms between the hyrax screw and first molar bands are flexible [17,29]. The latter reduces the amount of dental

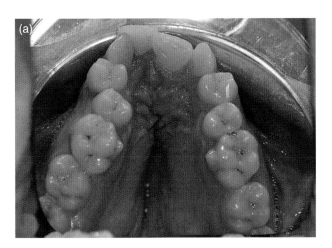
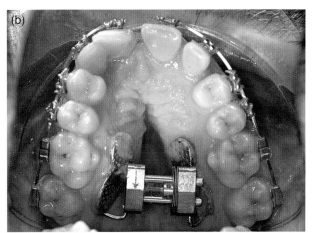

Figure 13.4 Palatal photographs of a patient unsuitable for midpalate sited anchorage. (a) The pretreatment photograph shows the extremely narrow, high-vaulted (cleft-like) palate with additional midarch constriction and multiple absent teeth. (b) Postexpansion views. Notably the maxillary dentition had to be provisionally aligned to enable any type of expander to be fitted. A bone-borne RME appliance was selected, with bilateral pairs of mini-implants in the palatal alveolar processes, and a SARME protocol was followed.

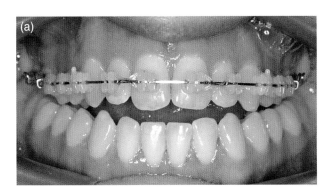
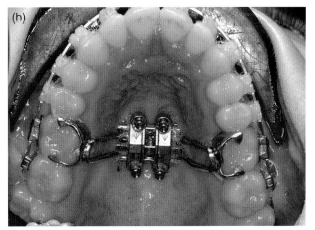

Figure 13.5 (a,b) Pre-expansion photographs of a 26-year-old female undergoing non-surgical expansion with an MSE type of hybrid appliance. The archwire has been sectioned in the midline. The MSE has been fixed to the midpalatal shelves using four 11 mm (total) length screws for bicortical engagement. (c,d) Views taken after two weeks of expansion. There has been obvious expansion of the screw, with an associated increase in the intermolar width and a diastema is now present. There appears to have been constrictive movement of the wires connecting the molars and hyrax screw. *Source:* Case illustrations kindly provided by Dr Lars Christensen, Oxford, UK.

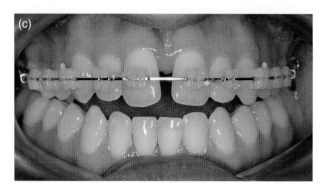

Figure 13.5 (Continued)

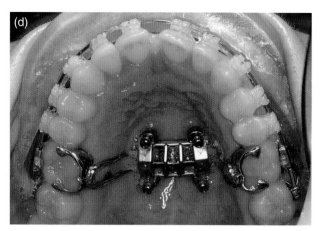

expansion and these palatal arms may even be removed once the MSE appliance has been fitted (where they act solely as positioning guides). Initial results indicate that this bicortical mini-implant anchorage results in improved mini-implant stability, decreased mini-implant deformation and fracture, more parallel expansion in the coronal plane, and increased expansion in bone-borne palatal expansion [29].

> The addition of mini-implant anchorage to a conventional RME appliance offers a similar long-term amount of skeletal expansion to that provided by surgical expansion techniques, although surgical assistance may still be indicated in more mature adult patients.

Figure 13.6 A hybrid hyrax RME appliance on a demonstration model of the maxillary dentition and palate. The first molars form the tooth-borne component and parasagittal mini-implants are located under the caps, anterior to the hyrax screw.

13.8.2 Hybrid Hyrax RME Appliance

This alternative appliance appears simpler since it involves only two anterior (parasagittal) palatal mini-implants and molar bands, although it requires precise connection of the metal framework onto the mini-implants (Figure 13.6). This appliance has been popularised by the innovative team of German orthodontists led by Drs Pieter Dietrich, Bjorn Ludwig and Benedict Wilmes. Initially, they demonstrated the benefits of hybrid anchorage in conjunction with early Class III facemask correction [30], but it has subsequently been applied to more extensive expansion goals in older patients. This hybrid design is especially favourable in young patients where alveolar bone support is much less than the midpalatal sites, and insertion of mini-implants distal to the upper first molars is impractical (due to the unerupted second molars). However, a randomised con-trolled trial of 25 adolescent patients (mean age 14 years) treated with this version of hybrid RME compared with conventional RME appliances showed little difference in skeletal outcomes between the two groups [31]. In addition, similar levels of buccal bone loss occurred adjacent to the anchor teeth (upper first molars) in these groups.

From a practical perspective, Toklu et al. [31] also commented that insertion of anterior palatal mini-implants may be difficult in patients with palatally displaced upper lateral incisors and those with a narrow palate (which in many caseloads tends to be the group of patients most in need of expansion!) [31]. Arguably, the cases most successfully treated with this hybrid RME appliance have been young Class III patients where the primary objective is to provide bone anchorage for facemask treatment. In my

Table 13.1 Mini-implant (OMI) anchored expander design options with practical advantages and limitations

Type of RME anchorage	Advantages	Disadvantages
Tooth only	Low cost, simple fabrication and non-invasive insertion	Significant dental side-effects, increasing with skeletal maturity Requires SARME post puberty Limited long-term patient tolerance due to occlusal position of appliance Simultaneous orthodontic tooth movements restricted
Hybrid – tooth and midpalatal OMI borne	Skeletal anchorage feasible in young patients (with immature alveolar tissues) Close proximity of OMIs to dental roots and palatal suture easily avoided	Access not feasible in narrow, high-arched palates Potential conflict in path of insertion onto teeth and OMIs Independent molar movements not feasible
Hybrid – tooth and alveolar OMI borne	Feasible (access) in high-arched palates	Less effective in young patients in terms of cortical anchorage Potential conflict in path of insertion onto teeth and OMIs Independent molar movements not feasible
Mucosa and OMI borne (hybrid Haas design)	Simple appliance design and insertion Simultaneous orthodontic tooth movements feasible	Risk of gingival devascularisation if insufficient margin of tissue between teeth and baseplate
OMI only	Facilitates gingival hygiene Simultaneous orthodontic tooth movements feasible	May be difficult to seat on four OMIs during insertion

OMI, orthodontic mini-implant; RME, rapid maxillary expansion; SARME, surgically assisted rapid maxillary expansion.

experience, it is simply not feasible to insert midpalatal mini-implants in patients with narrow and high-vaulted palate morphology (which is typically seen in patients with narrow maxillary widths and bilateral cross-bites). Therefore, several other design options should be considered, depending on the individual patient's morphology, dental status and age. These various design options are described below and summarised in Table 13.1.

An alternative option for hybrid anchorage involves molar bands and mini-implants inserted in the palatal alveolar sites, for example mesial or distal to the maxillary first molars (Figure 13.7). This appliance is suitable for the many patients with narrow high-vaulted palates in whom handpiece and appliance access to midpalatal sites is severely restricted. However, it still incorporates anchor teeth, with the resultant risk of dental side-effects although these are less problematic than tooth-borne appliances alone. This was demonstrated in a short-term prospective study of 20 12-year-old female patients who had either standard RME or a hybrid RME appliance involving molar bands and four palatal alveolar mini-implants [32]. Both appliances resulted in similar amounts of dental arch (molar and premolar) expansion, although the hybrid version produced a greater change in facial width and less buccal inclination of the molars.

13.8.2.1 Case Example

- A 31-year-old male presented with a Class III malocclusion and mandibular asymmetry with the chin displaced to the left side (Figure 13.7a–d). The maxillary arch and palate were very narrow and the lower centreline was significantly displaced to the left side, but there was only mild vertical facial asymmetry. Maxillary expansion was required so that arch co-ordination would be achieved following an asymmetrical mandibular setback osteotomy. Bone-borne expansion was preferred given the extent of generalised gingival recession and thin gingival biotype already present. However, the midpalate area was not accessible for midpalate mini-implant insertions and the palatal alveolar mucosa was abnormally thick in the anterior half of the palate. Therefore, SARME with a hybrid tooth-implant borne expander was chosen as the most feasible and effective option.

- The maxillary dentition was first aligned, in separate halves, with the inclusion of molar bands on the second molar teeth (Figure 13.7e). A dental impression was taken for fabrication of mini-implant guidance stents and the hybrid RME. This would incorporate wire mesh rests on top of the mini-implant heads, inserted in the intermolar space (Figure 13.7f). Anterior rests were bonded on the second premolar crowns.

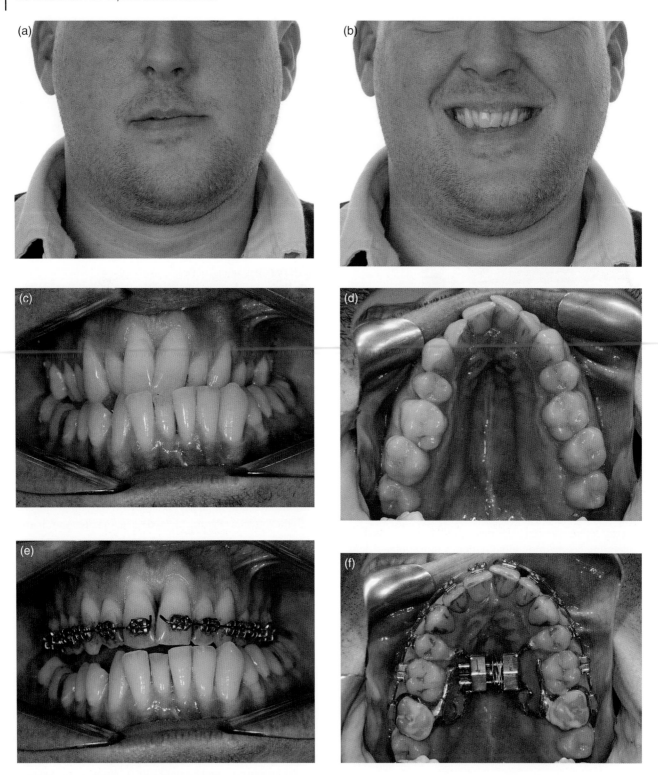

Figure 13.7   (a–d) Pretreatment photographs illustrating the Class III malocclusion and mandibular asymmetry (with the chin displaced to the left side) in this adult patient. (e,f) Treatment photographs showing initial alignment of the maxillary dentition, in two separate halves. The hybrid RME has been fitted, via molar bands on the second molars, bonded rests on the second premolars and the palatal alveolar mini-implants. (g,h) Intraoral radiographs showing the upper incisor area prior to expansion and after opening of the midpalatal suture. (i,j) Photographs taken after three weeks of expansion showing the widened screw of the hybrid RME and a midline diastema. (k–n) Preoperative photographs showing the decompensated Class III malocclusion and expanded upper arch. (o–r) Debond photographs, showing the corrected dental and facial midlines, and Class I occlusion. There had not been any worsening of the pre-existing gingival recession.

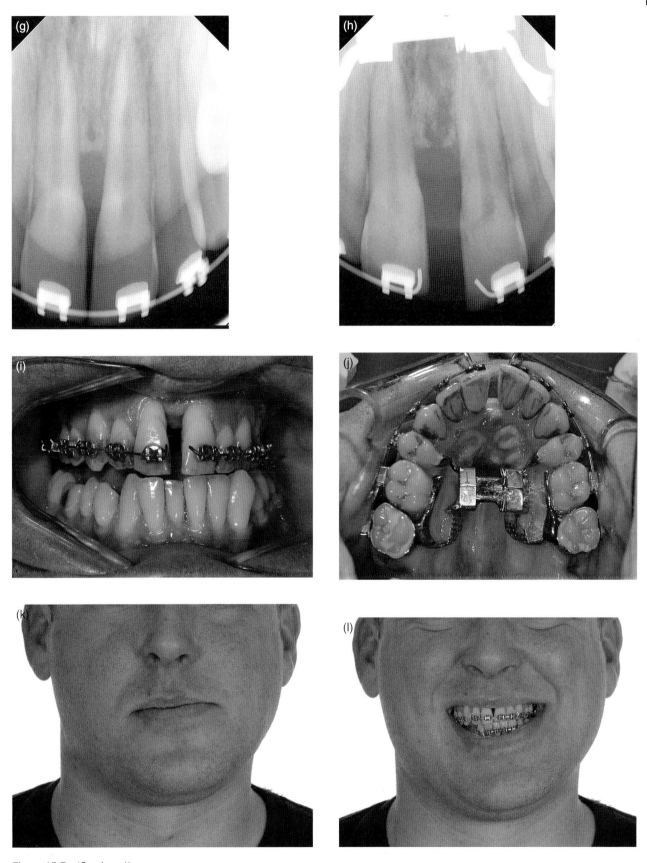

Figure 13.7 (Continued)

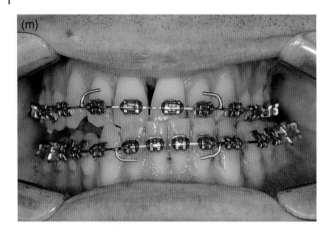

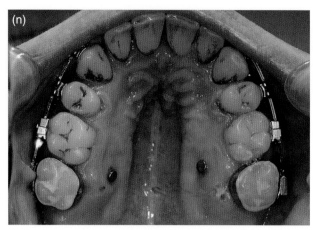

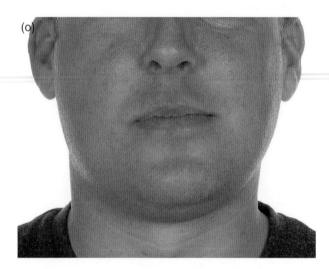

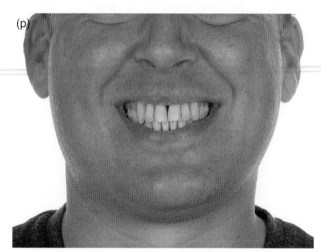

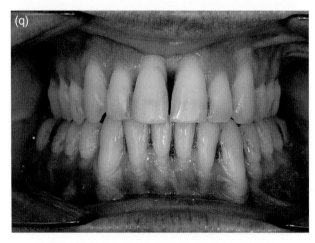

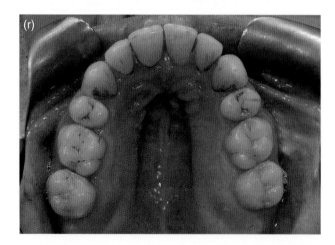

Figure 13.7 (Continued)

- Surgical corticotomies were performed, with the RME memory screw preactivated. This resulted in opening of the midpalate suture and a diastema within three weeks (Figure 13.7h–j).
- The archforms were then co-ordinated using full fixed appliances (following insertion of single archwires in the maxillary arch), ready for the mandibular surgery (Figure 13.7l–n). The hybrid expander was removed at this stage, after a nine-month passive period.
- Reasonable symmetry and occlusion were achieved following the osteotomy (Figure 13.7o–r).

13.8.3 Biomechanical Principles for Hybrid RME Appliances

- Midpalate insertion sites provide good cortical bone anchorage, but may not be accessible in patients with high-arched palates.
- Palatal alveolar insertion sites are accessible but unerupted posterior teeth may limit the use of these sites in younger patients, and the forces may not be transferred effectively to the circummaxillary sutures.
- Any conflict between the path of insertion of the molar bands and mini-implant connections needs to be minimised. This may be simplified, in the case of palatal alveolar mini-implants, by the use of wire mesh 'rests' rather than tight-fitting abutment caps. The mesh and mini-implant are then joined by composite resin (Figure 13.7f).

13.8.4 Clinical Steps for Hybrid RME

13.8.4.1 Preinsertion

1) For palatal alveolar sites, either select interproximal sites with sufficient space or diverge the roots of teeth adjacent to the planned insertion sites. This is achieved prior to expansion by bonding fixed appliance brackets with altered degrees of tip.
2) Take a dental impression or scan and fabricate both the RME appliance and the mini-implant stents together, or plan to insert the mini-implants prior to fabrication of the appliance.

13.8.4.2 Mini-implant Selection

3) 6 mm length, 2 mm diameter mini-implants are ideal for midpalate sites. 9 mm length, 1.5 mm diameter (long neck) sizes are more suitable for palatal alveolar sites.

13.8.4.3 Insertion

4) Insert 2–4 mini-implants. For palatal alveolar sites in adult patients, these are typically in mesial and distal positions relative to the upper first molars. Midpalatal

sites are at least 2–3 mm lateral to the midpalatal suture.

5) Seat the RME appliance onto the molar teeth and over the bilateral mini-implants. Then secure to the mini-implants according to the metal loop or cap design.
6) Expand the hyrax screw by at least 1 mm or until a midline diastema opens.

13.9 Non-tooth Borne Mini-Implant Only RME

Perhaps the most attractive design options centre on appliances which are independent of the teeth, although there is still the consideration of root proximity of palatal alveolar mini-implants. Non-tooth borne RME aims to deliver the expansion forces directly to the palatal skeletal complex and surrounding tissues, without eliciting dental side-effects. In particular, this avoidance of dental anchorage eliminates the side-effect of buccal crown tipping which is still observed with tooth-bone hybrid RME but not with mini-implant only RME designs [19,24,33]. Indeed, not only is the classic side-effect of buccal crown tipping of the anchor teeth avoided with these appliances, but palatal crown tipping may occur instead [19,24,33].

From a practical perspective, the exclusion of teeth from the appliance also allows orthodontic tooth movements to be undertaken independent of the expander, especially during a prolonged retention period of up to nine months. Such non-tooth borne RME appliances may be anchored solely on mini-implants (Figures 13.8, 13.9) or on a combination of mini-implants and a surrounding plastic Haas-type baseplate/flange (Figure 13.10). This typically requires four mini-implants rather than the customary two utilised in the simplest hybrid RME appliances. However, if the maxillary buccal teeth are unconnected then they may tip palatally during the expansion process. This may be most evident if occlusal locking with the lower buccal teeth prevents free movement of the upper molars. Therefore, Canan and Senısık [33] suggested the use of bite blocks to disengage the occlusion [33]. A simple alternative would be to fit a lower removable appliance with flat posterior biteplanes to free the buccal occlusion. It is also possible to stabilise the maxillary buccal teeth with either a modified fixed appliance or palatal arms extended from the appliance to the palatal aspect of the molar and premolar teeth.

13.9.1 Case Examples

1) **Mini-implant (only) borne RME (Figure 13.8)**

- A 22-year-old female presented with a Class I malocclusion and left-sided cross-bites (Figure 13.8a–d). There appeared to be a combination of mandibular (skeletal) asymmetry and functional displacement to the left side. The maxillary arch and palate were very narrow and the upper first premolars were absent. Maxillary expansion was required to correct the functional displacement and camouflage the underlying mandibular asymmetry.

- Bone-borne expansion was preferred given the extent of expansion required. However, the midpalate area was not accessible for midpalate mini-implant insertions so four mini-implants were inserted in palatal alveolar sites. A combination of SARME and a bone-borne expander was selected.
- The maxillary dentition was first aligned, in separate halves (Figure 13.8e,f). A dental impression was taken for fabrication of mini-implant guidance stents and the hybrid RME. This would incorporate abut-

ment caps on top of the mini-implant heads, secured with composite resin (Figure 13.8g).
- Surgical corticotomies were performed, with the RME memory screw preactivated. This resulted in an instant opening of the midpalate suture and a diastema (Figure 13.8g).
- Expansion continued by activation of the NiTi leaf springs until a sufficient diastema had opened (Figure 13.8i–k). The hybrid expander was removed after a nine-month retention period (Figure 13.8l,m).
- Good levels of maxillary expansion and arch co-ordination were achieved, accepting a minor residual shift of the lower centreline (towards the left side) due to the mandibular asymmetry (Figure 13.8n–q).

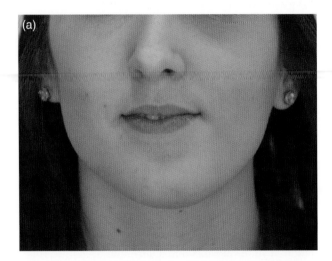
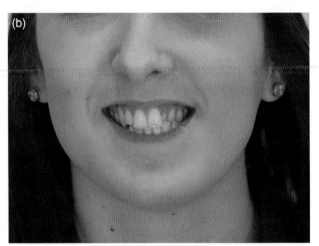
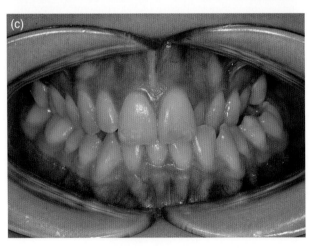
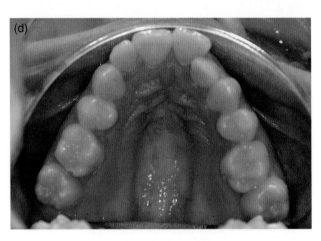

Figure 13.8 (a–d) Pretreatment photographs illustrating the Class I malocclusion and mandibular asymmetry (with the chin displaced to the left side) in this adult patient. (e,f) Treatment photographs, immediately prior to the maxillary corticotomy surgery, showing initial alignment of the maxillary dentition, in two separate halves. (g) Photograph taken during surgery, when the bone-borne RME has been fitted onto four mini-implants (in the palatal alveolus). The RME screw has just been released, resulting in the initial opening of a small diastema. (h,i) Intraoral radiographs showing the upper incisor area prior to expansion and after opening of the midpalatal suture. (j,k) Photographs taken after three weeks of expansion showing the widened screw of the hybrid RME and a midline diastema. (l,m) Photographs taken after nine months of retention, at which time the RME and mini-implants have been removed. (n–q) Debond photographs showing the Class I occlusion, with a small residual displacement of the lower centreline to the left side.

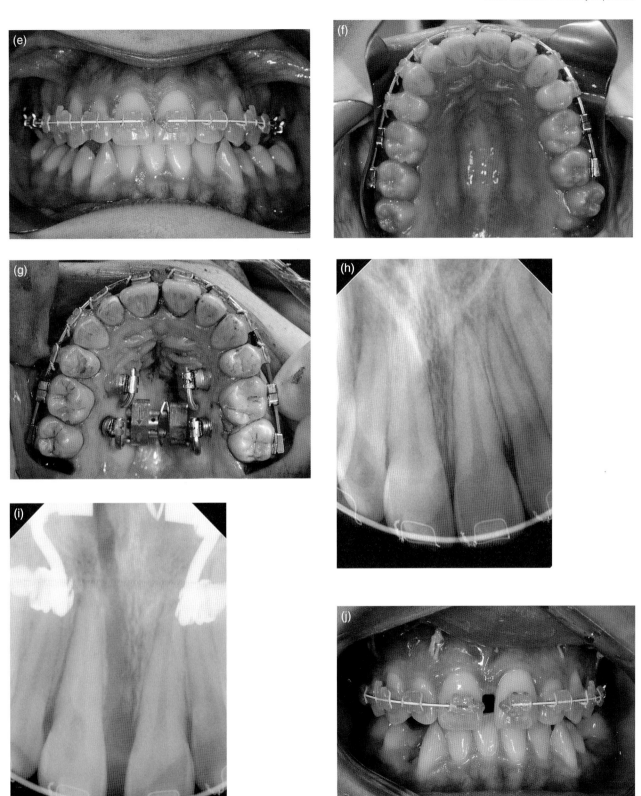

Figure 13.8 (Continued)

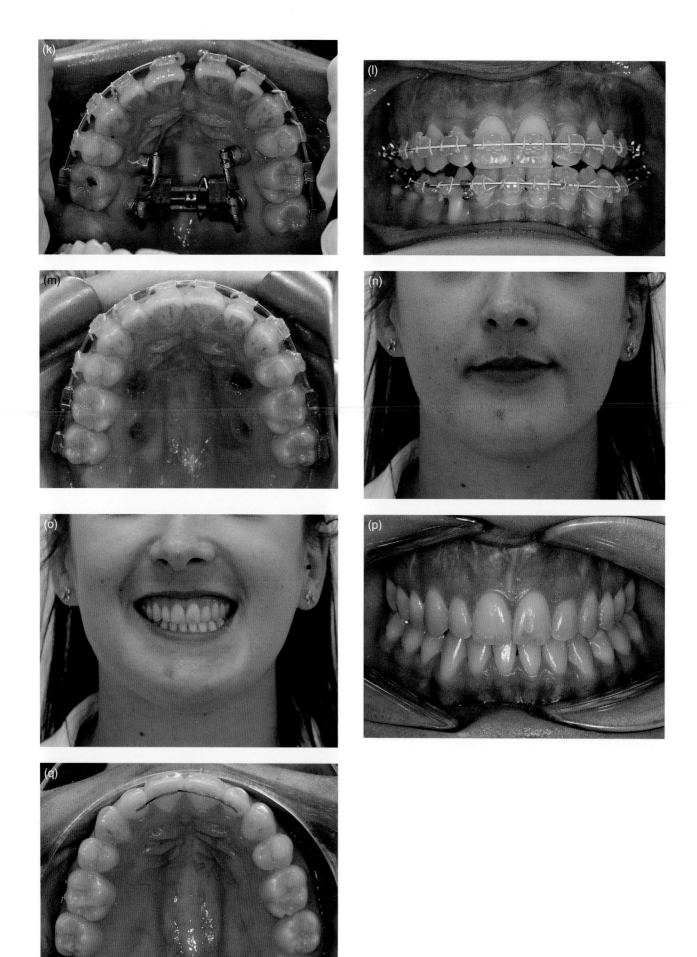

Figure 13.8 (Continued)

2) **Mini-implant (only) borne RME (Figure 13.9)**

- A 26-year-old male presented with a Class I malocclusion and anterior openbite (Figure 13.9a–d). There was an intact permanent dentition, but the maxillary arch was narrow and there was early generalised gingival recession. Maxillary expansion was required to co-ordinate the arches, especially after accounting for the risk of crossbites as the mandible rotated forwards during treatment.
- Non-surgical bone-borne expansion was preferred given the extent of expansion required. This utilised a combination of parasagittal and posterior palatal alveolar mini-implants (Figure 13.9e,f).
- A dental impression was taken for fabrication of mini-implant guidance stents and the RME appliance. The expander engaged the mini-implants via wire mesh rests on top of the posterior mini-implant heads and wire struts on the anterior mini-implants (Figure 13.9g).
- The midpalatal suture and interincisal space did not appear to open during the three weeks of this 'slow' expansion protocol (Figure 13.9g).
- Mucosal overgrowth occurred on the lateral aspect of the anterior palatal mini-implants after a further three weeks of expansion(Figure 13.9h,i). This meant that the RME had to be removed after several months and a quadhelix appliance used as partial retention (Figure 13.9j,k).
- Good levels of maxillary expansion and arch co-ordination were achieved, especially after allowing for the effects of anterior mandibular autorotation due to molar intrusion (Figure 13.9l–o).

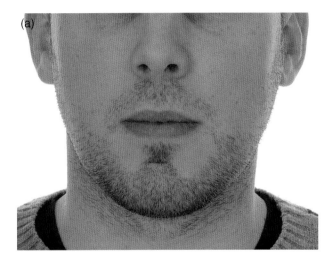

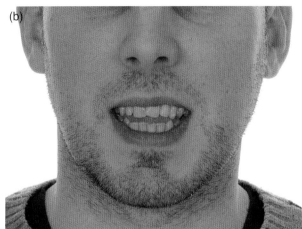

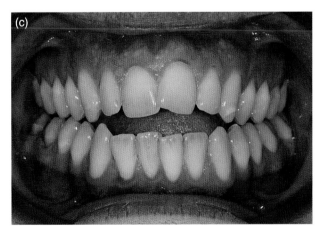

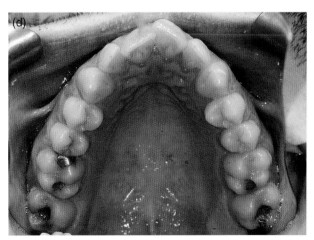

Figure 13.9 (a–d) Pretreatment photographs illustrating the Class II division 1 malocclusion and anterior openbite in this adult male. (e,f) Treatment photographs showing initial two parasagittal and two palatal alveolar mini-implants. The RME fitted onto these mini-implants, using composite resin to secure the mesh seats to the mini-implant heads. (g) Photograph showing the bone-borne RME appliance after the first two weeks of non-surgical expansion. The midpalatal suture remains closed. (h,i) Photographs taken after another two weeks of expansion showing the widened screw of the RME appliance, but no midline diastema. The right anterior mini-implant has become submerged in palatal mucosa. (j,k) Photographs taken after replacement of the RME appliance with a (tooth-borne) quadhelix. (l–o) Debond photographs, showing the expanded maxillary arch, and the corrected malocclusion and anterior openbite features.

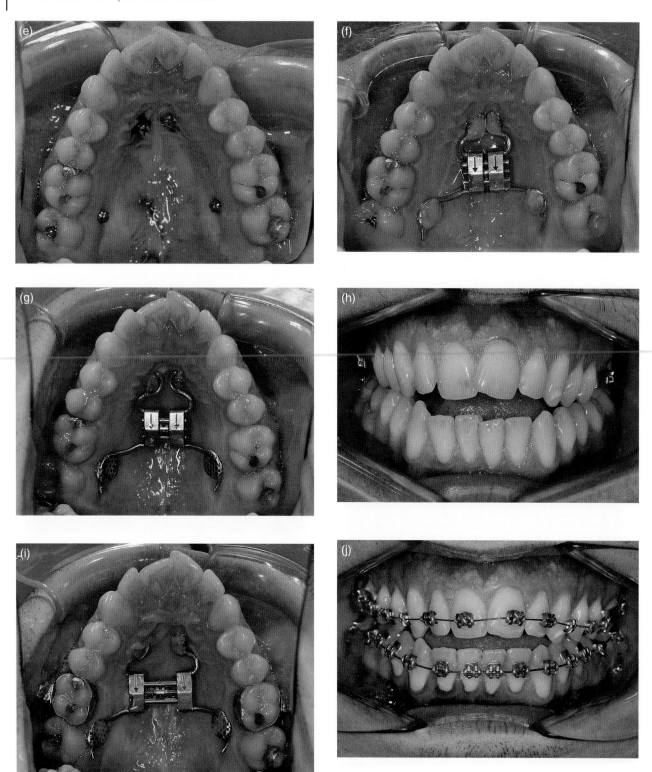

Figure 13.9 (Continued)

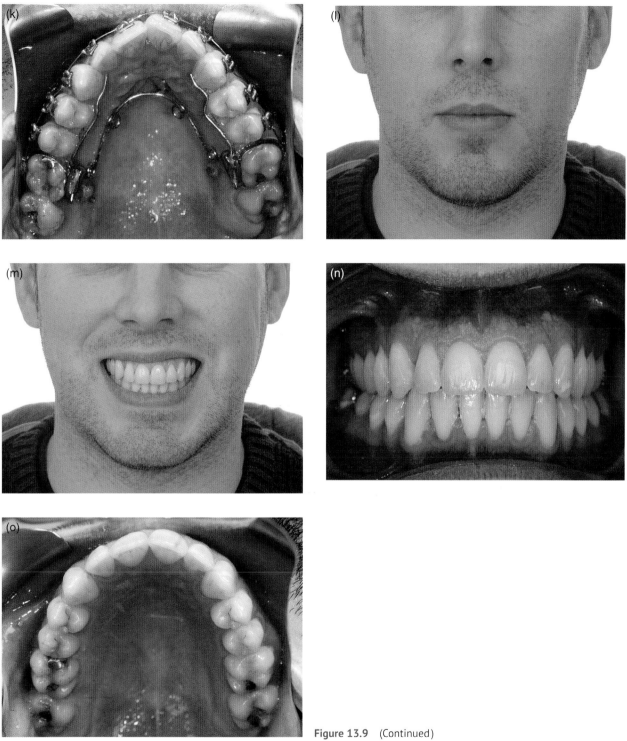

Figure 13.9 (Continued)

13.10   Biomechanical Principles

- Any conflict between the paths of insertion of the mini-implant connections needs to be minimised. One option is for the expander to be fabricated with the hyrax screw slightly opened and the screw is closed to facilitate placement of the expander onto the mini-implants.
- Midpalate insertion sites provide good cortical bone anchorage, but may not be accessible in patients with high-arched palates.
- Palatal alveolar insertion sites are accessible but unerupted posterior teeth may limit the use of these sites in younger patients.

13.10.1   Clinical Steps for OMI-borne RME

13.10.1.1   Preinsertion

1) For palatal alveolar sites, either select interproximal sites with sufficient space or diverge the roots of teeth adjacent to the planned insertion sites. This is achieved prior to expansion by bonding fixed appliance brackets with altered degrees of tip.
2) Take a dental impression or scan and fabricate both the RME appliance and the mini-implant stents together, or plan to insert the mini-implants prior to fabrication of the appliance.
3) Align mini-implants on each side as parallel as possible to one another, so that the path of appliance insertion is as simple as possible.
4) Ask the technician to fabricate the RME appliance with the hyrax screw preopened by 1 mm on the laboratory model. This will allow the screw to then be 'closed' in order to make it easier to fit over the mini-implants (and then expanded to fully seat it).

13.10.1.2   Mini-implant Selection

5) 6 mm length, 2 mm diameter mini-implants are ideal for midpalate sites. 9 mm length, 1.5 mm diameter (long neck) sizes are more suitable for palatal alveolar sites.

13.10.1.3   Insertion

6) Insert four mini-implants. For palatal alveolar sites, these are typically in mesial and distal positions relative to the upper first molars (in adult patients). Midpalatal sites are at least 2–3 mm lateral to the midpalatal suture.
7) Seat the RME appliance over the bilateral mini-implants and then secure according to the metal loop or cap design.
8) Expand the hyrax screw by at least 1 mm or until a midline diastema opens.

13.11   Haas-type (Mucosa) and Mini-implant RME

There appear to be differences in the effects of non-tooth borne expanders according to whether a Haas baseplate is involved. FEA research has suggested that the incorporation of acrylic baseplates produces truly horizontal expansion movements compared to hybrid and midpalate anchored mini-implant expanders [34]. The authors also suggested that the inclusion of Haas-type baseplates reduced the initial stress concentration (in the bone) around mini-implants and hence may enhance mini-implant stability, especially in young patients (with relatively less alveolar cortical support). It is therefore conceivable that palatal alveolar mini-implants have a clinically similar rate of stability to isolated midpalatal ones (despite the latter's insertion in thicker and denser palatal cortex) in RME cases. Similarly, another FEA study comparing tooth, hybrid (MARPE) and Haas-type OMI expanders demonstrated that the expansion force is concentrated in the immediate peri-implant bone around any directly loaded mini-implant [25]. Whilst the MARPE appliance's maximum stress level also occurred around the mini-implants, this was at a much lower level than in the Haas-type OMI expanders. Consequently, the theoretical advantage of bone-only supported RME is not upheld, although arguably this may not apply equally when low levels of force are applied, possibly via a 'memory' expansion screw.

The FEA findings reported by Lee et al. [34] have since been supported by a retrospective clinical study comparing a mini-implant supported Haas-type RME appliance with conventional tooth-borne appliances in patients with a mean age of 13 years [23]. It was shown that the combination of skeletal and soft tissue anchorage resulted in greater basal expansion, stable vertical parameters and an increase in the sella-nasion angle (SNA). At the same time, there was a small amount (3°) of indirect palatal (inwards) tipping of the upper first molars and modest (e.g. 1 mm) indirect expansion of the lower intermolar width. Hence, the authors recommended the use of this appliance in patients with increased vertical facial proportions, and that corticotomies may be required in adult patients.

The clinical effects of tissue mini-implant borne RME in young adult subjects have also been reported. Lin et al. [24] undertook a retrospective study of 28 postpubertal females (with a mean age of 18 years) in which a pretreatment CBCT scan showed almost or complete closure of the midpalatal suture. This study demonstrated twice as much skeletal expansion in the hybrid OMI group than with conventional RME (58% skeletal and 77.0% crown-level expansion relative to the screw opening in the mini-implant group, compared with 26% and 43% in the tooth-borne group). In addition, the midpalatal separation was greater posteriorly (more parallel) in the Haas mini-implant subjects, compared to the conventional V-shaped opening of the suture (wider anteriorly than posteriorly). Finally, as expected, there were fewer side-effects in this bone-anchored group – less buccal tilting of the dentoalveolar complex and less buccal alveolar bone loss.

13.11.1 Clinical Steps for Mucosa-OMI Borne RME

13.11.1.1 Preinsertion

1) Either select interproximal sites with sufficient space or diverge the roots of teeth adjacent to the planned insertion sites. This is achieved prior to expansion by bonding fixed appliance brackets with altered degrees of tip.

2) Take a dental impression or scan and fabricate both the RME appliance and the mini-implant stents together, or plan to insert the mini-implants prior to fabrication of the appliance.

3) Align mini-implants on each side as parallel as possible to one another, so that the path of appliance insertion is as simple as possible.

4) Ask the technician to fabricate the RME appliance with the hyrax screw preopened by 1 mm on the laboratory model. This will allow the screw to then be 'closed' in order to make it easier to fit over the mini-implants (and then expanded to fully seat it).

5) Ensure that there is sufficient distance between the coronal edge of the baseplate and the adjacent palatal gingival margins (to avoid the risk of reduced blood flow to the gingival margins).

13.11.1.2 Mini-implant Selection

6) 9 mm length, 1.5 mm diameter (long neck) sizes are more suitable for palatal alveolar sites.

13.11.1.3 Insertion

7) Insert four mini-implants, typically in mesial and distal positions relative to the upper first molars (in adult patients). However, a single mini-implant per side may be reasonable in adolescent patients where the sutural resistance is relatively low.

8) Add chlorhexidine gel either directly around the mini-implants or onto the fitting surface of acrylic baseplates around the mini-implant sites.

9) Seat the Haas baseplates over the bilateral mini-implants and then secure with cold-cure acrylic or composite resin.

10) Expand the hyrax screw by at least 1 mm or until light blanching of the adjacent mucosal margins occurs.

13.11.2 Case Example

1) **Haas and mini-implant hybrid RME (Figure 13.10)**
   - A 28–year–old male presented with a Class I malocclusion and anterior openbite (Figure 13.9a–d). There was an intact permanent dentition, but the maxillary arch was narrow and there was early generalised gingival recession. Maxillary expansion was required to co-ordinate the arches, especially after accounting for the risk of cross-bites as the mandible rotated forwards during treatment.
   - Non-surgical bone-borne expansion was preferred given the extent of expansion required. This utilised a combination of palatal alveolar mini-implants and Haas-type acrylic baseplates.
   - A dental impression was taken for fabrication of mini-implant guidance stents (Figure 13.10e) and the RME appliance (Figure 13.10f). The expander engaged the mini-implants via holes in the acrylic bases (Figure 13.10f–h). The gap between mini-implant and baseplate was sealed with composite resin.
   - The midpalatal suture and interincisal space did not appear to open during the three weeks of this 'slow' expansion protocol (Figure 13.10i,j).
   - The expander appliance was used following the expansion phase for molar intrusion, particularly involving elastomeric traction from distal hooks (embedded in the acrylic bases) and second molar palatal buttons (Figure 13.10k,l).
   - Good levels of maxillary expansion and arch co-ordination were achieved, especially after allowing for the effects of anterior mandibular autorotation due to molar intrusion (Figure 13.10m–p).

13.12 Summary of RME Design Selection

So how do we translate these FEA and clinical research studies into a practical range of solutions applicable to patients of varying ages? It's clear that there are differences between designs in terms of their practical application and clinical outcomes. These practical differences are summarised in Table 13.1, whilst the combined influences of age and RME design are highlighted in Figure 13.11. In effect, the older the patient, the greater their level of circummaxillary and palatal suture inertia and skeletal resistance to expansion, and hence the more beneficial it will be to involve mini-implant anchorage. Or, in other words, skeletal anchorage reduces the negative effects of increasing age and somatic maturity on RME effectiveness, and results in a greater proportion of skeletal change

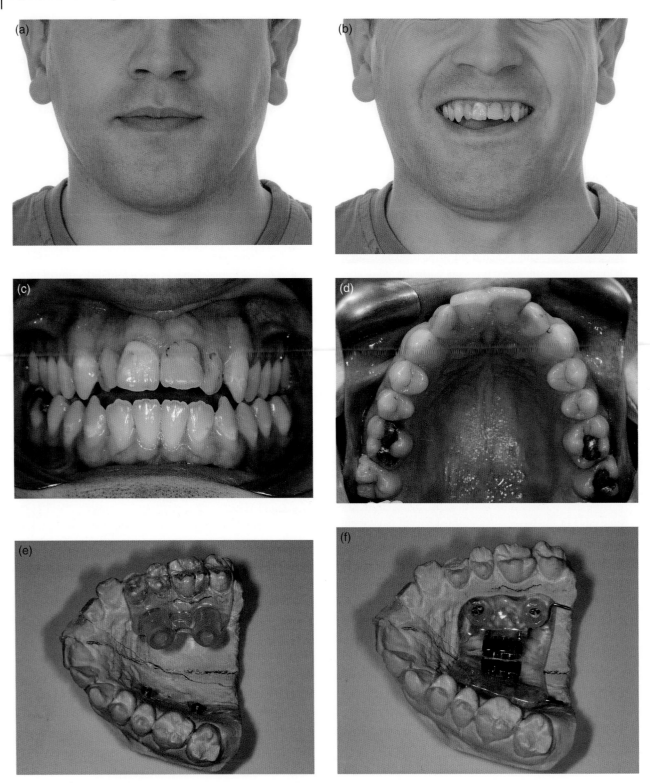

Figure 13.10 (a–d) Pretreatment photographs illustrating the Class II division 1 malocclusion and anterior openbite in this adult male. (e,f) Photographs of the mini-implant (palatal alveolar) stent and then Haas-type hybrid RME preparation on a working model of the maxillary dentition and palate. (g) Photograph showing three palatal alveolar mini-implants *in situ*. The right anterior mini-implant was not inserted due to limited interproximal space. (h) The Haas-type mini-implant RME appliance has been fitted, ready for composite resin infill of the acrylic baseplate holes. (i,j) Photographs taken after three weeks of non-surgical expansion. The midpalatal suture remains closed. (k,l) Photographs showing the molar intrusion phase, with the RME appliance *in situ* during its retention phase. Elastomeric traction has been applied, from hooks on the distal aspect of the acrylic baseplates to buttons on the second molars. (m–p) Debond photographs, showing the expanded maxillary arch, and the corrected malocclusion and anterior openbite features.

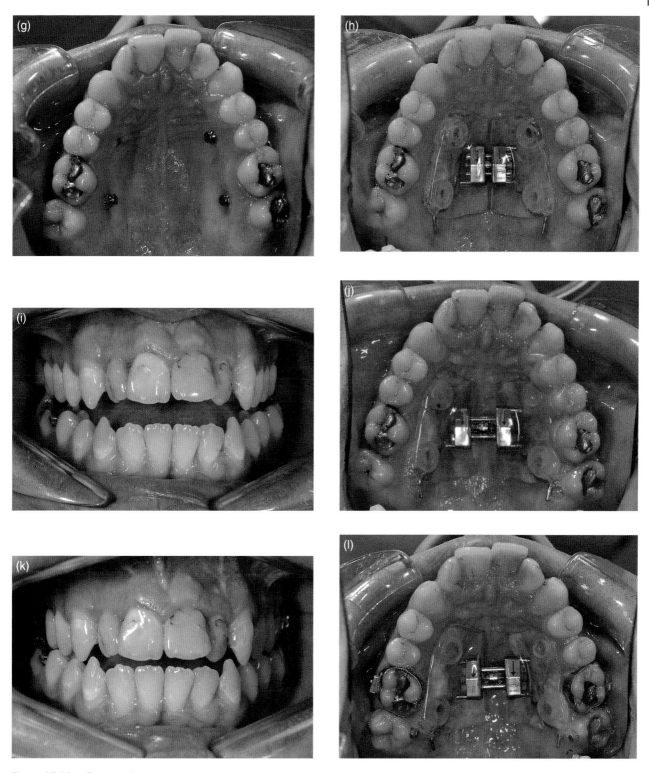

Figure 13.10 (Continued)

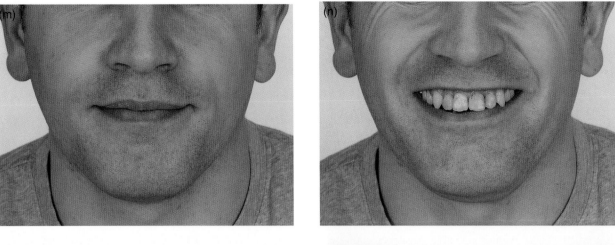

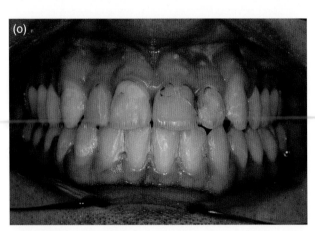
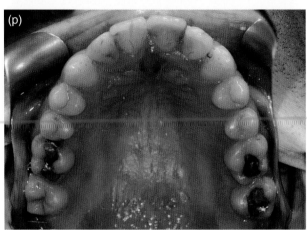

Figure 13.10 (Continued)

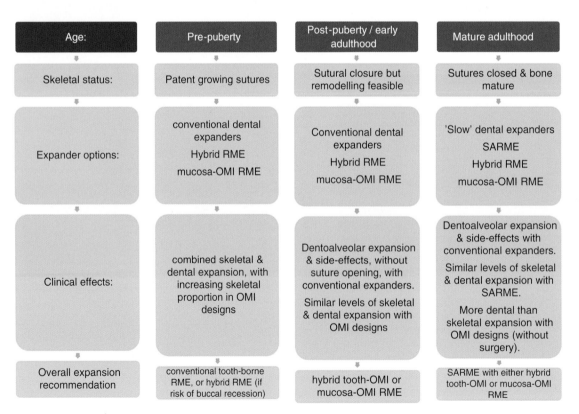

Age:	Pre-puberty	Post-puberty / early adulthood	Mature adulthood
Skeletal status:	Patent growing sutures	Sutural closure but remodelling feasible	Sutures closed & bone mature
Expander options:	conventional dental expanders Hybrid RME mucosa-OMI RME	Conventional dental expanders Hybrid RME mucosa-OMI RME	'Slow' dental expanders SARME Hybrid RME mucosa-OMI RME
Clinical effects:	combined skeletal & dental expansion, with increasing skeletal proportion in OMI designs	Dentoalveolar expansion & side-effects, without suture opening, with conventional expanders. Similar levels of skeletal & dental expansion with OMI designs	Dentoalveolar expansion & side-effects with conventional expanders. Similar levels of skeletal & dental expansion with SARME. More dental than skeletal expansion with OMI designs (without surgery).
Overall expansion recommendation	conventional tooth-borne RME, or hybrid RME (if risk of buccal recession)	hybrid tooth-OMI or mucosa-OMI RME	SARME with either hybrid tooth-OMI or mucosa-OMI RME

Figure 13.11 Flowchart summarising the relationship between patient age, skeletal maturity, RME design options and clinical effects.

being achieved. Therefore, whilst a hybrid hyrax (tooth and anterior mini-implant borne) RME appliance may be appropriate in a preadolescent patient, it will be much more prone to dental side-effects in postpubertal patients. Furthermore, tooth support should be avoided in patients with thin gingival biotypes and/or narrow alveolar ridges where periodontal losses may occur, either immediately or as a delayed response to arch expansion.

Consequently, the choice of expander design often depends on the patient age, and especially on their palate width, depth and shape. At the time of writing this edition, in 2019, the MSE type of expander, using posterior midpalate sites, may offer the most effective (basal) skeletal expansion in adults. However, this approach is not feasible in patients with narrow high-arched palates. In these cases, the combined mucosa and mini-implant borne appliance offers the best balance of simplicity of fabrication and fitting, plus the minimisation of dental movements and side-effects.

Newer types of 'memory' hyrax expansion screws may work well with mini-implant anchorage since they deliver relatively lower and more continuous force levels than traditional hyrax screws, without the conceptual need for high forces to negate tooth movements. However, in my experience, they are not powerful enough to separate the sutures in adult patients. Therefore, I would only recommend their use in very young patients or adults having surgical expansion. In the latter, the sutural resistance has already been overcome and the reduced patient compliance required for memory screw designs is helpful in the postoperative period.

References

1 Zhou, Y., Long, H., Ye, N. et al. (2014). The effectiveness of non-surgical maxillary expansion: a meta-analysis. *Eur. J. Orthod.* 36: 233–242.

2 Lo Giudice, A., Barbato, E., Cosentino, L. et al. (2018). Alveolar bone changes after rapid maxillary expansion with tooth-born appliances: a systematic review. *Eur. J. Orthod.* 40: 296–303.

3 Rinaldi, M.R.L., Azeredo, F., de Lima, E.M. et al. (2018). Cone-beam computed tomography evaluation of bone plate and root length after maxillary expansion using tooth-borne and tooth-tissue-borne banded expanders. *Am. J. Orthod. Dentofac. Orthop.* 154: 504–516.

4 Garib, D.G., Henriques, J.F., Janson, G. et al. (2006). Periodontal effects of rapid maxillary expansion with tooth-tissue-borne and tooth-borne expanders: a computed tomography evaluation. *Am. J. Orthod. Dentofac. Orthop.* 129: 749–758.

5 Lagravere, M.O., Major, P.W., and Flores-Mir, C. (2006). Dental and skeletal changes following surgically assisted rapid maxillary expansion. *J. Oral Maxillofac. Surg.* 35: 481–487.

6 Verquin, M., Daems, L., and Politis, C. (2017). Short-term complications after surgically assisted rapid palatal expansion: a retrospective cohort study. *Int. J. Oral Maxillofac. Surg* 46: 303–308.

7 Tonello, D.L., de Miranda Ladewig, V., Guedes, F.P. et al. (2017). Midpalatal suture maturation in 11- to 15-year-olds: a cone-beam computed tomographic study. *Am. J. Orthod. Dentofac. Orthop.* 152: 42–48.

8 De Miranda Ladewig, V., Capelozza-Filho, L., Almeida-Pedrin, R.R. et al. (2018). Tomographic evaluation of the maturation stage of the midpalatal suture in postadolescents. *Am. J. Orthod. Dentofac. Orthop.* 153: 818–824.

9 Mommaerts, M.Y. (1999). Transpalatal distraction as a method of maxillary expansion. *Br. J. Oral Maxillofac. Surg.* 37: 268–272.

10 Asscherickx, K., Govaerts, E., Aerts, J., and van de Vannet, B. (2016). Maxillary changes with bone-borne surgically assisted rapid palatal expansion: a prospective study. *Am. J. Orthod. Dentofac. Orthop.* 149: 374–383.

11 Pulver, R.J., Campbell, P.M., Opperman, L.A., and Buschang, P.H. (2016). Miniscrew-assisted slow expansion of mature rabbit sutures. *Am. J. Orthod. Dentofac. Orthop.* 150: 303–312.

12 Moon, W. (2018). Class III treatment by combining facemask (FM) and maxillary skeletal expander (MSE). *Semin. Orthod.* 24: 95–107.

13 Walter, A., Wendl, B., Ploder, O. et al. (2017). Stability determinants of bone-borne force-transmitting components in three RME hybrid expanders – an in vitro study. *Eur. J. Orthod.* 39: 76–84.

14 Halicioglu, K. and Yavuz, I. (2014). Comparison of the effects of rapid maxillary expansion caused by treatment with either a memory screw or a hyrax screw on the dentofacial structures – transversal effects. *Eur. J. Orthod.* 36: 140–149.

15 Lanteri, C., Beretta, M., Lanteri, V. et al. (2016). The leaf expander for non-compliance treatment in the mixed dentition. *J. Clin. Orthod.* 50: 552–560.

16 Matsuyama, Y., Motoyoshi, M., Tsurumachi, N., and Shimizu, N. (2015). Effects of palate depth, modified arm shape, and anchor screw on rapid maxillary expansion: a finite element analysis. *Eur. J. Orthod.* 37: 188–193.

17 Cantarella, D., Dominguez-Mompell, R., Mallya, S.M. et al. (2017). Changes in the midpalatal and pterygopalatine sutures induced by microimplant-supported skeletal expander analyzed with a novel 3D method based on CBCT imaging. *Prog. Orthod.* 18: 34.

18 Lione, R., Ballanti, F., Franchi, L. et al. (2008). Treatment and posttreatment skeletal effects of rapid maxillary expansion studied with low-dose computed tomography in growing subjects. *Am. J. Orthod. Dentofac. Orthop.* 134: 389–392.

19 Celenk-Koca, T., Erdinc, A.E., Hazara, S. et al. (2018). Evaluation of miniscrew-supported rapid maxillary expansion in adolescents: a prospective randomized clinical trial. *Angle Orthod.* 88: 702–709.

20 Lee, K., Park, Y., Park, J., and Hwang, W. (2010). Miniscrew-assisted nonsurgical palatal expansion before orthognathic surgery for a patient with severe mandibular prognathism. *Am. J. Orthod. Dentofac. Orthop.* 137: 830–839.

21 Lee, S.C., Park, J.H., Bayome, M. et al. (2014). Effect of bone-borne rapid maxillary expanders with and without surgical assistance on the craniofacial structures using finite element analysis. *Am. J. Orthod. Dentofac. Orthop.* 145: 638–648.

22 Bazargani, F., Magnuson, A., and Ludwig, B. (2018). Effects on nasal airflow and resistance using two different RME appliances: a randomized controlled trial. *Eur. J. Orthod.* 40: 281–284.

23 Yilmaz, A., Arman-Ozcirpici, A., Erken, S., and Polat-Ozsoy, O. (2015). Comparison of short-term effects of mini-implant-supported maxillary expansion appliance with two conventional expansion protocols. *Eur. J. Orthod.* 37: 556–564.

24 Lin, L., Ahn, H., Kim, S. et al. (2015). Tooth-borne vs bone-borne rapid maxillary expanders in late adolescence. *Angle Orthod.* 85: 253–262.

25 Seong, E., Choi, S., Kim, H. et al. (2018). Evaluation of the effects of miniscrew incorporation in palatal expanders for young adults using finite element analysis. *Korean J. Orthod.* 48: 81–89.

26 Choi, S., Shi, K., Cha, J. et al. (2016). Nonsurgical miniscrew-assisted rapid maxillary expansion results in acceptable stability in young adults. *Angle Orthod.* 86: 713–720.

27 Lim, H., Park, Y., Lee, K. et al. (2017). Stability of dental, alveolar, and skeletal changes after miniscrew-assisted rapid palatal expansion. *Korean J. Orthod.* 47: 313–322.

28 Park, J.J., Park, Y., Lee, K. et al. (2017). Skeletal and dentoalveolar changes after miniscrew assisted rapid palatal expansion in young adults: a cone-beam computed tomography study. *Korean J. Orthod.* 47: 77–86.

29 Lee, R.J., Moon, W., and Hong, C. (2017). Effects of monocortical and bicortical mini-implant anchorage on bone-borne palatal expansion using finite element analysis. *Am. J. Orthod. Dentofac. Orthop.* 151: 887–897.

30 Wilmes, B., Nienkemper, M., and Drescher, D. (2010). Application and effectiveness of a mini-implant and tooth-borne rapid palatal expansion device: the hybrid hyrax. *World J. Orthod.* 11: 323–330.

31 Toklu, M.G., Germec-Cakan, D., and Tozlu, M. (2015). Periodontal, dentoalveolar, and skeletal effects of tooth-borne and tooth-bone-borne expansion appliances. *Am. J. Orthod. Dentofac. Orthop.* 148: 97–109.

32 Mosleh, M.I., Kaddah, M.A., El Sayed, F.A.A., and El Sayed, H.S. (2015). Comparison of transverse changes during maxillary expansion with 4-point bone-borne and tooth-borne maxillary expanders. *Am. J. Orthod. Dentofac. Orthop.* 148: 599–607.

33 Canan, S. and Senısik, N.E. (2017). Comparison of the treatment effects of different rapid maxillary expansion devices on the maxilla and the mandible. Part 1: evaluation of dentoalveolar changes. *Am. J. Orthod. Dentofac. Orthop.* 151: 1125–1138.

34 Lee, H.K., Bayome, M., Ahn, C.S. et al. (2014). Stress distribution and displacement by different bone-borne palatal expanders with micro-implants: a three-dimensional finite-element analysis. *Eur. J. Orthod.* 36: 531–540.

14

Orthognathic Surgical Uses

Orthodontic mini-implants provide a variety of novel applications for adult patients undergoing orthognathic surgical correction of their dentoskeletal deformity. For instance, some patients have traditionally been viewed as unsuitable for orthognathic treatment because their dental status is inadequate, due to either insufficient teeth or periodontal support. A suboptimal dentition contraindicates conventional intraoperative intermaxillary fixation (IMF) and postoperative elastic traction, or even pre- and postsurgical fixed appliance phases. However, it has been feasible since at least 2005 to effectively manage such patients during the perioperative period using mini-implants, either as an alternative to fixed appliance surgical hooks, whereby heavy elastic traction is avoided on vulnerable teeth, or in lieu of an orthodontic (labial) appliance altogether [1]. In particular, the relatively small body diameters and head sizes of mini-implants (Figure 14.1a) mean that they pose less risk to dental roots and cause less trauma to the soft tissues, respectively, than conventional surgical IMF screws (Figure 14.1b) [1–4].

However, despite their smaller body dimensions, mini-implants still need to be inserted with guidance and precision. This has been demonstrated recently by a retrospective study of 50 orthognathic cases where there was considerable variation in the surgical mini-implant insertion angles and a very high proportion (41%) of these had some degree of root contact, even after allowing for the overestimating effect of this on panoramic radiographs [5]. Therefore, orthodontists should consider providing surgical colleagues with guidance stents for intraoperative mini-implant insertions, as described in Chapter 3.

Mini-implant anchorage also works very usefully in patients with a healthy dentition who do not need extensive presurgical tooth movements. These patients may now be treated using 'alternative' orthodontic treatment approaches/appliances, such as lingual fixed appliances, orthodontic aligners (rather than labial brackets) and 'surgery first' treatment. In these scenarios, it is possible for a patient to undergo surgery and even have postoperative traction without any labial orthodontic attachments. From the orthodontist's perspective, the use of mini-implants in 'surgery first' cases avoids the need to bond a potentially vulnerable fixed appliance and prepare passive archwires, immediately prior to surgery (which in my mind means that the surgery isn't truly first!). From the patient's perspective, the mini-implants are very discrete and there is no interference with hygiene around the dentition and gingival margins. The fixed appliances may then be bonded within weeks of surgery for efficient tooth alignment and settling of the occlusion whilst the dentition is in a 'fluid' state and there is still a regional acceleratory phenomenon (RAP) effect. This is consistent with the dramatically reduced treatment times of 'surgery first' treatment [6]. Therefore, the various pre- and postsurgical orthognathic treatment scenarios and phases suitable for the adjunctive use of mini-implants are described in this chapter, under the headings shown in Table 14.1.

> Mini-implants can be used either as an alternative to fixed appliance surgical hooks, whereby heavy elastic traction is avoided on vulnerable teeth, or in lieu of an orthodontic (labial) appliance altogether.

14.1 Clinical Objectives

The range of orthognathic treatment problems which may be overcome by the adjunctive use of mini-implants includes patients with the following.

- Large centreline discrepancies where mini-implant anchorage will enable full correction of the dental component, facilitating surgical correction of the skeletal asymmetry (Figure 14.2).
- Absence of the lower first or second molars such that the mandibular third molar should ideally be protracted and preserved, rather than sacrificed as part of a mandibular surgery plan (Figure 14.3).

The Orthodontic Mini-Implant Clinical Handbook, Second Edition. Richard Cousley.
© 2020 John Wiley & Sons Ltd. Published 2020 by John Wiley & Sons Ltd.

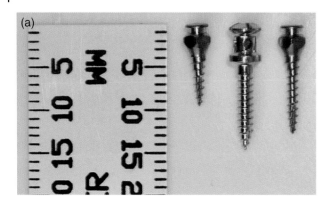
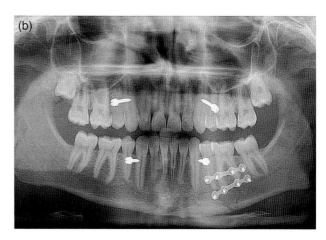

Figure 14.1 (a) Photograph of 6 mm (*left*) and 9 (*right*) mm length IMT mini-implant versions with an IMF screw in the centre. (b) Panoramic radiograph showing close root proximity and poor angulation of IMF screws in a mandibular trauma case.

Table 14.1 Different time points (stages) of the orthognathic treatment pathway when mini-implants may be used to supplement the treatment

Orthognathic stage	Mini-implant applications	Illustration
Preoperative orthodontics	Decompensation and centreline correction	Figure 14.2
	Molar protraction (from the potential osteotomy site)	Figure 14.3
	Occlusal cant correction (unilateral intrusion)	Figure 14.4
	Reduction of excess vertical face height/anterior openbite (bilateral molar intrusion)	Figure 14.5, 14.6
At surgery	Intermaxillary fixation for 'surgery first', compromised dentitions, aligner and lingual orthodontics	Figure 14.7, 14.8
Immediate postoperative traction	Traction for mandibular displacement/'callus moulding'	Figure 14.9
	Elimination of premature contacts by tooth intrusion	Figure 14.10
Surgical relapse 'rescue'	Elimination of premature contacts by tooth intrusion	
Postoperative orthodontics	Finishing dental movements, e.g. molar distalisation and final centreline correction	Figure 8.13

- Large arch spaces where there is a contradiction between incisor decompensation (involving proclination) and space closure (which classically retroclines the incisors). Molar protraction is then indicated.
- Facial asymmetry which is primarily transverse, but where presurgical levelling of an associated occlusal cant will optimise the transverse and anteroposterior surgical correction (Figure 14.4).
- Excessive face height and/or anterior openbite (AOB) where preoperative molar intrusion will convert their treatment from a bimaxillary surgical plan to a single jaw (mandible-only) osteotomy (Figure 14.5). Alternatively, it may make a differential surgical impaction movement more feasible in a large AOB case, by levelling the maxillary occlusal plane preoperatively and hence reducing the amount of posterior surgical movement required (Figure 14.6). This approach reduces surgical costs and

morbidity, especially in terms of unfavourable nasal changes. In my experience, this has been very successful and something that patients are keen to consider (and avoid maxillary surgery when feasible), especially if their primary concern is their occlusion rather than facial features.
- An insufficient number of teeth, teeth with vulnerable root lengths, or periodontal tissue support to tolerate intermaxillary forces.
- Teeth at risk of extrusion due to short roots (during the use of intermaxillary traction) (Figure 14.7).
- 'Surgery first' cases where a reasonable occlusion is feasible at surgery and fixed appliances may be avoided altogether or added postoperatively (Figure 14.8).
- Treatment with lingual or aligner orthodontic appliances, requiring a means of fixation on the labial side.
- An incomplete or unsatisfactory immediate or longer term surgical outcome, where further surgery is contraindicated

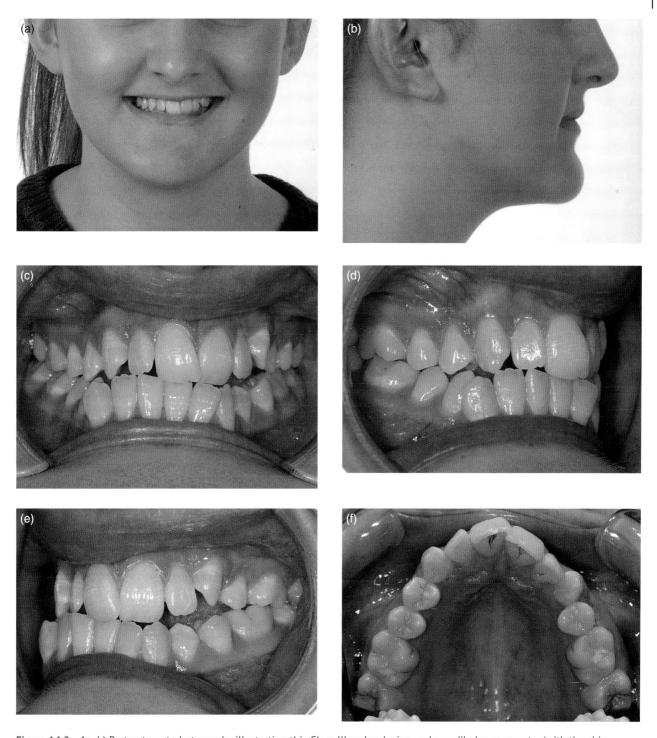

Figure 14.2 (a–h) Pretreatment photographs illustrating this Class III malocclusion and mandibular asymmetry (with the chin displaced to the right side). The upper left first premolar is absent and the upper centreline is significantly displaced to the left side whilst the lower centreline is to the right. (g,h) Pretreatment radiographs confirming absence of the upper left first premolar and the compensated skeletal III features. (i,j) Photographs showing upper and lower fixed appliances and a buccal mini-implant. There is elastomeric traction connecting it to a crimpable powerarm (mesial to the upper right canine bracket). (k–p) Preoperative photographs and lateral cephalogram showing the decompensated Class III malocclusion and corrected upper dental centreline. The maxillary cant is now more evident. (q,r) Immediate postoperative radiographs. (s–v) Debond photographs, showing the corrected dental and facial midlines, and Class I occlusion.

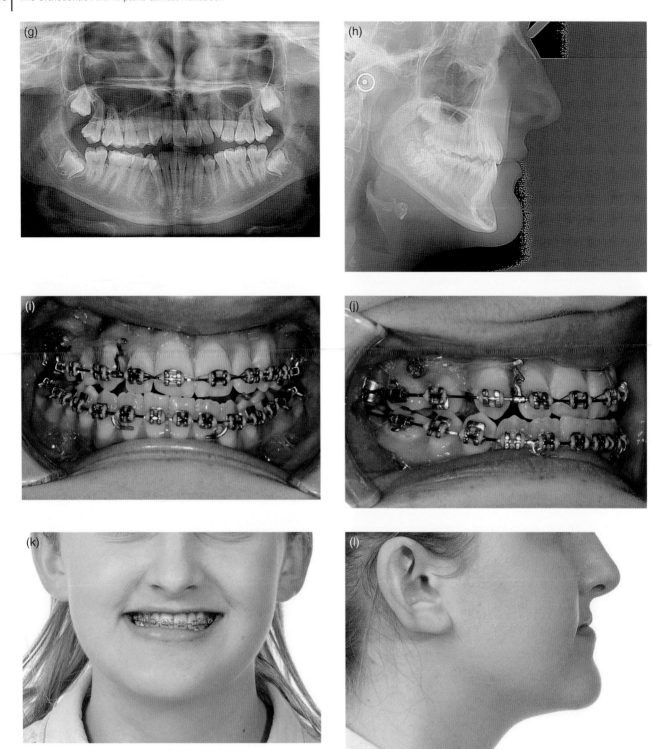

Figure 14.2 (Continued)

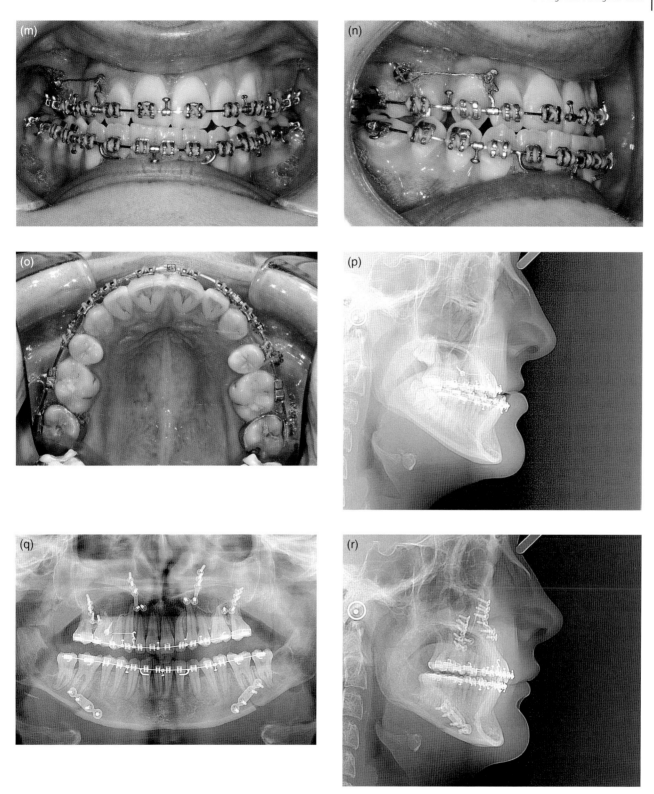

Figure 14.2 (Continued)

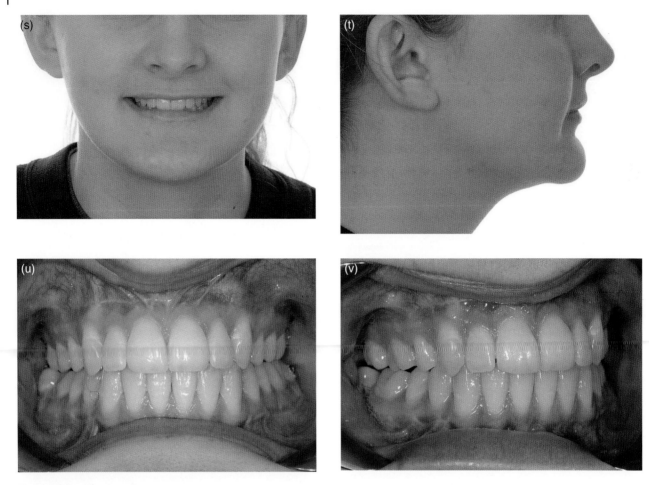

Figure 14.2 (Continued)

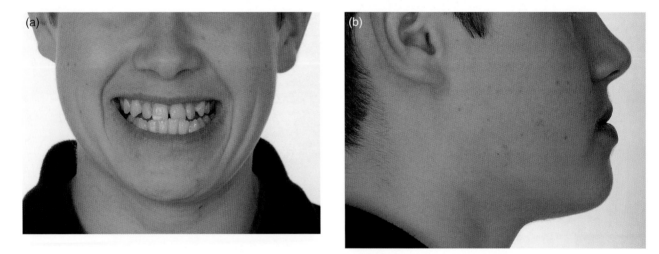

Figure 14.3 (a–e) Pretreatment photographs illustrating this compensated Class III malocclusion. There is severe upper arch crowding with displacement of both centrelines to the left side. The latter was associated with mandibular asymmetry. (f) This pretreatment panoramic radiograph confirms absence of the lower right first molar and the adjacent, immature, unerupted third molar. (g) This panoramic view was taken after 10 months of molar protraction into the edentulous lower right first molar space. The third molar had spontaneously moved mesially during this time. The mini-implant is seen between the lower right premolar roots. (k–p) Preoperative photographs and lateral cephalogram showing the decompensated Class III features and preservation of the lower centreline displacement to the left side. The lower right third molar was partially erupted, adjacent to the second molar. (q,r) Immediate postoperative radiographs. (s–w) Debond photographs, showing the corrected dental and facial midlines, and Class I occlusion. The partially erupted lower right third molar is also seen.

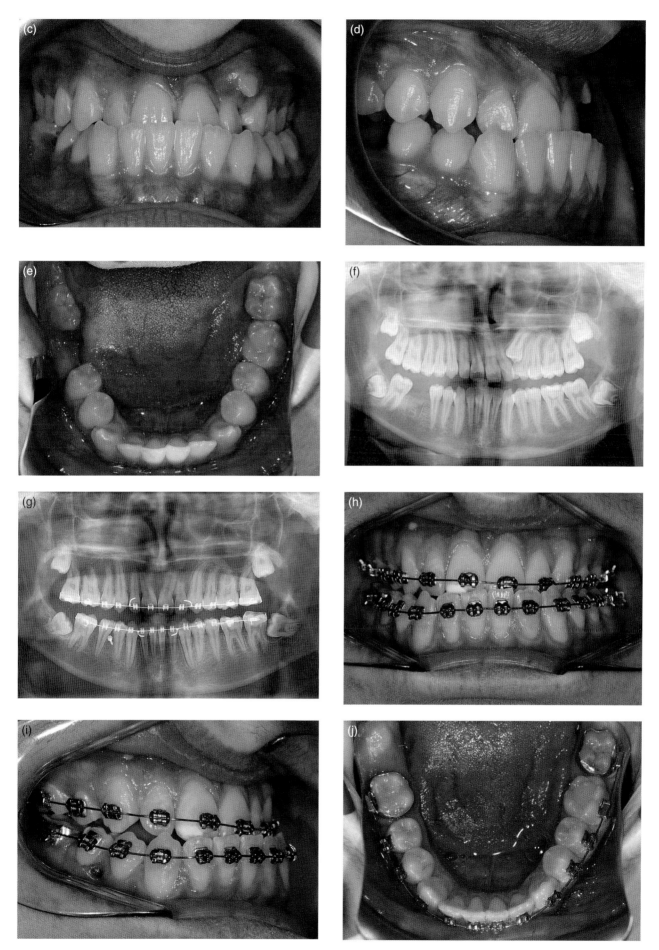

Figure 14.3 (Continued)

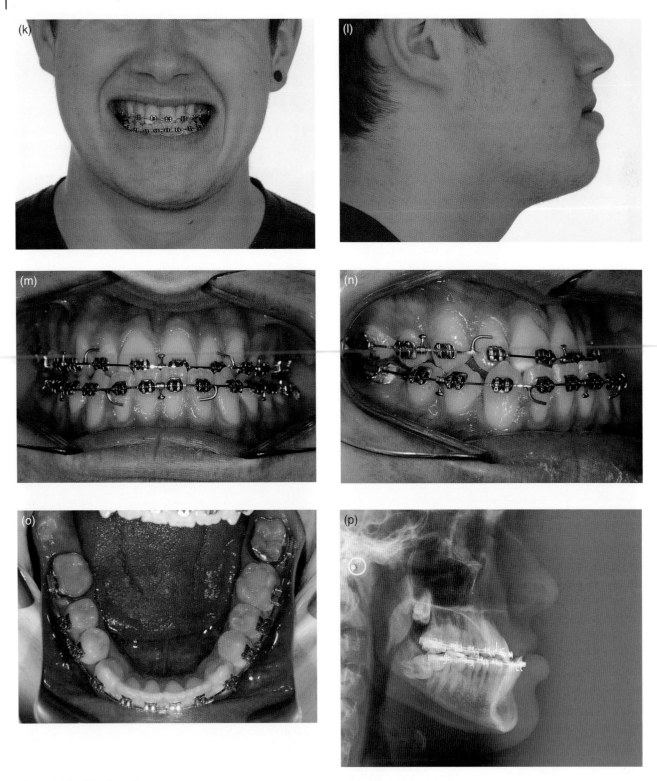

Figure 14.3 (Continued)

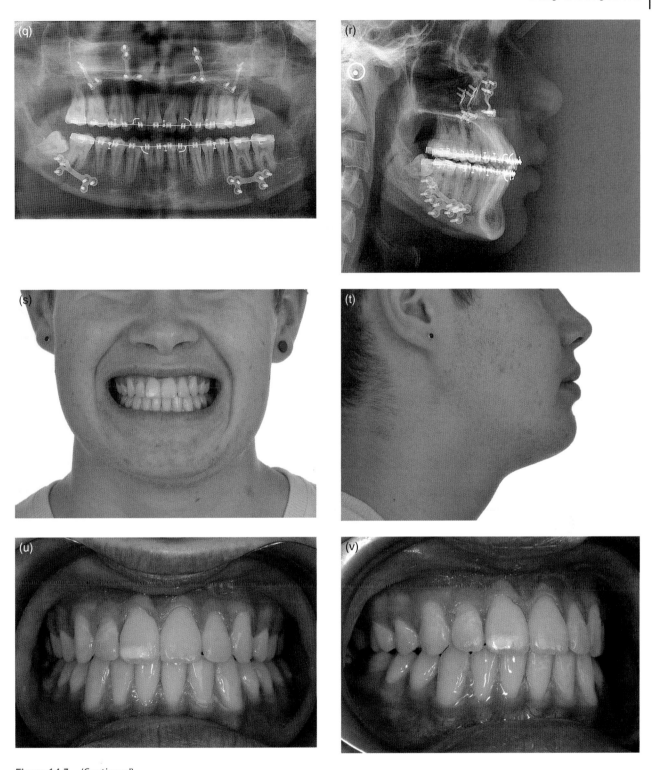

Figure 14.3 (Continued)

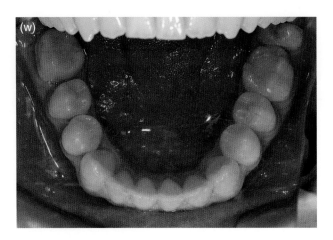

Figure 14.3 (Continued)

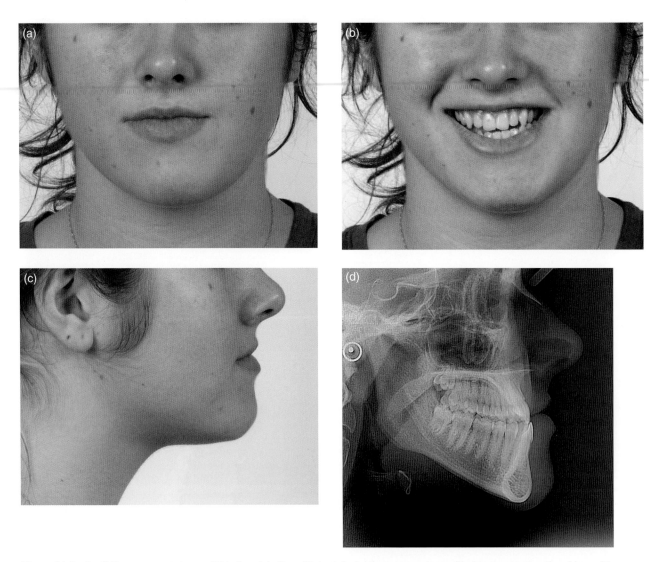

Figure 14.4 (a–f) Pretreatment views of this female's Class III dentofacial features and mandibular asymmetry; the chin and lower centreline are displaced to the left and the occlusal plane is higher on the left side. (g,h) A right lateral openbite beginning to develop with right maxillary intrusion, using a mini-implant sited buccal and mesial to the first molar. (i–n) A large lateral openbite has developed preoperatively, eliminating potential occlusal interferences when the mandible is surgically repositioned. (o–t) Postoperatively, the Class III and asymmetry problems have been corrected, and the mini-implant traction stopped. (u–w) Debond facial views and the occlusion (x,y) 18 months after debond.

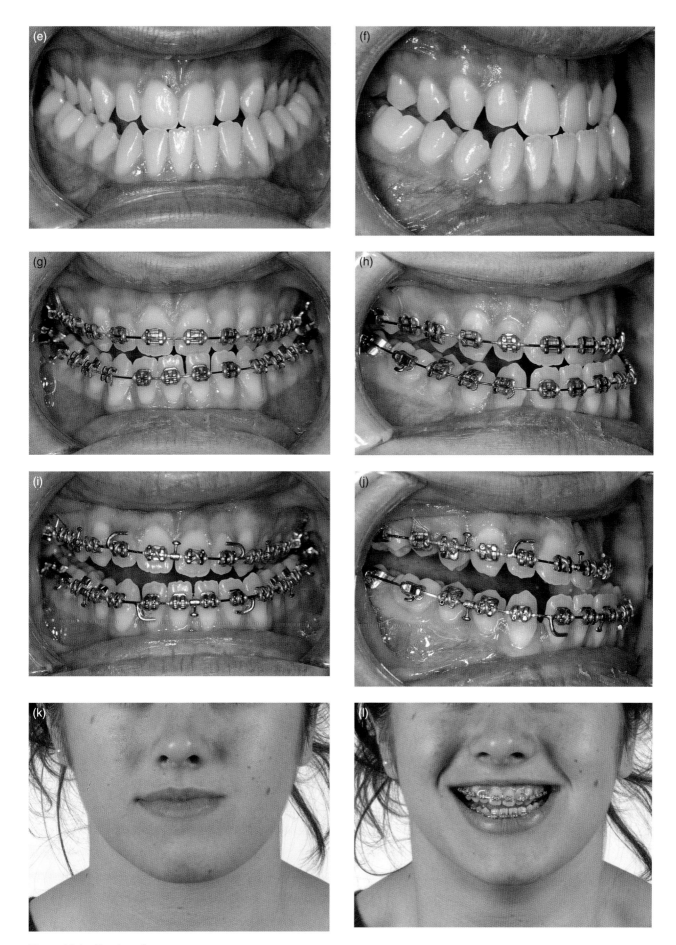

Figure 14.4 (Continued)

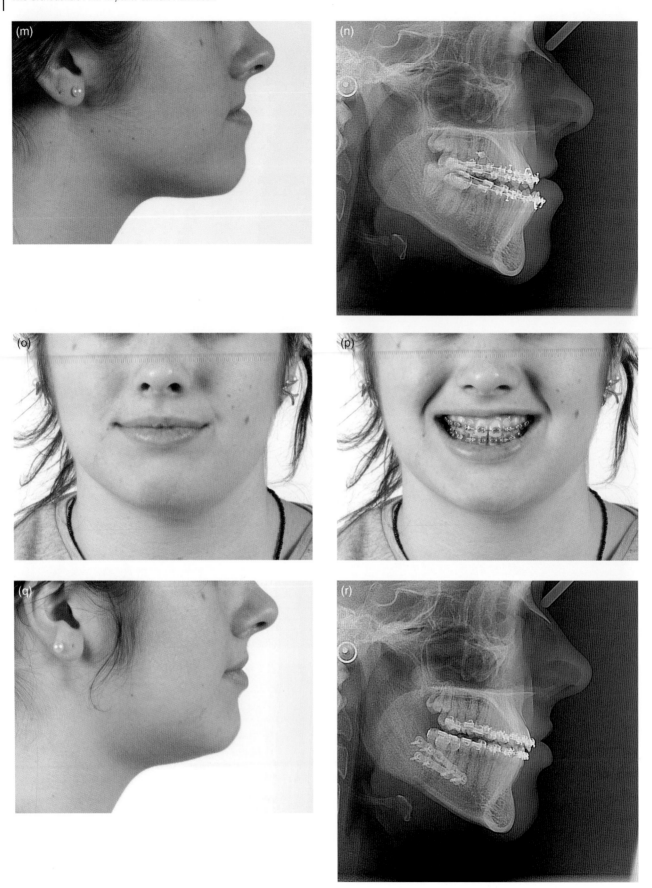

Figure 14.4 (Continued)

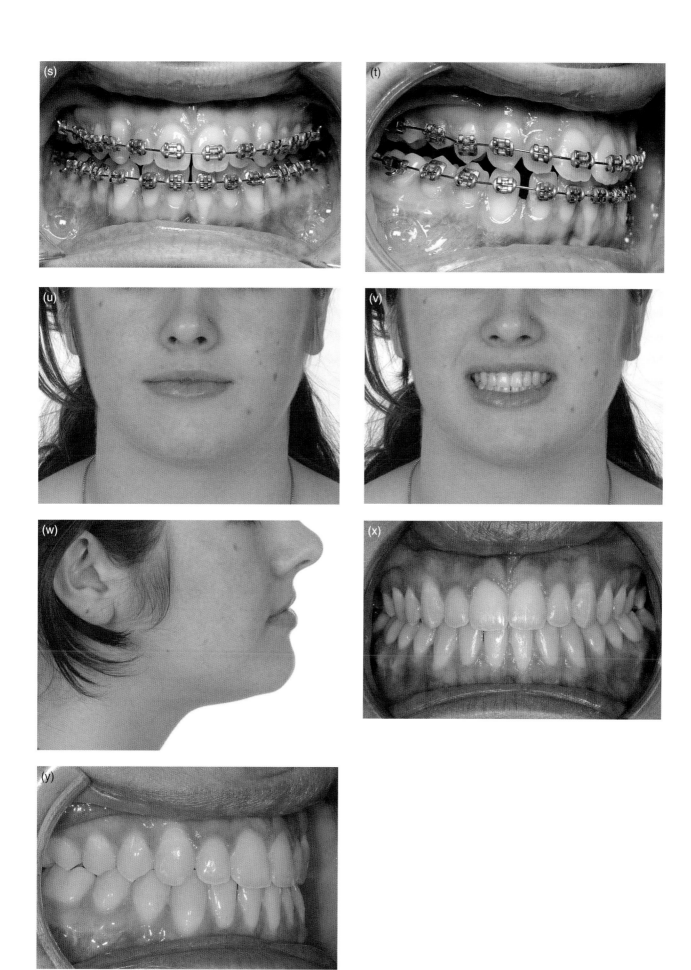

Figure 14.4 (Continued)

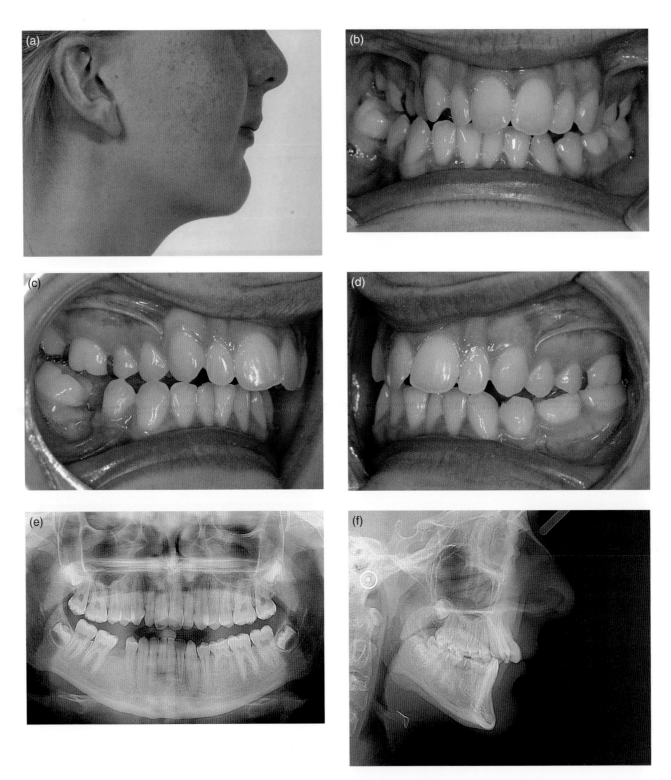

Figure 14.5 (a–d) Pretreatment photographs of this 16-year-old female, illustrating her Class II division 1 malocclusion and Class II facial profile. (e,f) Pretreatment radiographs confirm the increased mandibular plane angle, retroclined lower incisor feature, and absence of both lower second premolars absent. The retained lower left second deciduous molar has short root lengths. (g–l) Photographs and a lateral cephalogram taken at the start of the molar intrusion phase. Upper 0.019 × 0.025 and lower 0.018 in. steel archwires were *in situ*. Space was being created for alignment of both lower central incisors prior to their bonding and then banding of the lower second molars. Bilateral palatal mini-implants (1.5 mm diameter, 9 mm length) had just been inserted mesial to the upper second molars and elastomeric traction applied to the quadhelix arms and hence to the first molars. At the same time, elastomeric traction was applied across the mandibular second deciduous molar spaces. (m–q) Photographs and a lateral cephalogram taken at the preoperative planning stage, after 10 months of molar intrusion. A deep overbite has been created and the lower second deciduous molar spaces closed. (r) Cephalometric superimposition of the preintrusion and preoperative lateral cephalograms. This shows the reduction in lower face height and skeletal Class II associated with counter-clockwise mandibular rotation. It also shows some incisor retroclination, especially in the maxillary arch, accompanied by modest upper incisor extrusion. (s,t) Immediate postmandibular advancement radiographs. (u) Cephalometric superimposition of the pre- and immediate postoperative lateral cephalograms showing the mandibular advancement changes: a 6 mm advancement with a 4 mm increase in the lower anterior face height. (v–z) Photographs and a lateral cephalogram taken at debond, after a total of 26 months treatment. These show the full correction of her Class II malocclusion, AOB and hypodontia features.

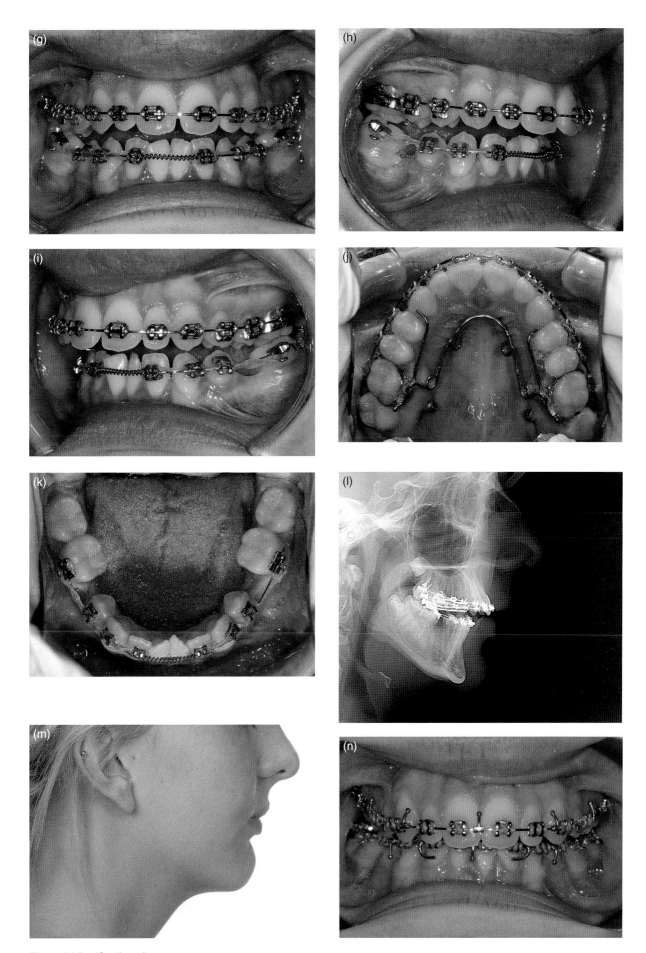

Figure 14.5 (Continued)

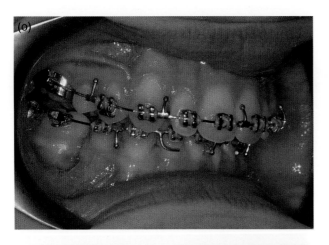

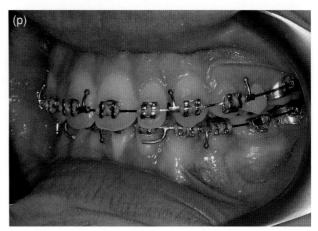

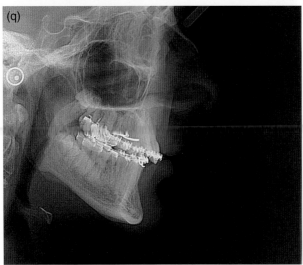

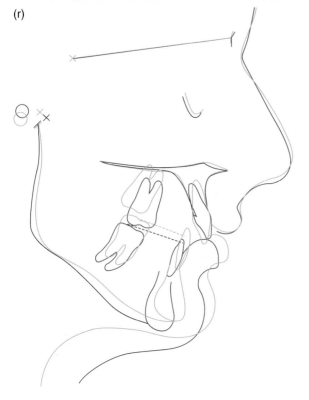

SKELETAL			SOFT TISSUES		
SNA	°	0.5	Lip Sep	mm	−1.0
SNB	°	1.0	Exp UI	mm	2.0
ANB	°	−0.0	LS-E	mm	−1.5
SN/MxP	°	−1.5	LI-E	mm	−0.0
MxP/MnP	°	−4.5	NLA	°	12.5
LAFH	mm	−4.0	LLA	°	−1.0
UAFH	mm	−0.5	Holdaway	°	−3.0
LAFH/TAFH	%	−1.5			
LPFH	mm	2.0	**NOSE PROMINENCE**		
UPFH	mm	2.0			
PFH	mm	1.5	Nose tip	mm	1.0
Wits	mm	−1.5	Nose angle	°	2.0

TEETH			CHIN PROMINENCE		
Overjet	mm	−1.5	Chin tip	mm	5.0
Overbite	mm	6.5	B-NPo	mm	−2.0
UI/MxP	°	−12.5	LADH	mm	0.5
LI/MnP	°	−2.0			
Ilangle	°	19.0			
LI-APo	mm	−0.5			
LI-NPo	mm	−1.5			

Figure 14.5 (Continued)

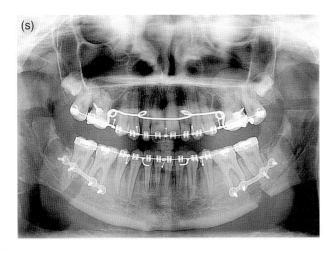

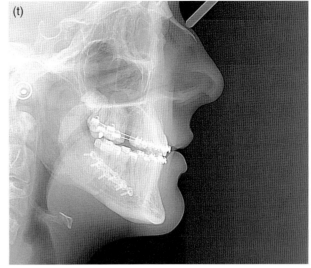

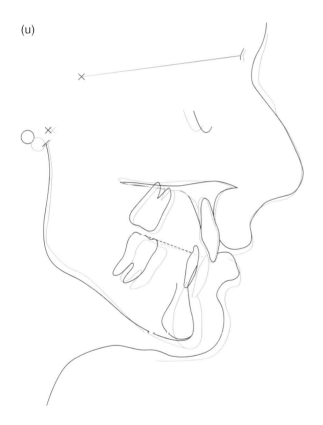

SKELETAL			SOFT TISSUES		
SNA	°	−0.0	Lip Sep	mm	0.5
SNB	°	3.0	Exp UI	mm	−1.5
ANB	°	−3.5	LS-E	mm	−0.5
SN/MxP	°	2.0	LI-E	mm	0.5
MxP/MnP	°	2.5	NLA	°	−15.5
LAFH	mm	4.0	LLA	°	14.0
UAFH	mm	0.5	Holdaway	°	−3.5
LAFH/TAFH	%	1.5			
LPFH	mm	−2.0	NOSE PROMINENCE		
UPFH	mm	−1.5			
PFH	mm	−4.5	Nose tip	mm	−3.0
Wits	mm	−3.0	Nose angle	°	−2.5
TEETH			CHIN PROMINENCE		
			Chin tip	mm	−1.0
Overjet	mm	−6.0	B-NPo	mm	3.0
Overbite	mm	−1.5	LADH	mm	0.0
UI/MxP	°	2.5			
LI/MnP	°	−1.0			
IIangle	°	−4.0			
LI-APo	mm	3.0			
LI-NPo	mm	2.0			

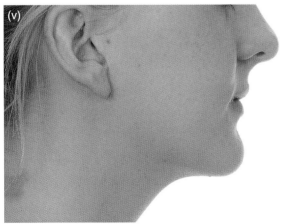

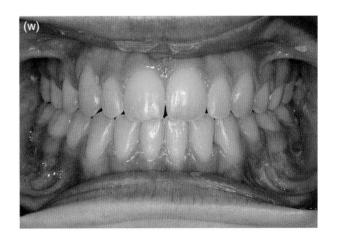

Figure 14.5   (Continued)

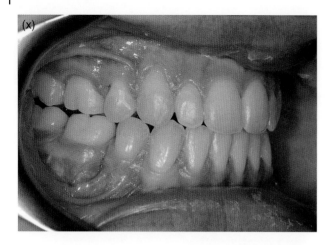

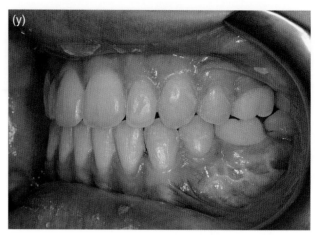

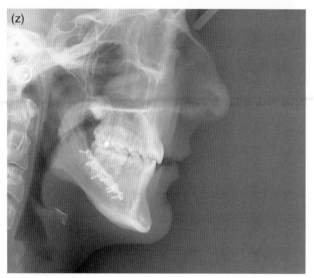

Figure 14.5 (Continued)

or declined. In my experience, it is possible to 'save' some patients from secondary surgery by the correction of premature contacts (especially on molar teeth). This may be through bite closing traction applied to mini-implants (rather than extruding teeth) (Figure 14.9) or through mini-implant intrusion (Figure 14.10).

14.2 Treatment Options

- Maxillary or bimaxillary orthognathic surgery, for asymmetry or AOB cases, where the occlusal plane is levelled or impacted (respectively) by the maxillary osteotomy.
- Conventional surgical hooks for fixation and traction from a (labial) fixed appliance.
- Surgical fixation using archbars.
- Surgical anchorage using IMF screws (Figure 14.1).
- Orthodontic mini-implants for intraoperative fixation and postoperative traction.

14.3 Relevant Clinical Details

As shown in Table 14.1, the stages during the orthognathic treatment pathway when mini-implants may be utilised are as follows.

- Presurgical orthodontics.
- Orthognathic surgical episode, when IMF is required.
- Immediate postoperative phase, when intermaxillary traction is required.
- Postsurgical orthodontics.
- Long term after surgical relapse has occurred.

The most relevant clinical details in determining mini-implant usage in this group of patients are the:

- vertical face height parameters, such that mini-implant intrusion is appropriate in patients with excessive face height/AOB features, but extrusive mechanics are more suitable for short-face patients

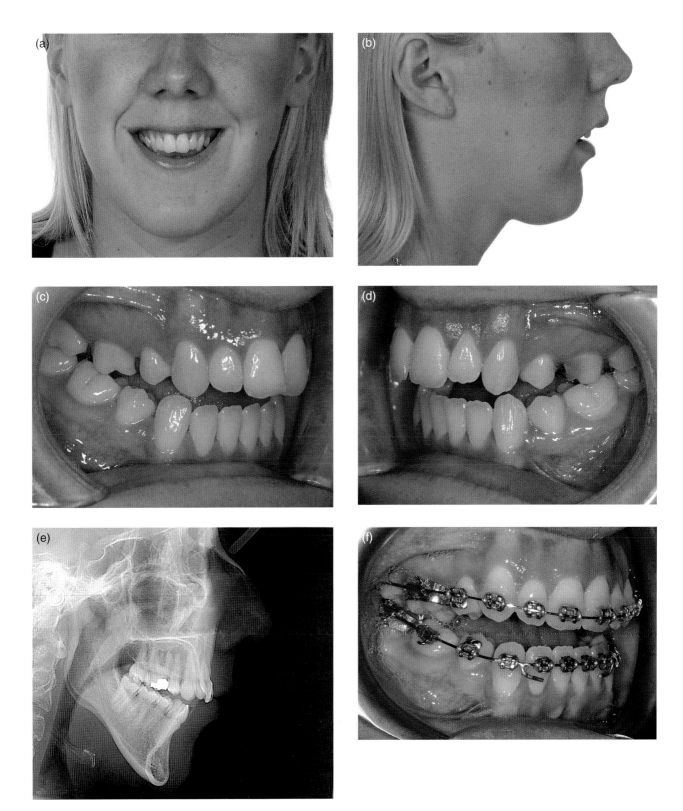

Figure 14.6 (a–e) Pretreatment photographs and lateral cephalogram of this 22-year-old female illustrating her Class II division 1 malocclusion and AOB. She has a Class II facial profile, incompetent lips and a narrow maxillary archform. All the first premolars were absent. (f–i) Photographs and a lateral cephalogram taken on insertion of bilateral palatal alveolar mini-implants sited distal to the upper first molars. Elastomeric traction was applied to the modified quadhelix appliance. (j–o) Photographs and a lateral cephalogram taken at the preoperative stage, after seven months of maxillary molar intrusion. The patient now had a positive overbite and improved Class II malocclusion features. (p) Superimposition of the pre- and postintrusion lateral cephalograms, showing the upper molar intrusion changes, negligible movement of the upper incisors, and a counter-clockwise mandibular rotation. (q,r) Immediate postoperative lateral cephalogram and a superimposition of this on the preoperative cephalogram. These show that the 6 mm 'even' maxillary impaction had been undertaken, with an associated favourable mandibular autorotation. (s–u) Photographs taken one month after surgery, after removal of the quadhelix and the traction from the palatal mini-implants. (v–y) Photographs taken at debond, after a total treatment time of 26 months. (z) Superimposition of the pretreatment and postdebond cephalograms showing the total treatment (intrusion and impaction) changes due to the substantial vertical and rotational changes.

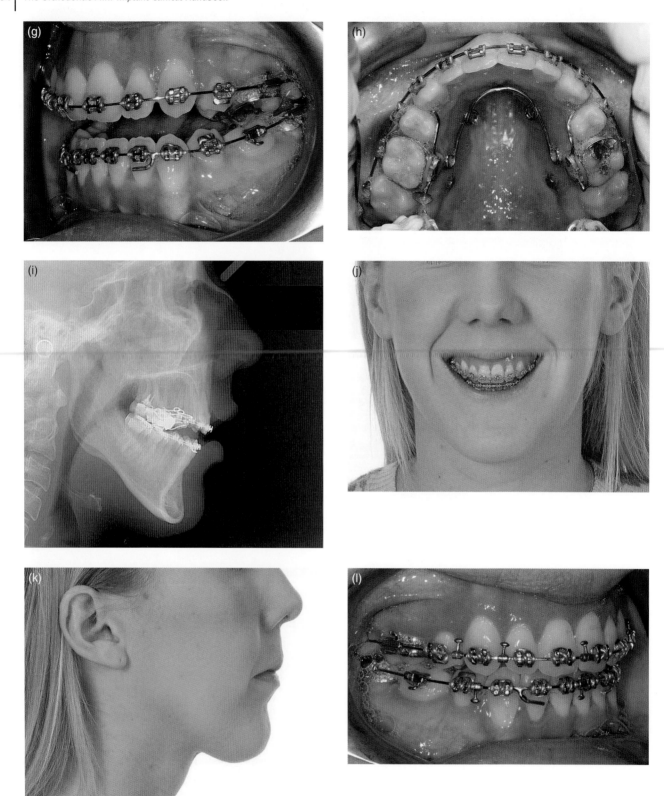

Figure 14.6 (Continued)

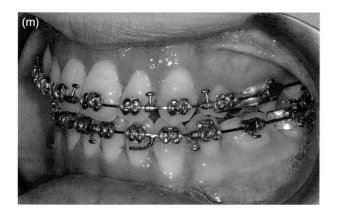

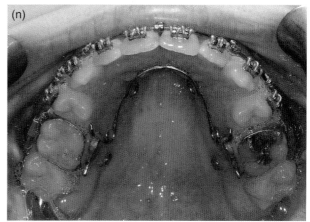

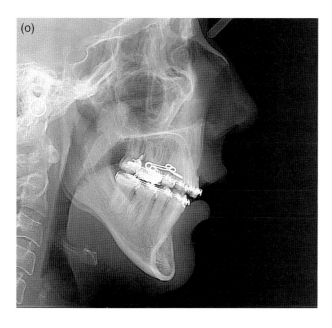

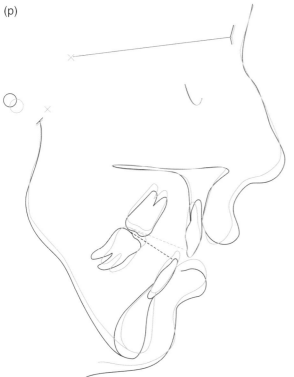

SKELETAL			SOFT TISSUES		
SNA	°	0.5	Lip Sep	mm	−4.0
SNB	°	0.0	Exp UI	mm	0.5
ANB	°	0.5	LS-E	mm	−1.0
SN/MxP	°	−1.0	LI-E	mm	−0.5
MxP/MnP	°	−2.0	NLA	°	4.5
LAFH	mm	−2.0	LLA	°	−2.0
UAFH	mm	−0.5	Holdaway	°	−2.5
LAFH/TAFH	%	−0.5			
LPFH	mm	−1.5	NOSE PROMINENCE		
UPFH	mm	0.0			
PFH	mm	−1.5	Nose tip	mm	−0.5
Wits	mm	12.5	Nose angle	°	1.0

TEETH			CHIN PROMINENCE		
Overjet	mm	2.0	Chin tip	mm	2.5
Overbite	mm	4.5	B-NPo	mm	−1.0
UI/MxP	°	6.5	LADH	mm	1.0
LI/MnP	°	0.5			
IIangle	°	−5.5			
LI-APo	mm	−1.5			
LI-NPo	mm	−2.5			

Figure 14.6 (Continued)

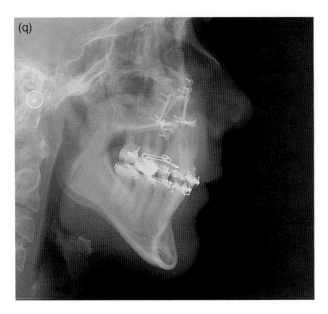

(q)

(r)

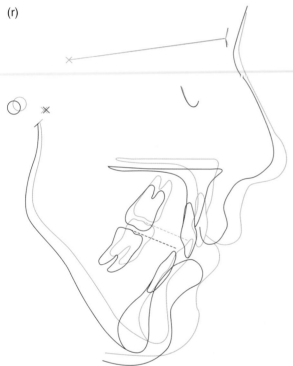

SKELETAL			SOFT TISSUES		
SNA	°	3.8	Lip Sep	mm	−7.6
SNB	°	3.0	Exp UI	mm	−5.3
ANB	°	0.8	LS-E	mm	0.2
SN/MxP	°	1.7	LI-E	mm	−3.1
MxP/MnP	°	−2.9	NLA	°	15.7
LAFH	mm	−0.3	LLA	°	6.7
UAFH	mm	−4.5	Holdaway	°	3.4
LAFH/TAFH	%	2.0			
LPFH	mm	1.5	NOSE PROMINENCE		
UPFH	mm	−1.5			
PFH	mm	−0.7	Nose tip	mm	3.1
Wits	mm	−4.2	Nose angle	°	0.7
TEETH			CHIN PROMINENCE		
Overjet	mm	−1.9	Chin tip	mm	9.4
Overbite	mm	1.6	B-NPo	mm	-0.7
UI/MxP	°	−2.5	LADH	mm	1.6
LI/MnP	°	4.6			
IIangle	°	0.9			
LI-APo	mm	1.2			
LI-NPo	mm	0.5			

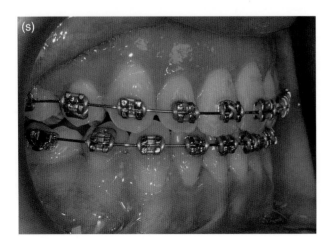

(s)

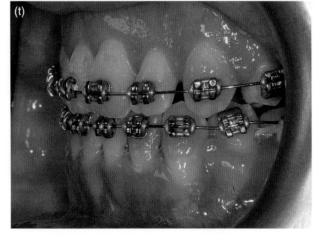

(t)

Figure 14.6 (Continued)

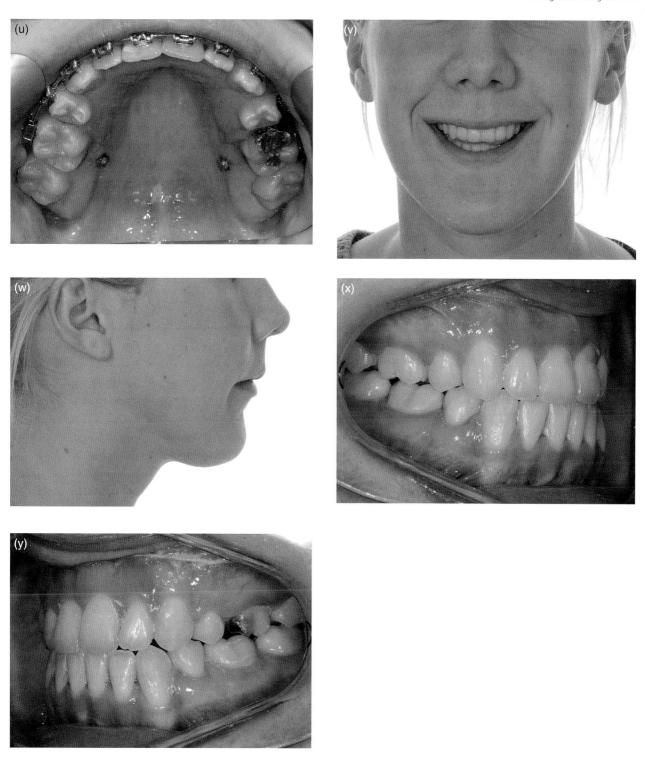

Figure 14.6 (Continued)

(z)

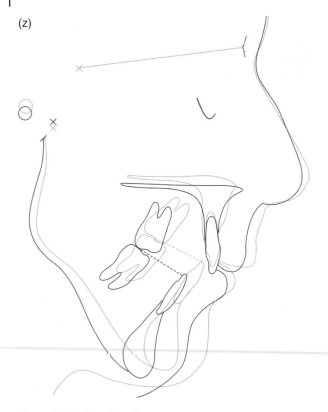

SKELETAL			SOFT TISSUES		
SNA	°	1.3	Lip Sep	mm	−1.0
SNB	°	3.3	Exp UI	mm	−0.9
ANB	°	−2.0	LS-E	mm	−0.1
SN/MxP	°	2.2	LI-E	mm	−3.1
MxP/MnP	°	−9.0	NLA	°	2.0
LAFH	mm	−1.2	LLA	°	−11.9
UAFH	mm	−1.4	Holdaway	°	0.2
LAFH/TAFH	%	0.2			
LPFH	mm	1.0	**NOSE PROMINENCE**		
UPFH	mm	−2.0			
PFH	mm	−0.8	Nose tip	mm	4.2
Wits	mm	1.2	Nose angle	°	5.9

TEETH			CHIN PROMINENCE		
Overjet	mm	−4.9	Chin tip	mm	8.4
Overbite	mm	6.2	B-NPo	mm	−1.1
UI/MxP	°	3.5	LADH	mm	2.1
LI/MnP	°	6.5			
Iiangle	°	−1.0			
LI-APo	mm	0.7			
LI-NPo	mm	−0.8			

Figure 14.6 (Continued)

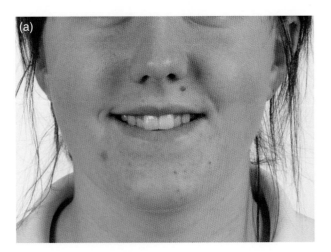
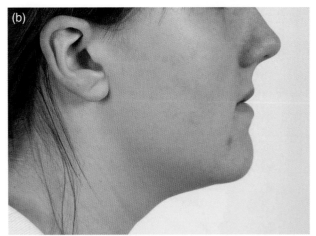

Figure 14.7 (a–f) Pretreatment views showing the combination of Class III and multiple short maxillary root problems. The upper first premolars are also absent. (g–k) Preoperative views following limited alignment and decompensation of the maxillary arch. No surgical hooks have been placed in the upper labial segment because of the short incisor roots. (l,m) Three upper and seven lower mini-implants inserted (free-hand) intraoperatively and used for wire IMF. (n,o) Postoperative radiographs showing several of the mini-implants close to the roots of teeth and the projection of the anterior ones. (p,q) Mucosal overgrowth of several lower mini-implants, sited at the MGJ, resolved by easing the tissue off these heads and then explantation, under local anaesthesia. (r–u) Debond views.

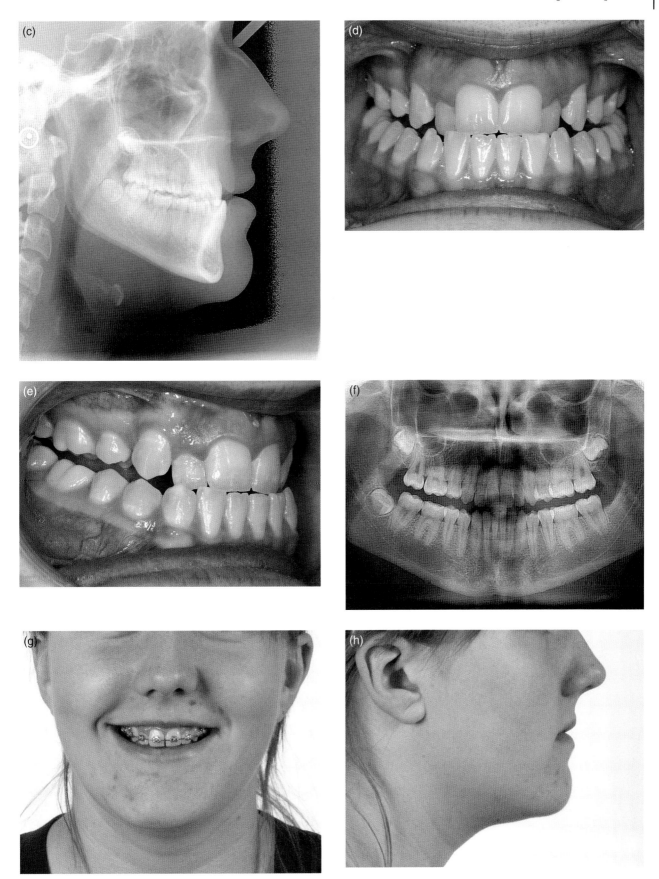

Figure 14.7 (Continued)

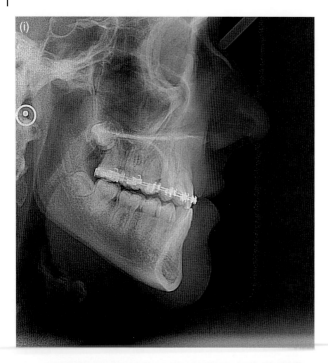

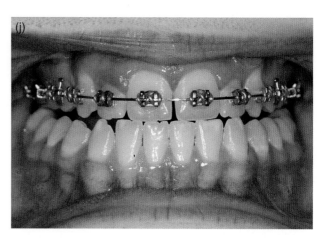

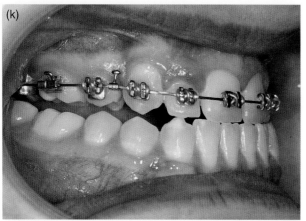

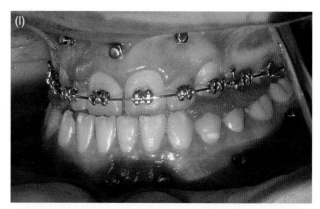

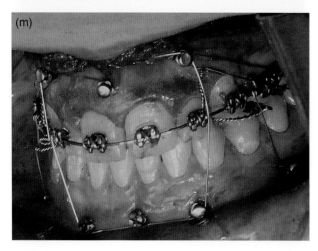

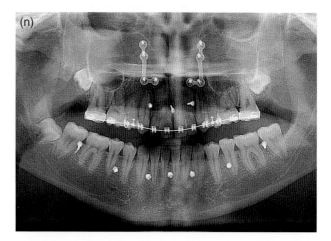

Figure 14.7 (Continued)

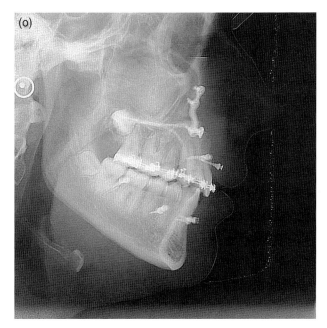

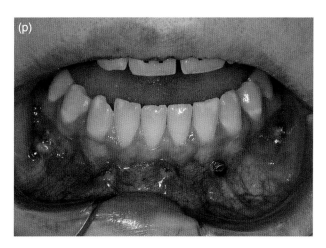

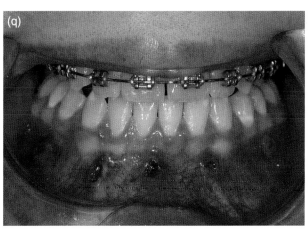

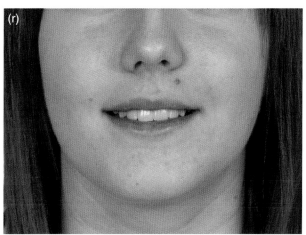

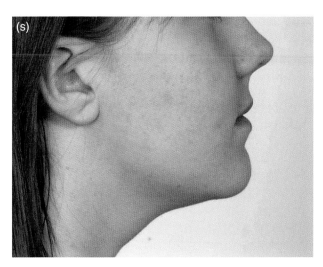

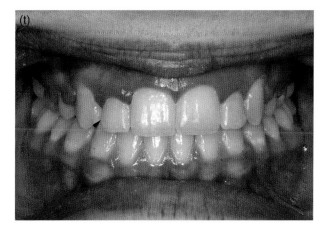

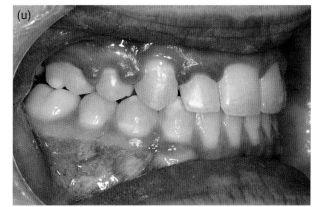

Figure 14.7 (Continued)

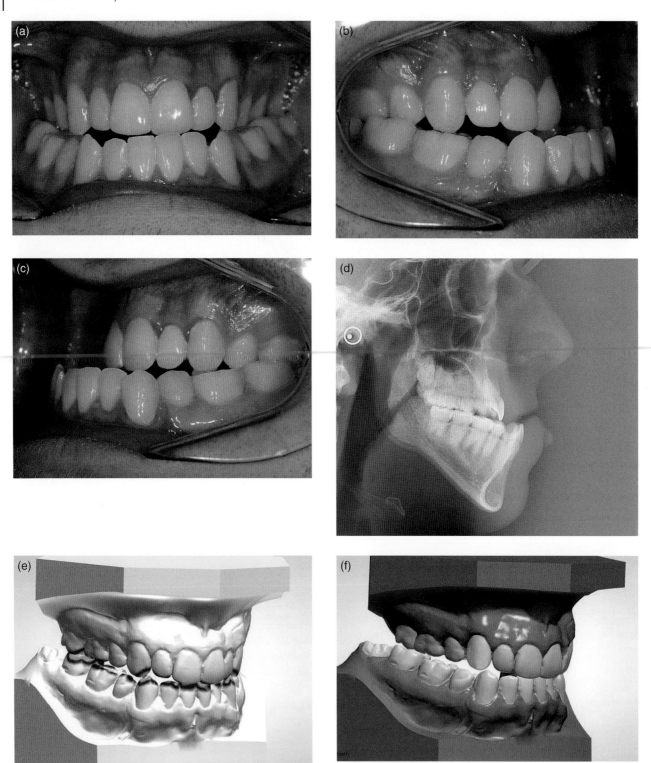

Figure 14.8 (a–d) Presurgical photographs and lateral cephalogram of the severe Class III malocclusion, and absent first premolars, in this 20-year-old male. (e) Digital model simulation of the proposed immediate postoperative occlusion, highlighting premature contact on the canines and second molars. (f) Digital simulation where the right maxillary canine has been intruded to assess the effects on the potential postoperative occlusion. (g–i) Photograph and radiographs taken within two weeks of bimaxillary surgery, showing the corrected Class III dentofacial positions and the nine IMT mini-implants which had been used for IMF. (k–m) Photographs taken eight weeks after surgery, after removal of the mini-implants and bonding of both arches. (n–p) Debond photographs, after seven months of orthodontics and overcorrection of the right second molar premature contacts.

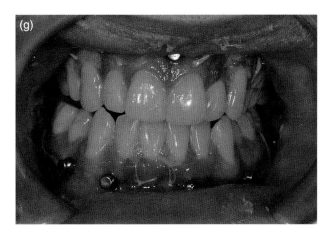

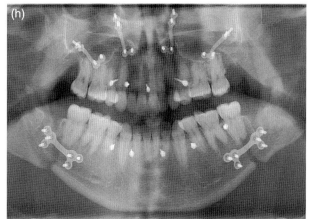

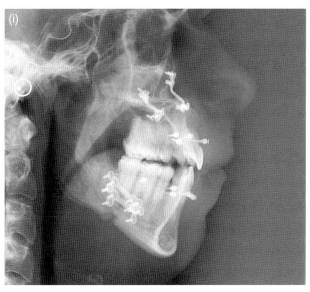

(j)

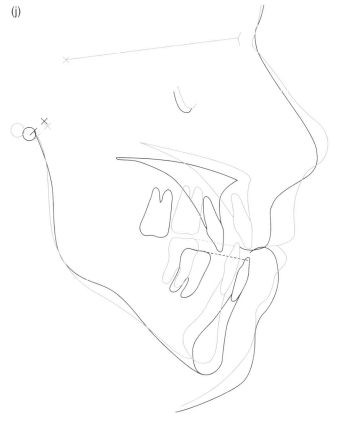

SKELETAL			SOFT TISSUES		
SNA	°	10.0	Lip Sep	mm	1.5
SNB	°	−1.5	Exp UI	mm	0.0
ANB	°	11.0	LS-E	mm	9.0
SN/MxP	°	7.5	LI-E	mm	4.5
MxP/MnP	°	−9.5	NLA	°	1.5
LAFH	mm	−2.0	LLA	°	−6.5
UAFH	mm	−4.0	Holdaway	°	19.0
LAFH/TAFH	%	1.0			
LPFH	mm	10.5	NOSE PROMINENCE		
UPFH	mm	0.5			
PFH	mm	0.5	Nose tip	mm	5.0
Wits	mm	16.5	Nose angle	°	6.0
			CHIN PROMINENCE		
TEETH					
			Chin tip	mm	7.5
Overjet	mm	16.0	B-NPo	mm	−1.0
Overbite	mm	1.5	LADH	mm	1.5
UI/MxP	°	7.0			
LI/MnP	°	−0.0			
IIangle	°	2.5			
LI-APo	mm	−11.5			
LI-NPo	mm	−3.0			

Figure 14.8 (Continued)

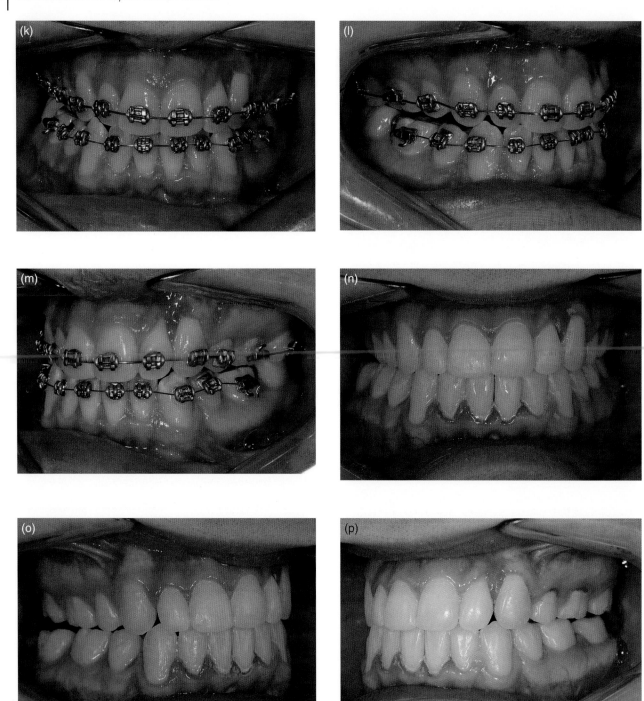

Figure 14.8 (Continued)

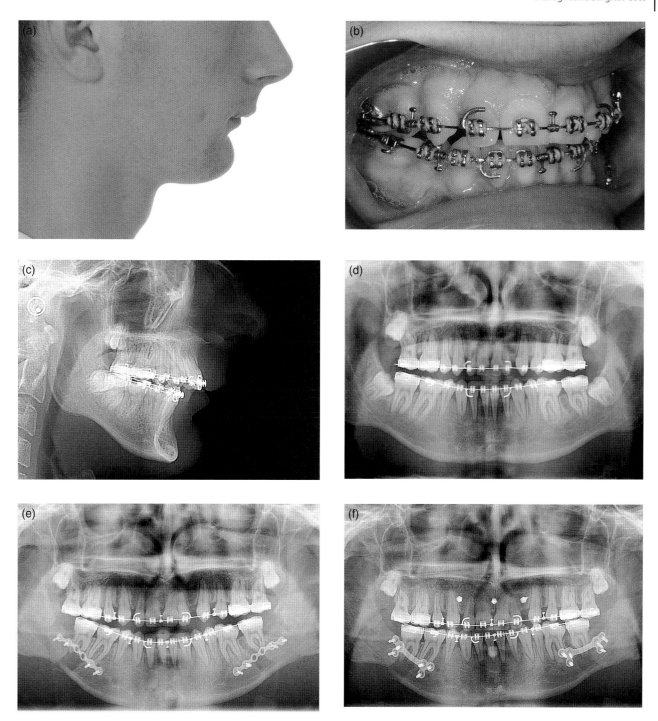

Figure 14.9 (a–d) Preoperative photographs and radiographs showing this 19-year-old male's Class II dentofacial features, although the patient has habitually postured his mandible anteriorly as in the intraoral photograph. (e) A panoramic radiograph taken following a 10 mm mandibular advancement osteotomy. There has been vertical collapse of the right mandibular height and premature contact of the right molars. The short upper incisor root lengths are also shown. (f) A panoramic radiograph taken four weeks after the osteotomy, showing new fixation plates and similar levels of the dentition on both sides. Three upper anterior mini-implants are present. (g–i) Photographs and a lateral cephalogram taken two weeks after the secondary surgery. An anterior 'box'(intermaxillary) elastic connects the mini-implants and the lower fixed appliance. (j) A panoramic radiograph taken six weeks after the secondary surgery and showing reasonable parallelism of the occlusal planes, although the right mandibular gonial angle is more pronounced than the left side. (k,l) Photographs taken at debond, six months after the secondary surgery.

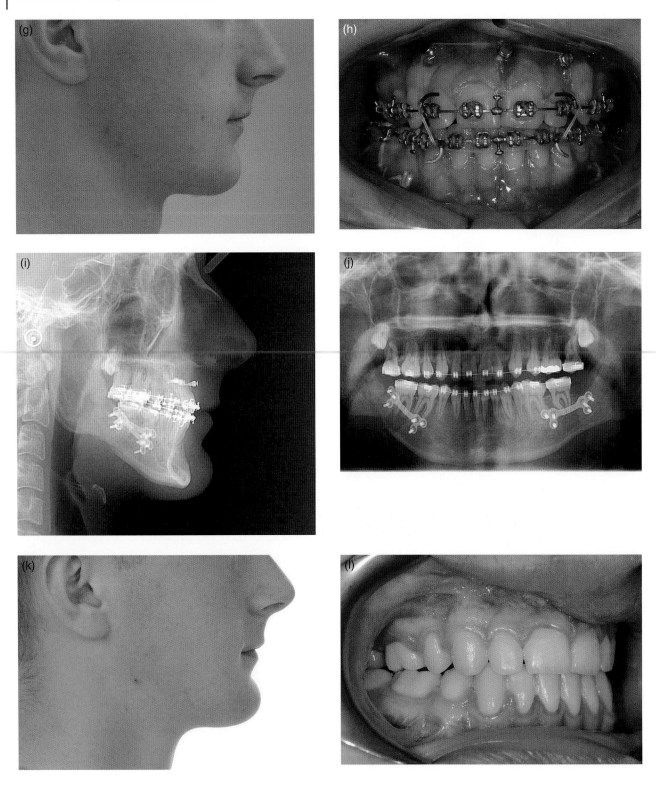

Figure 14.9 (Continued)

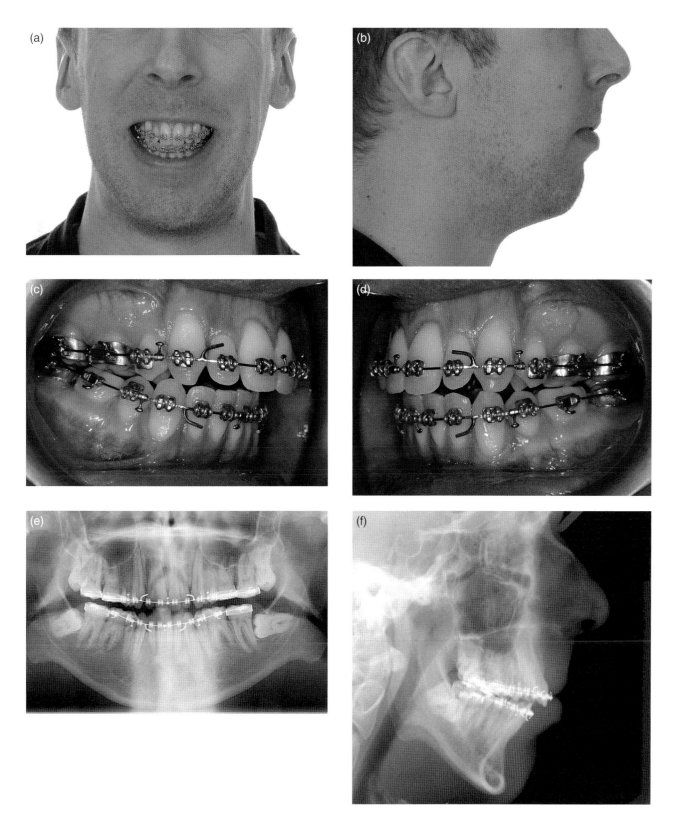

Figure 14.10 (a–g) Preoperative photographs, radiographs and cephalometric figures showing this patient's Class II malocclusion, moderate skeletal II base, increased vertical facial parameters and increased upper incisor display. (h,i) Early postoperative radiographs showing the outcomes of the combined maxillary impaction osteotomy and advancement genioplasty. (j) Cephalometric superimposition of the pre- and postoperative radiographs, indicating favourable maxillary impaction but also advancement movements. Consequently, the mandible had rotated in a counter-clockwise direction, but with only a small reduction on the overjet. (k–m) Photographs taken four months after surgery, when a right palatal mini-implant had been inserted and traction applied to the adjacent first molar sheath. There is a 7 mm overjet and Class II canine relationships (right side worse than left side). (n–p) Photographs taken eight months after surgery, when the canine relationships were almost Class I bilaterally and the maxillary occlusal plane had levelled to the point of premature contact on left molar palatal cusps. A left palatal mini-implant was inserted at this stage. (q,r) A left lateral intermaxillary traction elastic was commenced after four months of bilateral traction, when the Class II malocclusion features had been corrected. (s–x) Debond photographs and lateral cephalogram showing the Class I occlusion and skeletal position with a normal amount of upper incisor vertical display. (y,z) Photographs of the occlusion 30 months after debond, showing the stable Class I finish and settled molar positions.

(g)

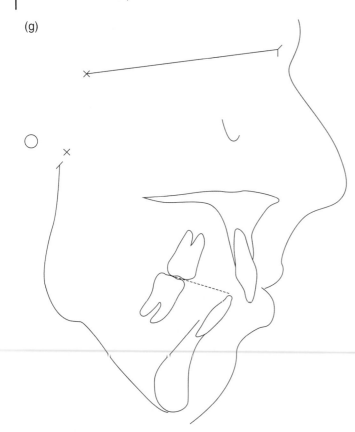

SKELETAL			SOFT TISSUES		
SNA	°	75.0	Lip Sep	mm	−0.5
SNB	°	66.5	Exp UI	mm	5.5
ANB	°	8.5	LS-E	mm	−3.0
SN/MxP	°	7.5	LI-E	mm	1.0
MxP/MnP	°	41.0	NLA	°	150.5
LAFH	mm	83.0	LLA	°	142.5
UAFH	mm	58.5	Holdaway	°	16.0
LAFH/TAFH	%	58.5			
LPFH	mm	53.5	**NOSE PROMINENCE**		
UPFH	mm	53.5			
PFH	mm	87.0	Nose tip	mm	23.0
Wits	mm	10.0	Nose angle	°	28.5

TEETH			CHIN PROMINENCE		
Overjet	mm	8.0	Chin tip	mm	−22.0
Overbite	mm	0.0	B-NPo	mm	−3.0
UI/MxP	°	10.0	LADH	mm	45.5
LI/MnP	°	91.5			
IIangle	°	127.5			
LI-APo	mm	1.5			
LI-NPo	mm	6.5			

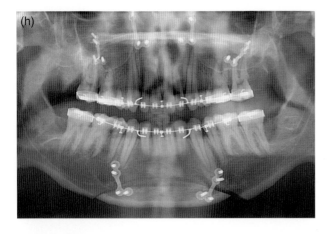

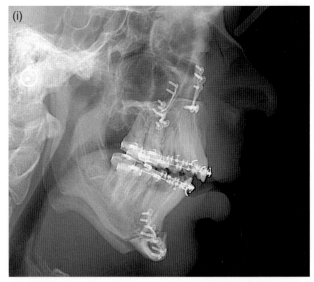

Figure 14.10 (Continued)

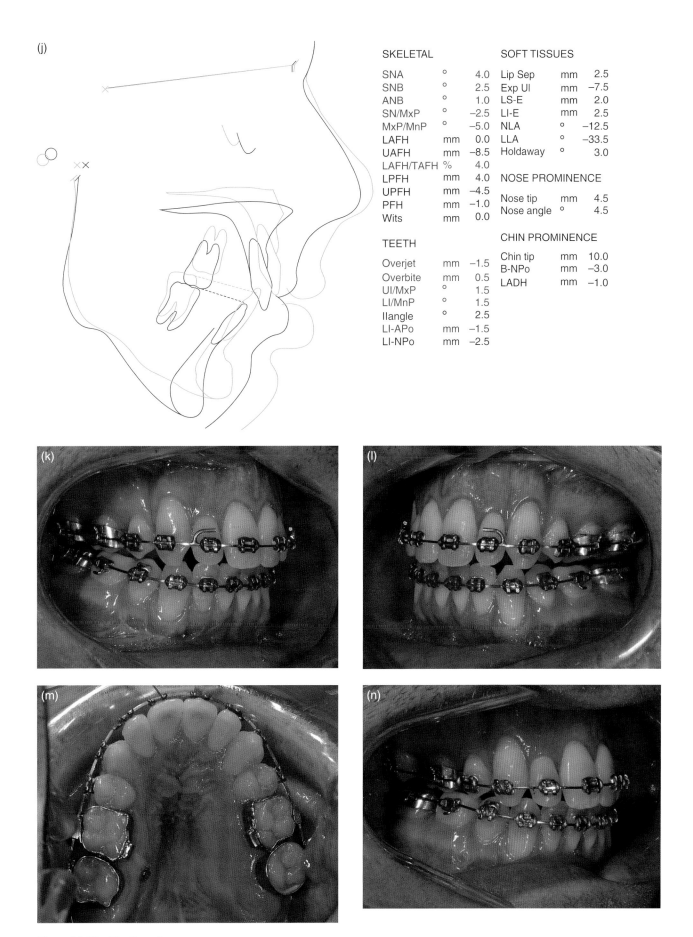

(j)

SKELETAL			SOFT TISSUES		
SNA	°	4.0	Lip Sep	mm	2.5
SNB	°	2.5	Exp Ul	mm	−7.5
ANB	°	1.0	LS-E	mm	2.0
SN/MxP	°	−2.5	LI-E	mm	2.5
MxP/MnP	°	−5.0	NLA	°	−12.5
LAFH	mm	0.0	LLA	°	−33.5
UAFH	mm	−8.5	Holdaway	°	3.0
LAFH/TAFH	%	4.0			
LPFH	mm	4.0	NOSE PROMINENCE		
UPFH	mm	−4.5			
PFH	mm	−1.0	Nose tip	mm	4.5
Wits	mm	0.0	Nose angle	°	4.5

TEETH			CHIN PROMINENCE		
Overjet	mm	−1.5	Chin tip	mm	10.0
Overbite	mm	0.5	B-NPo	mm	−3.0
UI/MxP	°	1.5	LADH	mm	−1.0
LI/MnP	°	1.5			
IIangle	°	2.5			
LI-APo	mm	−1.5			
LI-NPo	mm	−2.5			

Figure 14.10 (Continued)

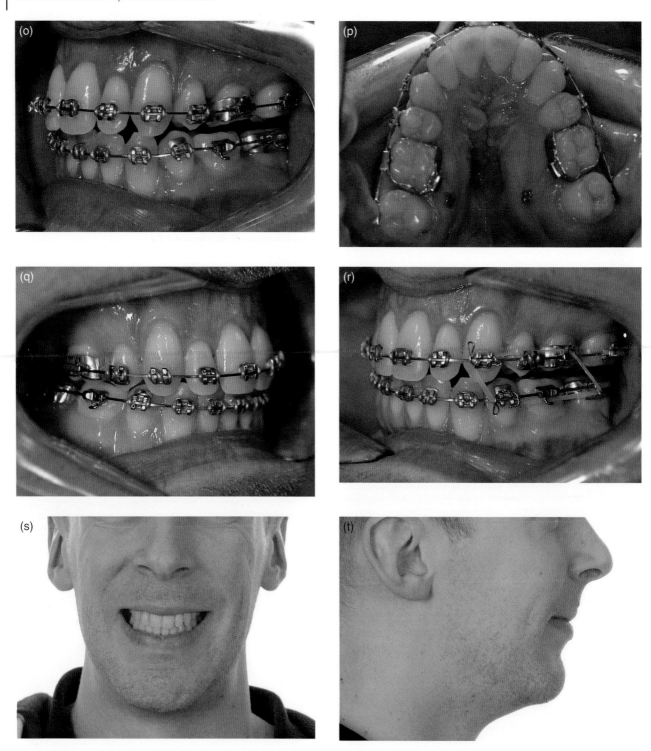

Figure 14.10 (Continued)

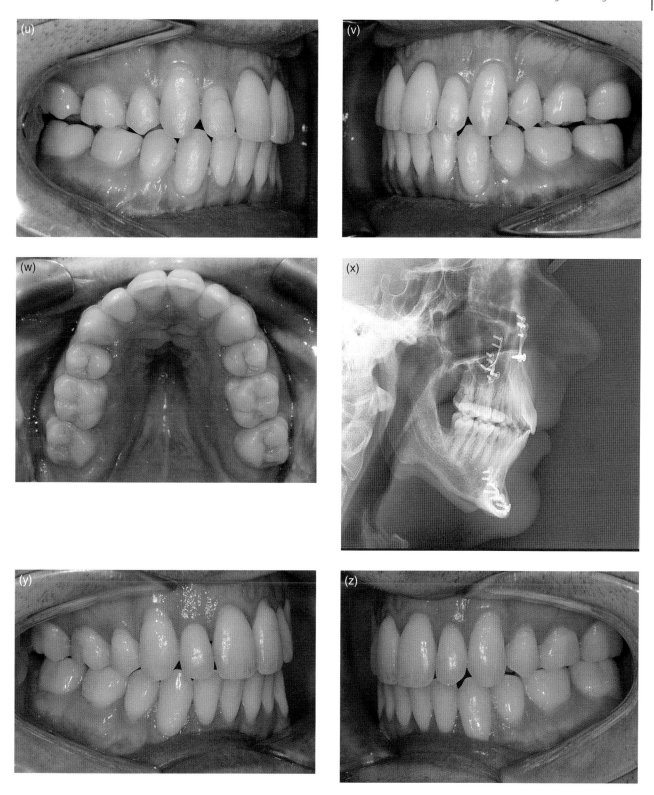

Figure 14.10 (Continued)

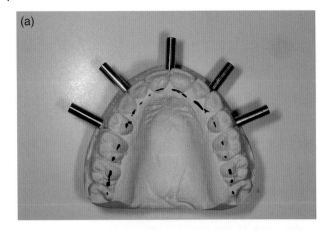

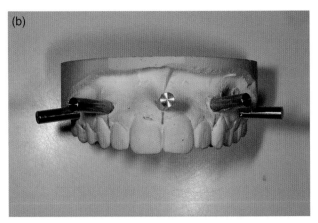

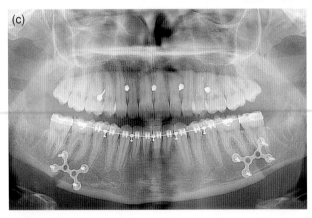

Figure 14.11 (a,b) Photographs of a preoperative working model of the maxillary arch, showing five mini-implant abutments *in situ*. These reflect the positions and angles of insertion for the intraoperative insertion of mini-implants for IMF purposes. (c) A postoperative panoramic radiograph which confirms that the planned positioning of the mini-implants was achieved by the surgical team, through the use of a guidance stent.

- presence of vertical facial asymmetry manifesting as a maxillary occlusal cant
- periodontal status and root lengths of teeth since prolonged and/or heavy intermaxillary traction will have a deleterious effect on such teeth
- height of buccal/labial attached gingiva in areas where mini-implants are indicated
- root proximity of teeth adjacent to the planned insertion sites
- potential occlusal interferences and hence suitability for 'surgery first' treatment.

14.4   Biomechanical Principles

- Ideally, insert the mini-implants in sufficient numbers (e.g. three for anterior and five for full arch support, respectively), in both dentate and edentulous sites, where they will provide fixation points consistent with the planned occlusion and hence lines of traction.

- Elastics are less likely to be dislodged from a mini-implant which has been inserted in a horizontal direction (parallel to the occlusal plane) rather than at an oblique angle.
- Some surgeons appear to have a 'tent peg' concept where they insert IMF screws at incorrect (coronally inclined) vertical angles in the belief that they will resist IMF and traction forces better. However, this places the screw body in a site with less bone and closer to the coronal aspect of the roots! Therefore, it is important to either advise the surgical team on the precise location and angles of insertion (perpendicular to the alveolar surface or apically inclined) or to provide them with a guidance stent (Figure 14.11). The process of producing a surgical guidance stent is similar to the standard orthodontic one described in Chapter 3.
- Traction to 'settle' an unsatisfactory postoperative occlusion should be applied before maturation (solidification) of the osteotomy site callus. This may be indicated when the stability of the 'rigid' fixation is suboptimal. It is appropriate if extrusive/bite closing forces are ideal and is often referred to as 'callus moulding'.

14.5 Clinical Tips and Technicalities

- Remember that orthodontic mini-implant insertion is different from the two bone screw techniques which maxillofacial surgeons are familiar with: maxillofacial bone fixation and dental implantology. Therefore, it is essential that whoever places the mini-implants must understand their apparently innocuous but fundamental differences, and familiarise themselves with the relevant clinical instruments and steps. In particular, mini-implant insertion is a gentle technique using light forces, and one where the angles of insertion are carefully defined. These details can be critical since mini-implants typically remain *in situ* for months, relying on secondary stability, not just primary stability at the time of surgery.

- Orthognathic surgical usage is further complicated by access problems since it can be surprisingly difficult to line up the correct path of insertion when the patient is supine and surgical drapes restrict lateral access. Unfortunately, it is not unusual, in such circumstances, for fixation and surgical IMF screws to be inserted with incorrect posteriorly directed angulation. This can still be the case for posterior mini-implant insertions, as illustrated in Figure 14.12 where the mini-implants were inserted through the maxillary first molar furcations rather than the adjacent interproximal spaces. Consequently, all clinicians involved in surgical cases should be aware of this directional problem, and if in doubt then consider advance fabrication of a guidance stent (Figure 14.11).

- If the labial frenum is prominent then minimise patient discomfort, and soft tissue interference or overgrowth (over the mini-implant head), by either avoiding mini-implant insertion in the midline or performing a frenectomy.

- Horizontal angles of insertion (i.e. parallel to the occlusal plane) and full insertion of the mini-implants also help to minimise irritation of the lip/cheek soft tissues. Conversely, overinsertion makes it more likely that the intermaxillary wires/elastics may impinge on the adjacent gingival tissues.

- Consider presurgical root divergence to create interproximal space at the ideal mini-implant insertion sites. For example, limited fixed appliance alterations of the root alignment may be undertaken to facilitate mini-implant surgical usage. This may be particularly beneficial for sites such as the mandibular incisor region where the interproximal widths are typically narrow and the roots closely approximated.

- The anterior alveolar depth can be measured on a lateral cephalogram (Figure 14.13) or a cone beam computed tomography (CBCT). This will indicate whether the midline area provides sufficient depth for a long (e.g. 9 mm) body length mini-implant when it is inserted horizontally (parallel to the occlusal plane).

- Ideally, use a mini-implant head with a rounded contour and low profile, e.g. the Infinitas IMT version (Figure 14.14) with its mushroom-shaped head (http://www.dbortho.com/collections/infinitas-mini-implants/products/infinitas-imt-screws). This ensures patient comfort when the mini-implants are inserted in relatively remote sites and are more likely to rub against the

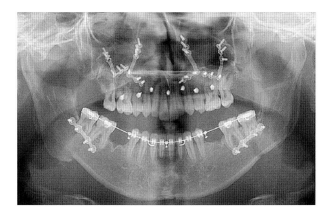

Figure 14.12 Panoramic radiograph showing mini-implants inserted in an orthognathic case, including two located in the maxillary first molar furcation areas.

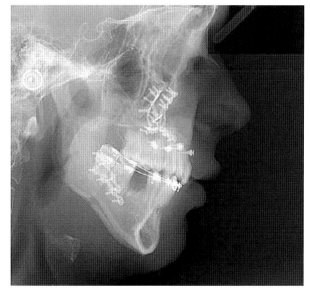

Figure 14.13 A lateral cephalogram showing the alveolar depth in the anterior maxillary and mandibular regions. The posteriorly directed angle of mini-implants inserted in theatre at the time of the osteotomy is also seen.

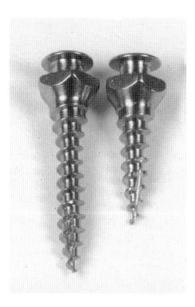

Figure 14.14 Close-up views of the IMT mini-implants showing their head's large external undercut and mushroom-shaped top.

cheeks and lips (without a nearby fixed appliance to buffer the soft tissue contact). The generous undercut of the Infinitas IMT mini-implant head also helps the patient to place and retain elastics used for traction.

Remember that orthodontic mini-implant insertion is different from the two bone screw techniques which maxillofacial surgeons are familiar with: maxillofacial bone fixation and dental implantology.

14.6 Clinical Steps

14.6.1 Preinsertion

1) Determine the insertion sites and number of mini-implants required.
2) Consider presurgical divergence of the roots of teeth adjacent to the insertion sites where the interproximal space is narrow and an alternative adjacent site not suitable. This may be the case particularly in the lower incisor area, where the limited height of attached gingiva also limits the option of avoiding the roots by using an apical insertion level. Divergence is achieved by bonding the brackets at altered tips; for example, for insertion mesial to the canine root then add mesial tip to the lateral incisor bracket and distal tip to the canine one.
3) If the patient has vulnerable tooth roots then consider presurgical orthodontics for alignment purposes only,

specifically to eliminate potential occlusal interferences at surgery (Figure 14.7). A rigid (e.g. 0.019×0.025in. steel) orthodontic archwire and surgical hooks can then be avoided since mini-implants will be used for IMF and traction purposes.

14.6.2 Mini-implant Selection

4) A narrow-diameter mini-implant, such as 1.5mm, is appropriate for interproximal sites.
5) Select a mini-implant with a sufficiently long neck to reduce the risk of the intermaxillary wire/elastic catching on the gingival tissues.
6) If there is sufficient height of the attached gingiva then the insertion should be perpendicular to the surface. Consequently, a long mini-implant body (e.g. 9mm length Infinitas version) should be used in posterior maxillary sites (distal to the canine) and also anteriorly, provided that there is sufficient depth of palatal alveolus to accommodate this. This can be verified on a CBCT or a lateral cephalogram (Figure 14.13). A short body length (e.g. 6mm Infinitas version) is appropriate for mandibular sites and in patients with a narrow anterior maxilla where there is a risk of perforating through to the palatal tissues.

14.6.3 Insertion

7) Superficial anaesthesia of the insertion sites, unless the insertions occur when the patient is under general anaesthesia.
8) Insert the mini-implants through attached gingiva on the buccal side of the alveolus, close to or at the mucogingival junction (MGJ) (to help in avoiding the tooth roots).
9) A small (10–30°) *apical* inclination is appropriate where the attached gingival height is limited, and surgeons should remember that the 'tent peg' principle (where screw insertions are coronally directed) is not appropriate here.
10) Use a mucotome for any insertions through loose mucosa.
11) Use a cortical punch to perforate dense cortex in the posterior mandible sites.
12) Avoid overinsertion, by stopping the screwdriver once its tip touches the mucosa and then inserting further by a few turns at a time, if appropriate.
13) Take an intraoral radiograph (postoperatively) if close root proximity is suspected clinically.
14) Complete insertion to the point where the mini-implant neck is partially submerged yet the head is fully accessible.

14.6.4 Postinsertion

15) Apply IMF or elastic traction from the mini-implants to surgical hooks or other mini-implants in the opposing arch. Postoperative intermaxillary elastic traction is variable and dependent on the amount of mouth opening achievable. However, it is appropriate to use similar elastics and force levels to those utilised for conventional intermaxillary traction.

16) Keep the mini-implants *in situ* until it is clear that further anchorage is not required.

14.7 Case Examples

1) **Presurgical centreline correction (Figure 14.2)**
   - A 17-year-old female presented with a Class III malocclusion and mandibular asymmetry (chin displaced to the right side). The upper left first premolar had previously been extracted to enable the adjacent canine to erupt, and the upper centreline was significantly displaced to the left side (Figure 14.2a–h).
   - Bimaxillary surgery was planned, involving a maxillary advancement osteotomy (with a small differential impaction on the left side) and an asymmetrical mandibular setback osteotomy. Presurgical correction of the upper dental centreline would be ideal to facilitate subsequent surgical planning and correction of the facial asymmetries.
   - The maxillary arch was aligned and levelled and then a buccal mini-implant (1.5 mm diameter, 9 mm length) was inserted mesial to the upper right first molar (Figure 14.2i,j). Elastomeric traction was applied to a crimpable powerarm (mesial to the upper right canine bracket).
   - This traction corrected the upper centreline preoperatively and a passive ligature wire was then attached from the mini-implant to the powerarm (Figure 14.2k–p).
   - Final space closure was performed postoperatively, after removal of the mini-implant and planned anchorage loss. The patient then had coincident dental centrelines and a more symmetrical facial appearance (Figure 14.2s–v).

2) **Presurgical molar protraction (Figure 14.3)**
   - A 17-year-old male presented with a Class III dentofacial deformity, which required orthodontics and bimaxillary surgery (Figure 14.3a–f). He required maxillary premolar extractions for relief of crowding and incisor decompensation, but ideally would be treated on a non-extraction basis in the mandibular arch. Therefore, treatment was complicated by recent loss of the right mandibular first molar. Conventional

closure of this space would involve slippage of the lower centreline to the right side, but this was contraindicated since the dental centreline matched the asymmetrical chin position (which was displaced to the left side). The lower right third molar was present and ideally would be preserved at surgery, but this would be problematic given the mandibular setback movement required on this side.
   - The dental arches were aligned and levelled to reach the stage of 0.019 × 0.025 in. steel archwires. The lower right second premolar was tipped mesially for root divergence during this phase. A buccal mini-implant (1.5 mm diameter, 9 mm length) was then inserted between the lower right premolar roots. Elastomeric traction was applied directly to the second molar hook to protract this tooth.
   - This traction protracted the lower right second molar tooth preoperatively, and the unerupted third molar moved mesially at the same time (Figure 14.3g). At the same time, decompensation of the anterior teeth was progressing. Several brackets were repositioned, including the lower right second premolar when the mini-implant was explanted (Figure 14.3h–j).
   - The lower right third molar was partially erupted, adjacent to the second molar, when the patient reached the stage for his bimaxillary surgery (Figure 14.3k–o). Hence it did not interfere with the mandibular setback osteotomy (Figure 14.3q,r).
   - The patient was debonded prior to full eruption of the lower right third molar, due to work commitments (Figure 14.3s–w). This left the option of limited treatment to upright it at a later stage.

3) **Presurgical unilateral intrusion (Figure 14.4)**
   - A 16-year-old female presented with a Class III malocclusion featuring asymmetrical mandibular prognathism (chin displaced to the left side) and a mild occlusal cant (higher on the left side) (Figure 14.4a–f).
   - An asymmetrical mandibular setback osteotomy was planned, and intrusion of the upper right buccal segment was indicated to facilitate optimal surgical positioning of the mandible.
   - The maxillary arch was aligned and levelled and then a buccal mini-implant (1.5 mm diameter, 9 mm length) was inserted mesial to the upper right first molar (Figure 14.4g,h). Elastomeric traction was applied to the adjacent second premolar bracket and first molar hook.
   - This traction created a right lateral openbite such that the amount of intrusion had been overcorrected preoperatively (Figure 14.4i–n).
   - The mandible was surgically repositioned with the freedom to select an optimal vertical level on the right

side, such that a right lateral openbite was still present one month postoperatively (Figure 14.4o–s).

- The patient's Class III malocclusion was corrected and her dental and facial asymmetries were improved without the need for a maxillary osteotomy. The right lateral openbite overcorrection settled during the postoperative orthodontic phase, accepting a small residual centreline discrepancy (Figure 14.4t–y).

4) **Bilateral molar intrusion combined with a mandibular osteotomy (Figure 14.5)**

- A 16-year-old female presented with a Class II division malocclusion on a moderate skeletal II base with an increased mandibular plane angle and retroclined lower incisors. She had hypodontia with both lower second premolars absent, but all third molars present (Figure 14.5a–f). The retained lower left second deciduous molar had short root lengths.

- A mandibular advancement osteotomy was planned but this would have resulted in an AOB, given the 'downwards' trajectory of mandibular advancement. Therefore, upper molar intrusion was indicated to reduce the vertical face height and mandibular plane angle prior to mandibular surgery (rather than performing a maxillary osteotomy since the upper incisor display was satisfactory and the patient was keen to avoid any extra morbidity).

- Initial maxillary arch expansion and alignment of both arches were undertaken. Bilateral palatal mini-implants (1.5 mm diameter, 9 mm length) were then inserted mesial to the upper second molars (Figure 14.5g–l). Elastomeric traction was applied to the quadhelix arms and indirectly to the first molars. At the same time, elastomeric traction was applied across the mandibular second deciduous molar spaces.

- This 10-month molar intrusion traction created a deep overbite and a reduction in the lower face height during the preoperative phase (Figure 14.5m–q). The lower second deciduous molar spaces were closed at the same time.

- The mandible was then surgically advanced by 6 mm with an associated increase in the lower anterior face height, but without recurrence of the original AOB (Figure 14.5s–u).

- The patient completed her treatment after a total of 26 months, with full correction of her Class II malocclusion and hypodontia features (Figure 14.5v–z).

5) **Bilateral molar intrusion combined with a maxillary osteotomy (Figure 14.6)**

- A 22-year-old female presented with a Class II division 2 malocclusion on a skeletal II base with an increased mandibular plane angle and an associated AOB (Figure 14.6a–e). The patient's lips were incompetent and there was an increased upper incisor/gingival display. The maxillary arch was narrow and all the first premolars were absent.

- A maxillary osteotomy was considered, but it was felt that the amount of differential posterior impaction required may be difficult to achieve and that this would have a negative effect on the patient's nasal morphology. A large clockwise rotation of the maxilla would also have left the maxillary incisors appearing retroclined since it was going to be difficult to over-torque them given their pretreatment retroclination and the absent premolar teeth. Therefore, it was agreed that molar intrusion should be used to level the maxillary dentition preoperatively, followed by an equal (anterior and posterior) maxillary impaction movement.

- Both arches were aligned and levelled, plus the maxillary arch was expanded. Bilateral palatal alveolar mini-implants (1.5 mm diameter, 9 mm length) were then inserted distal to the upper first molars (Figure 14.6f–i). Elastomeric traction was applied to the modified quadhelix appliance.

- The maxillary molar intrusion corrected the AOB and improved the Class II malocclusion features, whilst maintaining the upper incisor level, preoperatively (Figure 14.6j–o).

- The maxilla was surgically impacted by 6 mm anteriorly and posteriorly, and with a modest advancement movement (Figure 14.6p–r). This maxillary movement, coupled with mandibular autorotation, resulted in the achievement of a Class I malocclusion, with competent lips and normal upper incisor display (Figure 14.6s–u).

- The patient completed her postoperative orthodontics after a total of 26 months (Figure 14.6v–y). In this time the maxillary dentition had undergone substantial vertical and rotational changes due to the combined intrusion and impaction stages (Figure 14.6z).

6) **IMF: vulnerable dentition (Figure 14.7)**

- A 15-year-old female presented with a Class III malocclusion on a moderate skeletal III base due to maxillary hypoplasia (Figure 14.7a–c). The upper first premolars had been extracted during an earlier course of orthodontic treatment, and there was generalised shortness of the maxillary dental roots (Figure 14.7d–f). The mandibular arch was reasonably well aligned.

- The maxillary root problems severely restricted the scope for orthodontics in this arch to simple alignment (Figure 14.7g–k). A reasonable occlusion could be achieved without further mandibular arch orthodontics.

- A maxillary osteotomy was undertaken four months into treatment, with IMF achieved by the use of three maxillary and seven mandibular mini-implants (Figure 14.7l–o). An upper labial frenectomy was also performed.

- The mandibular mini-implants were sited apical to the MGJ, in loose mucosa and subsequently underwent tissue overgrowth (Figure 14.7p). They were not required for postoperative traction and were easily removed after the soft tissues were eased off their heads, under local anaesthesia (Figure 14.7q).

- The lower fixed appliance was debonded eight months postoperatively, accepting dental centreline discrepancies because of the limited orthodontic feasibility (Figure 14.7r–u).

7) **IMF: surgery first (Figure 14.8)**

- A 20-year-old male presented with a severe Class III malocclusion and facial deformity. He had a history of four premolar extractions and fixed appliance treatment (Figure 14.8a–d).

- A reasonable occlusion could be achieved without preoperative orthodontics, accepting that there would be premature contact on the right canines and second molars (Figure 14.8e) which could be corrected by relatively minor tooth intrusion postoperatively (Figure 14.8f). Therefore, bimaxillary osteotomies were undertaken with the aid of nine upper and lower mini-implants for IMF (Figure 14.8g–j). An upper labial frenectomy was also performed.

- The mini-implants were not required for postoperative traction and were easily removed without local anaesthesia.

- The upper fixed appliance was bonded four weeks after surgery, then the lower arch another four weeks later (Figure 14.8k–m).

- Treatment was completed after seven months of fixed appliance usage, accepting the need for occlusal molar settling in the longer term (Figure 14.8n–p). The patient was then offered an advancement genioplasty to complete his treatment by balancing his facial profile, but declined this for personal reasons.

8) **IMF and intermaxillary traction (Figure 14.9)**

- A 19-year-old male who had presented with a severe degree of mandibular retrognathia was prepared for a mandibular osteotomy (Figure 14.9a–d). He underwent a 10 mm BSSO advancement and surgical removal of the mandibular third molars. However, it was clear after one week that the rigid fixation was failing on the right side of the mandible. This resulted in loss of right vertical ramus-body height and premature contact of the right molars (Figure 14.9e).

- IMF and 'heavy' elastic traction were contraindicated because of the short root lengths of the four upper incisors, especially the right central incisor. Therefore, the patient returned to surgery after four weeks for the fixation plates to be replaced and the occlusion re-established.

- At the same time, three IMT mini-implants were inserted in the upper anterior area, and intermaxillary elastic traction applied between these and the lower fixed appliance (Figure 14.9f–i). This postoperative traction continued for six weeks, until the occlusion appeared to be stable and the mini-implants were removed (Figure 14.9j).

- The fixed appliances were debonded six months later, without the need for further elastic traction (Figure 14.9k,l).

9) **Postoperative relapse and molar intrusion correction (Figure 14.10)**

- A 26-year-old male presented with a Class II malocclusion on a moderate skeletal II base with an increased mandibular plane angle and increased upper incisor display. The first premolars were absent and the maxillary arch was narrow.

- The arches were aligned and decompensated with fixed appliances, ready for a combination of a maxillary osteotomy and genioplasty (Figure 14.10a–g).

- A maxillary impaction and advancement genioplasty movements were performed, but soon after surgery there appeared to be a maxillary cant with premature occlusal contact on the right molars. Cephalometric superimposition indicated that the maxilla had been inadvertently advanced (Figure 14.10j), resulting in a Class II malocclusion (Figure 14.10k,l).

- Given that the patient had presented with an increased face height, it was prudent to avoid tooth extrusions by the use of intermaxillary elastic traction. Therefore, rather than the patient having revisional surgery, it was decided to use molar intrusion to reduce the premature molar contacts and consequently cause a favourable mandibular autorotation.

- A mini-implant (1.5 mm diameter, 9 mm length) was inserted in the palatal alveolar area distal to the right first molar and elastomeric traction applied to the first molar (palatal sheath) (Figure 14.10m).

- After four months of intrusive traction, a similar mini-implant was inserted on the left side of the palatal alveolus and traction applied to the adjacent first molar (Figure 14.10n–p).

- After a further four months, a left-sided box elastic was added to level the mandibular occlusal plane (whilst traction was being applied to the opposing buccal segment) (Figure 14.10q,r).

- The fixed appliances were debonded 16 months after surgery, accepting minor molar openbites (overcorrections) and incomplete torque of these teeth (Figure 14.10s–x). The postoperative Class II features had been corrected.

- The intrusive changes remained stable, as evident at the patient's final review 30 months after debond (Figure 14.10y,z). One may speculate that extrusive mechanics, to close the incomplete occlusal contacts, would have resulted in an increase in tooth display and probably have been prone to relapse.

References

1 Gibbons, A.J. and Cousley, R.R.J. (2007). Use of mini-implants in orthognathic surgery. *Br. J. Oral Maxillofac. Surg.* 45: 406–407.

2 Coburn, D.G., Kennedy, D.W.G., and Hodder, S.C. (2002). Complication with intermaxillary fixation screws in the management of fractured mandibles. *Br. J. Oral Maxillofac. Surg.* 40: 241–243.

3 Fabbroni, G., Aabed, S., Mizen, K., and Starr, D.G. (2004). Transalveolar screws and the incidence of dental damage: a prospective study. *Int. J. Oral Maxillofac. Surg.* 33: 442–446.

4 Gibbons, A.J. and Hodder, S.C. (2003). A self-drilling intermaxillary fixation screw. *Br. J. Oral Maxillofac. Surg.* 41: 48–49.

5 An, J.H., Kim, Y.I., Kim, S.S. et al. (2019). Root proximity of miniscrews at a variety of maxillary and mandibular buccal sites: reliability of panoramic radiography. *Angle Orthod.* 89 (4): 611–616.

6 Peiro-Guijarro, M.A., Guijarro-Martinez, R., and Hernandez-Alfaro, F. (2016). Surgery first in orthognathic surgery: a systematic review of the literature. *Am. J. Orthod. Dentofac. Orthop.* 149: 448–462.

Index

The Orthodontic Mini-Implant Clinical Handbook, Second Edition. Richard Cousley.
© 2020 John Wiley & Sons Ltd. Published 2020 by John Wiley & Sons Ltd.